Health Informatics

Kathryn J. Hannah   Marion J. Ball
Series Editors

Springer
New York
Berlin
Heidelberg
Barcelona
Hong Kong
London
Milan
Paris
Singapore
Tokyo

Health Informatics Series
(formerly Computers in Health Care)

Series Editors
Kathryn J. Hannah   Marion J. Ball

(continued after Index)

Peter Ramsaroop   Marion J. Ball
David Beaulieu   Judith V. Douglas
Editors

Advancing Federal Sector Health Care

A Model for Technology Transfer

With 100 Illustrations

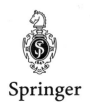

Springer

Peter Ramsaroop, MBA
Chairman and Founder
HealthCPR.com
6313 Fox Hunt Road
Alexandria, VA 22307, USA
formerly
Consultant
First Consulting Group
Baltimore, MD 21210, USA

Marion J. Ball, EdD
Adjunct Professor
Johns Hopkins University
   School of Nursing
Baltimore, MD 21205, USA
formerly
Vice President
First Consulting Group
Baltimore, MD 21210, USA

David Beaulieu
Vice President
Managing Director of the
   Government Practice
First Consulting Group
Avon, CT 06001, USA

Judith V. Douglas, MA, MHS
Adjunct Lecturer
Johns Hopkins University
   School of Nursing
Baltimore, MD 21205, USA
formerly
Associate
First Consulting Group
Baltimore, MD 21210, USA

Series Editors:
Kathryn J. Hannah, PhD, RN
Professor, Department of
   Community Health Science
Faculty of Medicine
The University of Calgary
Calgary, Alberta, Canada

Marion J. Ball, EdD
Adjunct Professor
Johns Hopkins University
   School of Nursing
formerly
Vice President
First Consulting Group
Baltimore, MD 21210, USA

Library of Congress Cataloging-in-Publication Data
Advancing federal sector health care: a model for technology transfer / editors, Peter Ramsaroop . . .
[et al.].
      p.   cm.—(Health informatics series)
      Includes bibliographical references and index.
      ISBN 0-387-95107-5 (alk. paper)
      1. Medicine, Military—Technological innovations—United States.   2. Medical innovations—United
States.   3. Medical informatics—United States.   4. Medical care—United States—Cost control.
5. Medical care—United States—Quality control.   I. Ramsaroop, Peter.   II. Health informatics
      [DNLM: 1. Delivery of Health Care—United States.   2. Medical Informatics Applications—United
States.   3. Biomedical Technology—United States.   4. Government Programs—United States.
5. Hospitals, Federal—organization & administration—United States.   6. Military Medicine—United
States.   W 26.5 A2447   2001]
RC971 .A28   2001
362.1 0973—dc21   00-059476

Printed on acid-free paper.

The following chapters were produced in whole or in part by officers or employees of the United States Government as
part of their official duties, and as such, the text is in the public domain: Chapters 4, 6, 8, 9, 10, 12, 13, 14, 15, 16, 17,
18, 19, 20, 22, and 23.

Production coordinated by Chernow Editorial Services, Inc., and managed by Tim Taylor; manufacturing
supervised by Joseph Quatela.
Typeset by Best-set Typesetter Ltd., Hong Kong.
Printed and bound by Maple-Vail Book Manufacturing Group, York, PA.
Printed in the United States of America.

9 8 7 6 5 4 3 2 1

ISBN 0-387-95107-5   SPIN 10774685

Springer-Verlag   New York Berlin Heidelberg
A member of BertelsmannSpringer Science+Business Media GmbH

A Dedication to Donald Allan Bror Lindberg, MD

It is unlikely that any one person in the federal government has contributed more to medical informatics than Donald A.B. Lindberg, the current Director of the National Library of Medicine. Lindberg's stature in the field and his contributions to medical informatics and to the National Library of Medicine have already been compared to those of John Shaw Billings. From 1865 to 1895, Billings, an Army medical officer, was the Director of the Army Surgeon General's Library, the forerunner of the National Library of Medicine created by congressional legislation signed by President Dwight Eisenhower in 1956.

Donald A.B. Lindberg received his A.B. *Magna cum Laude* in 1954 from Amherst College and his M.D. degree from Columbia University in 1958. After completing his training in pathology at the University of Missouri School of Medicine, he stayed on to become Professor of Pathology, Professor and Chairman of the Department of Information Science, Director of the Health Services Research Center and Health Care Technology Center, and Director of the Information Science Group.

In 1984, Donald Lindberg became the Director of the National Library of Medicine, a role he still plays with vision and strength. From 1992 to 1995, he took on an added task, serving as the first Director of the National Coordination Office for High Performance Computing and Communications, in the Office of Science and Technology Policy. Since 1996, he has been the United States Coordinator for the G-7 Global Healthcare Applications Project for the Global Information Infrastructure Initiative.

Through the years, Lindberg has served on many professional committees and boards of medical professional organizations. The recipient of dozens of honors and awards, including several honorary doctoral degrees, he was the first delegate from the American Medical Informatics Association to the International Medical Informatics Association. In addition to giving hundreds of invited lectures and talks throughout the world, he has published four books on medical informatics along with more than 200 scientific papers, technical reports, and book chapters.

The National Library of Medicine has made important contributions to medical informatics under Donald Lindberg's leadership. In the 1970s, the library initiated MEDLINE and began to offer extramural funding for medical informatics training programs. In 1980s, Lindberg launched two transformational efforts. The Integrated Academic Information Management System (IAIMS) program encouraged the use of computers and communication networks within healthcare institutions. The United Medical Language System (UMLS) project focused on access to machine-readable information located in a variety of sources, including the scientific literature, factual databanks, knowledge-based expert systems, and computer-based patient records. In the 1990s, the library supported projects in telemedicine, the human genome program, and the Visible Human project.

With such outstanding leaders as Donald A.B. Lindberg, the federal government has made substantial contributions to the domain of medical informatics that are improving health care for all.

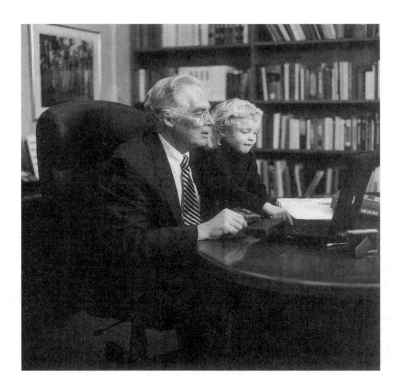

Foreword I

As a result of severe wounds received in World War II, I have spent many months in military hospitals, including 20 months in an Army hospital immediately after the war. I continue to use the Military Health System, as do many of my colleagues in Congress, because I firmly believe the quality of health care delivered in military and veterans hospitals is second to none.

The largest system of its type in the world, the U.S. military healthcare system is undergoing changes as dramatic as those experienced by the entire country. During Desert Storm, we saw new technologies, such as telemedicine, at work in the field. Since then, military medicine has continued to improve and develop innovations that often focus on healthcare issues of concern to society as a whole.

We already have seen technology transfer at work. Things we use in our everyday lives, from sunscreen to the Internet, have come to us directly from innovations developed by federal researchers. The private sector, working with the public agencies, has creatively adapted federal research. For example, the hemopump is used successfully by heart surgeons worldwide to save heart patients. This device, developed by Richard Wampler, was based on satellite technology information that was declassified in the early 1980s.

The chapters in this book focus on current federal sector efforts to shape health care and technology transfer. Many of the initiatives described involve some degree of partnering between the public and private sectors. Other initiatives aim to deliver top-quality care to populations that are microcosms of our society at large. These efforts strive to improve performance while containing costs. The solutions offered include redesigning processes and using technologies to do so.

The contributors to this book share their experiences from the federal sector health systems. The authors demonstrate successful technology programs that, in their opinion, have improved health care. They suggest ways to meet the demands of consumers who grow increasingly sophisticated and knowledgeable, and they offer valuable insights into the challenges of population-based health.

Both the private and public sectors can benefit from the collaborative wisdom of this book's editors and contributors. For policy makers and decision makers, this book provides a fresh look at technology transfer and innovation in health care—an area that is of profound concern to each and every one of us.
Aloha.

Daniel K. Inouye
Senior Senator (Democrat) from Hawaii
Ranking Minority Member
Defense Subcommittee of the Senate Appropriations Committee

Foreword II

As a long-time advocate of increased partnership between the Veterans Health Administration and the Military Health System, I strongly urge all healthcare professionals and every individual involved in the highest levels of policy making to read this most informative and timely book.

VA Medical Centers have long partnered with leading academic institutions throughout the country. Together, they have been responsible for cutting edge research and innovative clinical applications. Since 1984, the VA and DoD have had statutory authority to work together (VA/DoD Sharing Act). Although many projects, mostly local, have resulted, much more could be done to maximize the buying power and healthcare delivery capabilities of both organizations.

In my role as Chairman of the Congressional Commission on Service-members and Veterans Transition Assistance, I reported to Congress our recommendations to establish a joint VA/DoD healthcare policy office and create joint procurement activities. This experience, along with my other work in the federal sector, convinced me that partnering is critical.

Federal agencies and the private sector must expand and extend their collaborative efforts. Only then can technology and information transfer be maximized for the benefit of all Americans.

Anthony J. Principi
President, QTC Medical Services Inc.
Formerly Deputy Secretary of Veterans Affairs
Acting Secretary of Veterans Affairs
Under President George Bush

Foreword III

Health care for our citizens is of supreme importance to members of Congress. More than 200 years ago, Thomas Jefferson stated, "The health of the people is really the foundation upon which their happiness and all their power as a state depend." Congress funds the largest healthcare system in the world for active military personnel and for veterans. It funds research conducted by the National Institutes of Health and other federal agencies. It does this—and much, much more—to ensure that American health care will continue to improve. Only by changing can it remain the best in the world.

We are fortunate, as the chapters in this book document, to have a number of efforts ongoing in the federal sector to improve health care. Committed individuals are actively working to examine the healthcare services provided to our military and their dependents and to our veterans. They are developing new models for delivering quality services that contain costs, and they are exploiting the power of enabling technologies.

The work being done in our military health system and by the Veterans Administration holds great promise. The innovations tested in these two systems—the largest in the world—ultimately will serve us all. Among the initiatives reported on are projects designed to keep large numbers of people well and to know when and why they become ill. Others focus on making care available to patients wherever they, and their care providers, may be. From population-based health to telehealth, these are profound changes, changes that will eventually benefit us all.

To those who would doubt, I cite the impressive history of technology transfer, from public sector to private. It is not limited to the Internet and Teflon® pans—it extends to include the cardiac pacemaker, kidney transplants, and kidney and home dialysis techniques, to name just a few (all of them from the VA).

The individuals contributing to this volume are to be commended, for doing the work their chapters describe and for sharing that work with us. We owe them our gratitude for improving the service they provide within their respective organizations today, and for benefiting us all tomorrow. To them and their editors, our thanks.

Henry W. Foster, Jr., MD
Member, Board of Regents, National Library of Medicine
Senior Advisor to President Clinton
on Teen Pregnancy Reduction and Youth Issues
and
Professor Emeritus, Obstetrics and Gynecology
Meharry Medical College

Series Preface

This series is directed to healthcare professionals who are leading the transformation of health care by using information and knowledge. Launched in 1988 as Computers in Health Care, the series offers a broad range of titles: some addressed to specific professions such as nursing, medicine, and health administration; others to special areas of practice such as trauma and radiology. Still other books in the series focus on interdisciplinary issues, such as the computer-based patient record, electronic health records, and networked healthcare systems.

Renamed Health Informatics in 1998 to reflect the rapid evolution in the discipline now known as health informatics, the series will continue to add titles that contribute to the evolution of the field. In the series, eminent experts, serving as editors or authors, offer their accounts of innovations in health informatics. Increasingly, these accounts go beyond hardware and software to address the role of information in influencing the transformation of healthcare delivery systems around the world. The series also will increasingly focus on "peopleware" and the organizational, behavioral, and societal changes that accompany the diffusion of information technology in health services environments.

These changes will shape health services in the next millennium. By making full and creative use of the technology to tame data and to transform information, health informatics will foster the development of the knowledge age in health care. As coeditors, we pledge to support our professional colleagues and the series readers as they share advances in the emerging and exciting field of health informatics.

Kathryn J. Hannah
Marion J. Ball

Preface

The challenge in health care is to take what we know and what others know and put that knowledge into practice. The failure to act on existing knowledge is a serious and pervasive loss to our society as a whole. We now recognize this in the area of medical errors and patient safety. Our next task is to understand technology transfer within the context of the healthcare system as a whole and to leverage successful innovations between and across sectors.

No simple task, technology transfer involves both basic and social sciences. Take, for example, vaccine development and immunization programs, areas in which government plays a key role. In the words of Dr. Henry Foster, a long-time advocate of population health, the goal is not to spend millions of dollars on the vaccine and "have 40% of children unimmunized." The goal is to develop the vaccines—and to get them into those who are at risk.

The authors contributing to this volume report on their efforts to improve health care and contain costs by making judicious use of enabling technologies. We believe that their work will form a new generation of technology transfer and fulfill the promise of health informatics to us in this new millennium.

Moving into the future, we look to the past for guidance and reassurance. As Senator Daniel Inouye notes in his foreword and Drs. Morris Collen and Steven Phillips document in their chapters, there is clear and incontrovertible evidence that federal research and development initiatives have moved into the private sector and provided tangible benefits. Our other contributors set forth their experiences in collaborating to capitalize on existing and emerging technologies. To the instances of technology transfer they describe, we add still more.

The Veterans Health Administration, commonly referred to as the VA, has provided a host of innovations, including cardiac pacemaker monitoring, radioimmunoassay techniques for diagnostic testing, hepatitis vaccine, and kidney dialysis techniques. Add to this several firsts: the first successful drug therapies for tuberculosis, high blood pressure, and schizophrenia; and the first kidney transplant in the United States performed at a VA medical center. The VA has also developed a computerized fitness treadmill for wheelchairs, the light and responsive "Seattle Foot" for amputees, and computer-aided design and manufacture (CAD/CAM) applications for fitting and fabricating prostheses. Here its mission, to serve the nation's veterans, has clearly benefited others with very special needs. Other efforts have resulted in innovations that serve all of health care, notably research that led to the development of filmless radiology, computerized axial tomography (CAT), and magnetic resonance imagery (MRI).

Another agency to contribute greatly to the private sector is the Department of Agriculture. Research it has done has quite literally changed the way we live. We start with the discovery in 1941 of a superior strain of *Penicillium*, making large quantities of penicillin available. To this we add the development in 1953 of THPC, first used in military combat clothing, firefighters' uniforms, and hospital linens, and now used in children's nightwear. Work with *Taxus* plant cell cultures led to the industrial use of technology to produce taxol, now used to treat ovarian, breast, and other cancers. The insect repellent known as DEET, discovered more than 40 years ago, protected our troops assigned to Operation Desert Storm—and countless campers and picnickers—from mosquitoes and other disease-carrying pests. Lactaid makes milk and milk products digestible for lactose-intolerant individuals around the world, while databases at the National Agricultural Library (NAL) deliver information to consumers and professionals at www.nal.usda.gov and www.agnic.org on nutritional, environmental, and related issues.

We end our lists of successful technology transfer by highlighting the National Library of Medicine. Directed by Dr. Donald A.B. Lindberg, to whom this volume is dedicated, the Library and its scientific branch known as the Lister Hill Center have transformed health information. In the 1980s, the library foresaw the importance of integration in complex healthcare institutions, beginning the program now called Integrated Advanced Information Management Systems (IAIMS). It introduced Grateful Med software for MEDLINE searches to foster access outside the library walls and launched the Unified Medical Language System (UMLS) to bridge across different medical terminologies and provide a Rosetta Stone for sharing electronic patient records. In the 1990s, the library strengthened its national network, implemented Loansome Doc for requesting journal articles, expanded its information program in toxicology and environmental health, inaugurated its Web site (one of the first in the federal sector), and completed the Visible Human Project. As the 1990s ended, PubMed, MEDLINE*plus*, and PubMed Central were introduced to extend and ease access to biomedical literature housed in and indexed by the library. Early in 2000, the library launched www.ClinicalTrials.gov for patients and their families. Truly the library is playing a vital role in transferring technology and translating research into knowledge that directly impacts clinical care and each of us as consumers of healthcare information.

In the chapters that follow, contributors describe a host of activities under way in the areas of direct patient care, including those in the VA and the Department of Defense (DoD). The work ongoing in these two organizations, the largest of their kind in the world, is drawing upon and contributing to expertise in the private sector. For example, DoD relates its work in keeping a large fighting force fit and their families well, while the VA addresses care for a population over time. While DoD implements surveillance systems to detect outbreaks, the VA and DoD use telemedicine capabilities to provide care when and where it is needed. Meanwhile, individuals from the private sector working with DoD and the VA contribute their expertise in performance improvement through information management, and help to address issues of cost containment and return on investment in a fiscally demanding environment.

Both sectors learn; both sectors teach. This is, we believe, technology transfer at its best, and a source of pride to us as editors—and, much more importantly, as Americans.

Marion J. Ball and Judith V. Douglas

Acknowledgments

Putting together a contributed volume is no simple task, and we owe our thanks to our colleagues who helped us bring this book into print. Two come first to mind: Jennifer Lillis, the gifted, young, and tireless editor in our offices, and Nhora Cortes-Comerer, the supremely professional editor of the Health Informatics series at Springer-Verlag. There are many more: Patricia Carson, for furnishing us with Dr. Lindberg's picture and curriculum vitae; Dorsey Chescavage, for bringing our work to the attention of Senator Daniel Inouye and Mr. Anthony Principi for their forewords; Pamela André, for sharing the resources of the Agricultural Library; Dr. Morris Collen, for bringing his long friendship with Dr. Lindberg to the writing of the dedication; and Robert Maynard and Kathy Gardner Cravedi, for supplying information on the technology transfer theme.

As always, we thank our families for their love and support. From Peter Ramsaroop, thanks to his father, the late Dr. John Ramsaroop, his wife Anna, his son Shawn, and daughter Dawn. From Marion Ball, thanks to her husband John. From David Beaulieu, thanks to Bonnie, Ben, Zach, "and for the opportunity to do what I do." And from Judith Douglas, thanks to Paul.

Peter Ramsaroop, Marion J. Ball,
David Beaulieu, and Judith V. Douglas

Contents

PART 1 THE EMERGING FEDERAL SECTOR HEALTHCARE MODEL

PART 2 APPLYING NEW MODELS FOR IMPROVEMENTS AND COST CONTAINMENT

PART 3 ENABLING TECHNOLOGIES

ADVANCES IN FEDERAL SECTOR HEALTH CARE: A MODEL FOR TECHNOLOGY TRANSFER

Part 1
The Emerging Healthcare Model

Part 2
Performance Improvement and Cost Containment

Part 3
Enabling Technologies

Chapter 1
Moving to Population Health

Chapter 10
Managing Information, Not Technology

Chapter 17
Building a Unified Information Utility

Chapter 2
Caring for the Warfighter

Chapter 11
Demonstrating Return on Investment

Chapter 18
Supporting Shared Clinical Informatioin

Chapter 3
Nurturing Early Informatics

Chapter 12
Improving Access to Provider Information

Chapter 19
Tracking and Analyzing Symptoms from Afar

Chapter 4
Encouraging Technology Transfer

Chapter 13
Reducing Costs and Maintaining Mission

Chapter 20
Guarding Against Bioterrorism at Home

Chapter 5
Modeling the New DoD System

Chapter 14
Planning for the Integrated Enterprise

Chapter 21
Using Health Data to Serve All Americans

Chapter 6
Aligning Technology and Mission

Chapter 15
Improving Clinical Data for Decision Making

Chapter 22
Making Telemedicine a Reality

Chapter 7
Transforming the VA for Added Value

Chapter 16
Linking Financial and Utilization Data

Chapter 23
Serving Health Care in a Dot Com World

Chapter 8
Training Techno-Savvy Health Professionals

Chapter 9
Reallocating DoD Resources for Quality Care

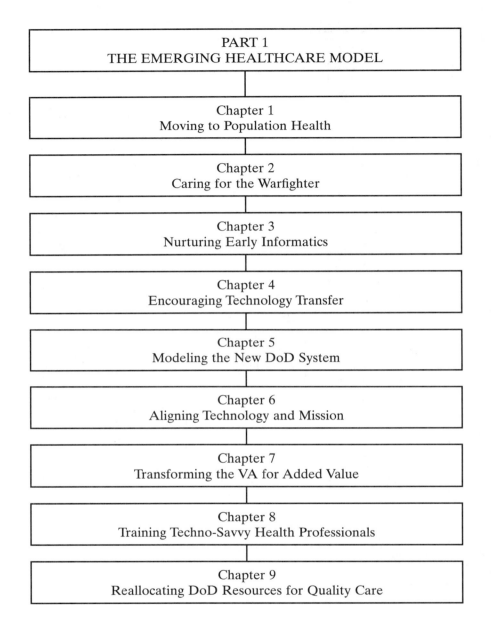

PART 1
THE EMERGING HEALTHCARE MODEL

Chapter 1
Moving to Population Health

Chapter 2
Caring for the Warfighter

Chapter 3
Nurturing Early Informatics

Chapter 4
Encouraging Technology Transfer

Chapter 5
Modeling the New DoD System

Chapter 6
Aligning Technology and Mission

Chapter 7
Transforming the VA for Added Value

Chapter 8
Training Techno-Savvy Health Professionals

Chapter 9
Reallocating DoD Resources for Quality Care

Part 1
The Emerging Federal Sector Healthcare Model

Chapter 9

1
The Longer View: Moving Toward Population Health in the Federal Sector

David Beaulieu

John Robbins begins his book *Re-claiming Our Health* (1998) with a fable about the current state of the U.S. healthcare industry. In the story, people head for the edge of a cliff and crash to the ground below, after which great care is taken to repair their injuries. Once they recover, however, they fall off the cliff again, and the cycle repeats itself. Few warnings are issued to prevent these catastrophes. Only after people are actually injured do they enjoy the best care and attention money can buy.

Like readers of Robbins' fable, we in health care are beginning to question whether we are spending money and resources in the right places. Health care is not just about repairing people when they fall off cliffs; it is also about involving the community in building fences to warn people about the danger. Investing in keeping people well is just as important as—if not more important than—spending money on health care after they become ill.

In the United States, we have yet to put this tenet into practice. The United States spends considerably more than the developed country average on health care, and the value we receive is questionable. Whether healthcare costs are measured as a percentage of the GDP, as the healthcare-burdened price of consumer products, or as a figure on an employee's pay stub, the cost of health care to consumers is extremely high given the services provided. Kindig lists specific factors for the high costs: rising physician incomes, a surplus of specialists, the aging population, an avalanche of paperwork and administration, "defensive medicine" in the malpractice climate, and an influx of new technology (Kindig 1997, p. 30). Adding to this list is the fact that healthcare professionals have been free to define what treatments are necessary—in fact, the power of the physician's pen determines more than 80% of healthcare costs. Attempts to curtail these trends have met a mountain of resistance.

5

Change Drivers: Consumerism and Shifting Demographics

In this new century, maintaining the wellness of populations will be key to increasing the value and managing the cost of health care. Two factors—the new era of healthcare consumerism and the shifting demographics of the U.S. population—underscore the importance of this new focus.

Consumers, who have learned to expect more from the products and services they purchase, are benchmarking their healthcare services against similar services they receive from the best organizations outside health care. They are using their experiences and observations to ask pointed questions. If a package shipping company can answer calls in one ring, why can't the insurance claim center? If an investment advisor can offer a convenient after-hours appointment within the week, why can't a physician? If a company will accept without question the return of a product that doesn't fit properly, why won't the triage center trust a consumer who shares information about medical symptoms?

Health care has not kept pace with the expectations of increasingly demanding consumers. Complaints about quality and access to care are common. Making convenient appointments with the "right" practitioner is still a challenge for the average consumer. Administrative minutiae have become more time consuming than the actual delivery of healthcare services, and stories of medication errors and the lack of patient safety in different care settings are increasingly prevalent. In the midst of this turbulence, organizations known for healthcare excellence and consumer satisfaction—e.g., Harvard Pilgrim and many Blue Cross Blue Shield plans—are falling on hard financial times.

Consumers concerned about how to avoid becoming ill or injured are attempting to patch health care's inadequacies through self-empowerment. They are making use of information sources readily available to them on the Internet—some useful and accurate, some misleading and potentially dangerous. They are asking medical providers to spend more time with them in appointments to explain new techniques, the rationale behind prescribing medications, and alternative treatments. Many of them are beginning to "shop" for better answers to their questions, having decided that traditional medical practitioners do not offer the best advice on how to stay healthy. This trend clearly illustrates our need for increased focus on population health and wellness.

Another challenge facing health care today is the shifting demographics of the U.S. population. As the number of elderly steadily increases, an unprecedented economic burden will be placed on working-age people. This phenomenon is already being seen in several European countries [Peterson's *Gray Dawn* (1999) discusses this in detail]. Increased comorbidities of the elderly will place more economic burden on the young and will revolutionize the family. According to economic estimates, the tax burden on younger generations is expected to double by the year 2030. Retirement also will be redefined as changes in employment law and practices require more flexibility in the workplace. People have been retiring earlier and using their time for more leisure activities; the Social Security Administration reported that the average retirement age decreased substantially from 66.5 years in 1960 to 63.6 in 1995. Staying healthy is an especially high priority for this active population.

Keeping people healthy early in life is key to avoiding large healthcare expenditures driven by care for the chronically ill. Without a dramatic change in healthcare policy to focus on maintaining wellness, the increased economic burden of traditional disease management will continue to hamper our society economically. Healthcare inflation will not be easily absorbed, and neither will the dramatic needs for long-term and skilled nursing care and assisted living arrangements. Many recent projections (Hewitt Associates Survey; Towers Perrin Survey) predict medical inflation will reach double digits in FY 2000. Generally, estimates project that older people will continue to consume three to five times more healthcare services per capita than younger people. As America "grays," a higher percentage of resources will need to be set aside for pensions and health care; OECD expects the GDP percentage to increase from 10.5% in 1995 to more than 17% in 2030.

Building Solutions Through Population Health

In *Purchasing Population Health*, David Kindig observes that throwing more money at our current healthcare problems will do little to solve them:

"There has long been a positive relationship between life expectancy and national per capita income but . . . a decreasing return begins to develop at higher expenditure levels (around $5,000 per capita in 1990). Diminishing marginal return is an important concept both in economics and in population health; it refers to lower increases in output for equivalent additional increases in input." (Kindig, pp. 36–37)

What, then, is the solution? As we shift to a population health mindset, it will be critical to

- Systematically implement new approaches to managing the health of populations
- Aggressively implement secondary prevention programs (disease management, case management, etc.) to help people with chronic illness maintain the highest quality of life possible
- Make progress in the use of pharmaceuticals within the context of access and affordability
- Complete research to identify the genetic basis of disease

The Public Sector's Role

Given its unique populations, employment longevity, and focus on fitness and readiness, the Department of Defense's Military Health System is well positioned to implement advances in population health and primary prevention. Similar opportunities in the private sector are few, given health plan enrollment "churn" and impact on the financial bottom line.

Major government agencies (e.g., the Department of Defense, Veterans Administration, Indian Health Service) control the three components of the healthcare system generally in competition within the private sector—the employer, the health plan, and the delivery system. This arrangement provides a unique opportunity to establish enterprises of cooperation and collaboration. The various healthcare systems under the public health system can be integrated to include larger numbers of individuals and establish broader financial risk.

The public health system must aggressively expand its role to improve the health of populations. As Kindig observes, "the challenge is to move to more complete vertical integration across the components of medical care, from prevention to acute care to long term care. This can be done in the private sector, as with the HMO sites, or in public sector activities, such as in the Veterans Administration, the Department of Defense, or the Indian Health Service healthcare systems" (Kindig, p. 128).

Eleven Worthy Aims

In 1994, Don Berwick introduced "eleven worthy aims" for "better outcomes, greater ease of use, lower cost, and more social justice in health status" (Berwick 1994, pp. 797–802). These aims, listed below, lay a good foundation for a population health program:

1. Reduce inappropriate surgery, admissions, and tests
2. Reduce underlying root causes of illness, such as smoking and injury
3. Reduce cesarean section rates below 10%
4. Reduce unwanted and ineffective end-of-life procedures
5. Adopt simplified formularies and streamline pharmaceuticals
6. Increase patient participation in decision making
7. Decrease delays and waiting of all types
8. Reduce inventory levels
9. Record only useful information, and only once
10. Reduce the total supply of high-technology medical and surgical care and consolidate it into regional centers
11. Reduce the racial gap in health status, beginning with infant mortality and low birth weight

Additional steps also must be taken to improve quality of life and avoid longer-term chronic illness. These steps include advances in smoking cessation, weight management, hypertension, women's health, prevention and treatment of asthma and diabetes, immunizations, cancer screening, and diagnosis and treatment of depression. In addition, the public health systems must prepare themselves to tackle the larger issues—namely, developing approaches to manage both the factors determining health and the responsible agents.

The Role of Genetics Research

Research into the genetic basis of disease will help individuals work with their care providers to develop specific, individualized approaches to maintaining health beginning from birth. Genetically identifying diseases will change the way they are classified from symptoms to genetic subtype. Thus, clinicians will be able to identify human genetic markers pointing to illnesses patients might be predisposed to acquire during their lifetime. Genetically linked syndromes like hypothyroidism, phenylketonuria (PKU), and cystic fibrosis can be identified early and treated. Drugs can be targeted on the basis of their likelihood of improving a specific individual's condition, and care providers will be better positioned to help consumers develop and implement targeted preventive care programs.

Obstacles to Population Health

There are several obstacles to implementing population health capabilities. One of these is the lack of accepted measures of healthcare outcomes—measurement needs to be made of the system, not the function. Other obstacles include consumer demands for what appear to be conflicting objectives: the desire for freedom of choice, universal access, high quality, and lower costs. As Joel Shalowitz observes, it is "impossible to fulfill all these demands simultaneously. The real challenge for the political process is to determine how we can achieve an optimal mix of these features, satisfy the most, disenfranchise the fewest, and return health insurance to its original purpose—indemnification against catastrophic loss" (Shalowitz 1999, p. 50).

As a society, we have not yet formed policies to reconcile conflicting consumer demands. What is missing, and what we need to clearly define, is a social ethic of what the nation wants to achieve in health care. Such an ethic will help shape methods of achieving better health in the population as a whole (Reinhardt 1997, pp. 1446–1447).

Achieving Population Health: Critical Success Factors

To accomplish population health goals, progress must be made in several key areas. Focused, deliberate work must be done to achieve these goals:

- Achieve clinical and information integration
- Establish common process frameworks
- Provide access to accurate information
- Introduce new approaches to technology development and insertion
- Understand the challenges of the new knowledge worker
- Leverage the value of partnering

Each of these key areas is discussed next.

Clinical and Information Integration

In 1996, First Consulting Group collaborated with the nonprofit Scottsdale Institute to survey 40 integrated delivery systems on their overall level of perceived integration in four areas: structural, operational, clinical, and information. Structural integration referred to the amount of legal and/or organizational integration, including having a single CEO and a board; offering primary, specialist, and hospital care; and running a health plan. Operational integration referred to refining the business processes of the organization, including common corporate processes, functions, budgets, and financial statements. Clinical integration referred to the ability to offer access to care throughout the organization in a systematic fashion, the ability to track outcomes for episodes of care across settings, and the delivery of wellness services. Information integration measured the extent of the organization's information infrastructure, communications, and applications to support operational and clinical integration (Drazen and Metzger 1999, pp. 16–21).

The results of the study were revealing. Most organizations had made the most progress in structural integration, while several reported significant progress in operational integration. Some were beginning to make progress in the areas of clinical and information integration, but they were only in the early stages. Figure 1.1 illustrates the overall results.

The conclusions of the study are critical to improving access to and delivery of health care, for chronic care as well as for population health. Drazen and Metzger concluded that "to deliver performance, integrated delivery networks (IDNs) must radically redesign core processes across the continuum and make significant investments in information systems" (p. 21). Only in this way can a healthcare system meet the needs of its consumers and purchasers while satisfying the needs of those who work within them. In accord with this realization, First Consulting Group began working with integrated delivery systems on new core process models to support the mission of these organizations.

Establishing a Common Process Framework

In *Strategies for Integrated Health Care*, Drazen and Metzger introduce a new process framework for the integrated delivery network of the twenty-

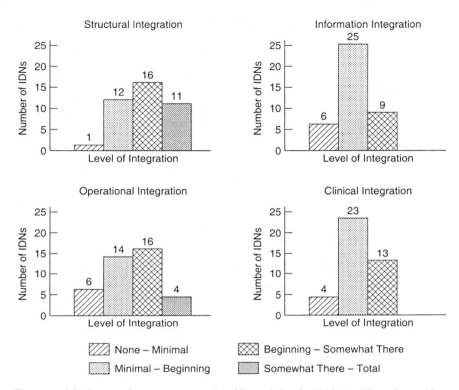

FIGURE 1.1. Integration survey results (Copyright © 1998 by First Consulting Group).

first century. They describe new processes that transform healthcare organizations, improving both business and clinical performance. Through collaboration with five integrating networks that were members of the Scottsdale Institute, the team made three observations:

- Although the organizations had a similar vision of the future, the path to achieve that vision was unclear.
- There was concern among all participants that without clarity about the path, many investments being made today might not be durable building blocks for the future.
- Communication was hampered by the lack of consistent terminology among the group—participants used terms such as *access to care, care management*, and *medical management* to mean quite different things. (Drazen and Metzger, p. 23).

This collaboration identified a need to provide a common framework for additional discussion. Drazen and Metzger developed a process framework,

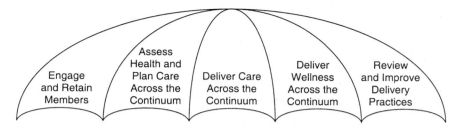

FIGURE 1.2. Integrated Delivery Network (IDN) process framework (Copyright © 1998 by First Consulting Group).

outlined in Figure 1.2, consisting of five core processes. Each of these was clearly delineated in the process model framework.

These new integrated models are improving access to care and cross-continuum care management. First Consulting Group has recently applied these models to delivery systems within the Department of Defense's Military Health System, with early successes.

The success of improvements in chronic disease management and implementation of population health capabilities will also depend on winning the information management battle. Successful reengineering projects must exploit information technology (IT) to deliver value quickly to the business, the consumers, and the providers. Connecting consumers to timely, accurate information is a key to future improvements in our healthcare system.

Information Access and Data Quality

The need for access to information is as critical as the need for access to care, and this is particularly true in working with population health. Because of the fragmentation of healthcare systems and their low information integration scores, there is an abundance of data but an absence of reliable, actionable information.

As more reliance is placed on partnerships across healthcare systems to achieve information and clinical integration, it will become more important to ensure that people are fully informed. This need will require fast access to enterprise-level information that is accurate, consistent, and available to all knowledge workers across the business, including trading partners. The issue of security will be a crucial one to resolve, because partnerships between patients and their care providers can be enhanced or corrupted by increased access to information via tools like the Web.

Technology Development and Insertion

Technology advances have made most of their mark on operations—the preservation of assets and cost control—rather than assisting executives with value creation. The reason behind the many recent technological failures is clear: executives have made massive investments with little attention to how people create knowledge and complete work. Often, information technology has obscured the fact that data must be organized and accessible to be transformed into information.

A tidal wave of executive discontent will result in significant changes in technology investments and a new focus on understanding the human side of work—specifically, how people learn and what they do at their jobs on a daily basis. Executives will continue to seek answers to two key questions: "What information do I need in order to lead?" and "What information do I need to provide to the coworkers on whom I depend?" Leaders will eliminate data that do not pertain to the information they need in order to act. They will understand that consumers and suppliers hold the most important information, and if necessary, they will go outside their organizations to get it.

Aligning technology investments with business outcomes has required IT executives to reevaluate their role within their organizations. James Cortada (1997) illustrates some of these behavior shifts in *Best Practices in Information Technology*. Historically, in the monopolistic, regulated environment, organizations were structured in a functional hierarchy, IT executives acted in a reactive instead of proactive capacity, mergers and acquisitions were strategic goals, and the focus was on a traditional sales approach. Now, with the emergence of the competitive, free market environment, the rules are changing. Teams and networks are replacing hierarchies, strategic alliances are replacing mergers, aggressive acquisition and market management are replacing the traditional sales approach, and IT executives must be proactive, reactive, and flexible to compete (Cordata, p. 21).

Perhaps the most important shift Cordata highlights is technology's transformation from an operational support tool to an enabler of the organization's strategic vision. To be effective, information technology must be fully integrated with the fundamental business purposes of the organization it serves—this means that information technology investments and ongoing costs must be tied to producing desired business outcomes. Technologies that do not synchronize with business objectives cannot be objectively supported by performance measures. Those that do synchronize with business objectives improve clinical quality and cost reduction. A good example is documented in the study by Glaser and Hsu (1999) at Brigham and Women's Hospital, which verified the positive financial impact of integrating various warnings with order entry systems.

One of the key thrusts in technology realignment to support business purposes is the need to change quickly. The introduction of speed requires new thinking about the life expectancy of technology investments. Old methods of application development and implementation are giving way to modular development approaches, faster depreciation of investments, and extremely fast deployment of new capabilities. Organizations are under pressure to change how new technologies are procured to avoid redundancy by the time users actually see the capability.

The information technology community is also under incredible pressure to communicate the IT strategic value to its constituencies. In the absence of agreement on the value information technology creates for the business and clinical community, discussions about its funding are a waste of time. IT value creation is a precursor to answering the key technology questions: Are we investing the right amount in the right areas? Do we have the right infrastructure to support the business, both short and long term? Communicating IT strategic value requires not only close relationships with business owners within an enterprise but also partnerships with customers and suppliers.

The role of the information technologist must change to respond to the new role of technology as an essential component of the organization's success. Technology management has changed; the new "whole view" technology management focuses on customer sales and service, aims to build customer satisfaction and loyalty through branding, focuses on developing new capabilities within more aggressive timeframes, and views technology as not just mission critical but also mission redefining (Modahl 1999, p. 156). Information technologists must adapt to these new ways of thinking that integrate external focus, speed, and strategic thinking to support the enterprise. They must also clarify their relationship to technology; as Modahl points out, it is often not in a consumer-driven company's interest to be a technology vendor. As a vendor, the IT department must continually innovate to stay ahead of competitors, struggle to reduce development costs, and market to achieve broad acceptance of proprietary technologists. In contrast, technology *users* buy the best of breed, pay the lowest market price for technologies, and benefit from industry-wide standardization (Modahl, p. 161).

Healthcare information technology leaders should keep some practical lessons in mind as they plan the implementation of new technologies.

- The capability created by the technology must enable business/clinical objectives.
- The new technology must be easier to use than the older technology or business process.
- The new technology should provide a new capability demanded by the users.
- Implementation of new technologies should be carefully planned, evolve incrementally, and become easier to use over time.

When used in the right way, information technology improves productivity for business operations and clinicians. Business advances enabled by technology insertion include labor reductions, automation of tasks, process simplification, and risk reduction. Technology insertion also enables greater flexibility, speed in adapting to new business demands, and overall reduction in costs. Cortada underscores the potential impact of compressing time through the use of information technology: productivity increases, investments can be recovered sooner, risks and expenses both decrease, corporate culture shifts, feedback is received faster, and agility and competitiveness improve.

Knowledge Workers

As people with deep expertise and strong self-confidence "volunteer" to work with specific healthcare organizations, enterprises are beginning to realize that they must satisfy the interests of these knowledge workers to stay competitive. In the future, businesses will thrive not on low labor costs, but on the ability of their workforce to attain the productivity made possible by new technologies and knowledge building.

Knowledge workers are assets because they own the means of production (unlike manual workers) and are committed to learning and delivering value. The success of an organization is directly tied to its ability to build the skills of more workers across the healthcare continuum so that they understand the larger picture (population health, wellness, community engagement). On the whole, manual skilled back office workers will be replaced with automated processes and administrative workers will move back into more highly specialized caregiving positions. The need will be for highly skilled customer service professionals in the front office, an especially critical step in the evolution from a disease-oriented to a population health-oriented system.

Transforming manual workers into knowledge workers admittedly is very expensive. For an organization to survive, however, it must invest in supplementary education to increase the productivity of autonomous, innovative knowledge workers. At the macro level, this is widely recognized as a national issue and has recently become the biggest presidential campaign issue for the 2000 election—62% of people polled rated this their number one concern in a recent survey. Significant investments will be required to enhance the skills of manual healthcare workers, who must increase their overall productivity to drive quality up and keep costs down.

Partnering

Highly competitive organizations understand that they must establish strong trading relationships to be successful. This means seeking partnerships, alliances, and joint ventures within and outside a specific business arena for capabilities that differentiate an organization from its competitors. Close, continuous, and "seamless" relationships with suppliers and full information integration with trading partners are essential to an organization's success and to its ability to adapt and change quickly.

To overcome economic and physical boundaries that impede growth, organizations must expand their scope and become more critical of investments in activities that no longer contribute to performance or produce results. The public sector healthcare community needs to carefully examine all existing relationships and create more selective partnerships. Organizations linked together must share purposes, and reward systems must be aligned to support the relationship. With common purposes and strong incentives in place, organizations will be positioned to overcome existing barriers to information and clinical integration.

References

Berwick, D.M. 1994. *Eleven Worthy Aims for Clinical Leadership of Health System Reform. JAMA* 272(10):797–802.

Cortada, J.W. 1997. *Best Practices in Information Technology: How Corporations Get the Most Value from Exploiting Their Digital Investments.* New York: Prentice Hall.

Drazen, E., Metzger, J. 1999. *Strategies for Integrated Health Care.* San Francisco: Jossey-Bass.

Glaser, J.P., Hsu, L. 1999. *The Strategic Application of Information Technology in Healthcare Organizations.* New York: McGraw-Hill.

Hewitt Associates Survey Indicates Companies and Consumers to Pay More for Health Care in 2000. Press Release: Business Wire, 2000.

Kindig, D. 1997. *Purchasing Population Health.* Ann Arbor: University of Michigan Press.

Modahl, M. 1999. *Now or Never: How Companies Must Change Today to Win the Battle for Internet Customers.* New York: Harperbusiness, pp. 156–157.

Peterson, P.G. 1999. *Gray Dawn: How the Coming Age Wave Will Transform America and the World.* New York: Times Books.

Reinhardt, W.E. 1997. *Wanted: A Clearly Articulated Social Ethic for American Health Care. JAMA* 248:1446–1447.

Robbins, J. 1998. *Reclaiming Our Health: Exploding the Medical Myth and Embracing the Sources of True Healing. Tiburon,* CA: H.J. Kramer.

Shalowitz, J. 1999. *Policy Challenges, The 21st Century Health Care Leader.* San Francisco: Jossey-Bass, p. 50.

Towers Perrin Survey Projects Double-digit Growth in Health Care Costs in 2000; Double-digit Increases Expected to Continue for Several Years. Press Release: Business Wire, January 10, 2000.

2
The Future of U.S. Military Health Care

COL. (RET.) ROBERT A. LEITCH AND PETER RAMSAROOP

It's time we steered by the stars, not by the lights of each passing ship.
—*General Omar Bradley*

The United States Military Health System (MHS) is a $16 billion organization providing comprehensive, state-of-the-art health care for a beneficiary population of 8.2 million servicemen and servicewomen, their dependents, and retirees. Care is provided though a worldwide network of 508 Medical Treatment Facilities (MTFs) and supporting structures, and the cost breakdown is approximately $12 billion for the MTFs and $3.5 billion for civilian support contracts through the TRICARE system. To undertake the difficult task of providing care to such an extensive population, the MHS employs 106,000 Active military and 48,000 civilian personnel. In addition to this large Active peacetime healthcare organization, there is a vast reserve organization made up of individuals and units in the National Guard and Reserve component that completes the entire Readiness structure of the MHS.

This complex organization is currently in the grip of two near simultaneous revolutions, the combined effects of which are set to bring about fundamental shifts in the way it delivers its services in peace and war. The first is the so-called healthcare revolution, an umbrella term for the recent influx of change in the way health care is practiced. The second, called the Revolution in Military Affairs (RMA) (Mazzar 1994), is a radical change in the way the warfighter conducts his business and in what he needs from his medical services. In this chapter, we discuss these two revolutions, examine their impact and what progress has been made to address them, and explore what future directions military health care might take.

Permanent Whitewater? Two Revolutions

Military health care is being shaped and redefined by a long list of powerful forces, some military specific, some shared by private sector health care. Such trends as the technology explosion, shifting demographics, diminishing manpower, and rising demands and expectations all add up to a future of maximum uncertainty. In the face of these profound and apparently continuous changes, it is not surprising that many in military health care feel as though they are "paddling their canoes in permanent whitewater" with no end in sight.

The Healthcare Revolution

Three key drivers, shown in Figure 2.1, are shaping the future of health care in the United States: demography, rising expectations, and technological innovation. A rapidly expanding population of persons over 65 will consume increasing amounts of healthcare resources in the decades to come. The warfighter is being challenged by imperatives like diminishing manpower, higher demands on the remaining numbers, rising expectations of the warfighter and the nation, and technological innovation. New technologies and practices like laparoscopic surgery are changing the practice of medicine and the patient experience: in the past 5 years, hospital bed stays have dropped from an average of 10 days to 6.5, while short stay admissions and outpatient procedures have caused hospital throughput to increase by 30% in the same period. At the same time, in the setting of limited budgets, these factors are exerting additional acute strains on the traditional "Iron Triangle" of defense spending (Figure 2.2).

At the core of current reforms is an attempt to limit spiraling costs while improving or at least maintaining quality and access by imposing managed care concepts. To fulfill this objective, health care is shifting away from traditional hospital-based medicine and toward primary care. This shift is only the beginning; in the next millennium, the Information Revolution is set to alter health care fundamentally. In a 1994 address to the Association of Military Surgeons of the United States, former U.S. Surgeon General C. Everett Koop described this future as "health care predicated upon customer-based responsibility, health promotion and preventive medicine, rather than the traditional 'sick care,' focusing on the treatment of

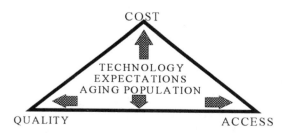

FIGURE 2.1. Shaping healthcare costs.

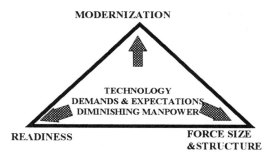

FIGURE 2.2. Straining the "Iron Triangle".

disease and injury, that has been the underpinning concept of medicine in the 20th century."

The Revolution in Military Affairs

The Revolution in Military Affairs (RMA) is technology-driven change. It requires armed forces to use state-of-the-art information technology and precision weapons to act rapidly and decisively on a high-tech battlefield. These future warfighting concepts will require much smaller armed forces, with the three services obliged to organize and train to operate jointly in operations that will normally be conducted in coalition with allies.

This doctrinal and organizational shift will require much less manpower, but much of the money potentially saved in "downsizing" will be needed to buy high-tech equipment. As technology advances, it both increases in cost and requires more highly skilled and trained operators, whose costs are also rising. The result is constant pressure to find money from so-called "savings in infrastructure costs," a euphemism for reducing personnel and personnel support structures. This core debate on the balance between modernization, readiness, and force structure (size) will remain a constant feature of military life.

Even as this "revolution" develops, another is hot on its heels: the shift from traditional warfighting toward Operations Other Than War (OOTW). In simple terms, OOTW refers to a spectrum of operations and conflict management short of conventional warfare. It encompasses operations as diverse as humanitarian relief, domestic security, counterterrorism, counternarcotics, and peacekeeping. The full effects of this shift are only now being realized.

The key questions raised by these revolutions in military thinking concern how to balance manpower needs, equipment, and training to meet all contingencies. In particular, serious doubts are being voiced about the utility of future armed forces designed primarily to operate on the high-tech battlefield of the type witnessed in the Gulf War.

Navigating the Whitewater: Effects and Current Progress

The net effect of these revolutions on the Military Healthcare Services System (MHSS) has been profound. Cold War medical plans required a large and complex medical structure reaching from Norway to Norfolk, Virginia, and from Seoul to San Diego, capable of providing comprehensive care to tens of thousands of military casualties. This requirement disappeared with the Berlin Wall, and the Gulf War experience confirmed that such a large and comprehensive medical structure was redundant. The operational structure of the military medical services required an urgent restructuring, and in 1993 it was subjected to intense scrutiny as part of the overall Department of Defense (DoD) review of the U.S. Armed Forces, called the 733 Study.

The 733 Study found that the peacetime primary care, occupational, and preventive medicine organizations (the basis of the operational readiness structures and the key elements of both First and Second Echelon care) were well maintained and adequate for their mission. However, strong reservations were expressed regarding the availability of relevant military medical training in a number of specialties and the clinical experience levels of medical personnel at the sharp end of operations, particularly the military "First Responders" or combat medics.

Military hospitals, for so long the "core business" of military medicine and consuming the lion's share of the military medical budget, were shown to be underutilized in many areas and profligate when compared with civilian organizations. Providing care for a young, fit community could neither fill beds nor provide the spectrum of medicine essential to train doctors, nurses, and other medical professionals. For many years, these hospitals had relied upon the care of military retirees to provide the spectrum of medical experience necessary for training and were increasingly forced to send military doctors and nurses to civilian hospitals to train in trauma management, the essential military medical skill. Even this option has limitations, as it cannot always provide training appropriate for war. Combat medicine produces peculiar training requirements; the wounds of war are often unique, such as those caused by shell and bomb splinters, landmines, and high-velocity, large-caliber small arms.

Moreover, as U.S. society continues to age dramatically, the numbers of military retirees using military healthcare facilities have continued to grow rapidly. Retirees represented 11% of total military beneficiaries in 1955. By 1998, this number had risen to 51%. The increases in cost that have accompanied this shift are considerable, and the results have been years of underfunding of the Defense Health Plan budget and the need to ask Congress for additional funding on an annual basis.

The military health services, at first ill prepared for so fundamental an examination, were slow to embrace the need for change. In addition, the warfighter, struggling to find clear direction in the middle of revolutionary change, was unable to describe what sort of medical organization would be needed to support future military operations across an ever widening spectrum. However, with budgets shrinking rapidly and with the experience of the Gulf War fresh in memory, military health services became convinced that future military victory must be achieved with minimal casualties. There were few incentives to spend money on "operational medical insurance."

Despite the turmoil created by interacting pressures, we are moving quickly to meet the challenges of the post-Cold War world. The Assistant Secretary for Defense (Health Affairs) and the Service Surgeons General have spent years navigating a turbulent and murky passage. Although there now appears to be a much clearer vision of the future and a genuine willingness to work toward a joint structure, they are still not out of the whitewater. Recent reviews may not have resulted in more major MHSS reductions, but more changes and some substantial reductions are inevitable as cost savings are enforced. Therefore, the restructuring of both peacetime and operational military health care must remain "a work in progress." Much hard work and innovative thinking are required to develop an organization that is fully able to meet the military's needs in the new century.

Steering a New Course: Future Directions in Military Health Care

What course should military health care take in the future? It is not possible to say precisely, nor is it wise or necessary to attempt to map a detailed course at this stage. A better plan of action is to decide on a general heading or direction and then "steer by the stars." We can then use the major principles and precepts of military health care as "waypoints" that enable us to maintain direction even when the events of the moment push us temporarily off course.

To decide our general heading, we must address two key questions:

- What will be the future business of military health care?
- Are we focusing on the right basic principles and precepts of military health care?

The Future Business of Military Health Care

To understand what the future business of military health care will be, we must first look at the "customer" or warfighter and attempt to determine his health needs. What will the future warfighter be like? What are the characteristics of the future battlefield on which he or she will fight? How must changes in military health care work to address emerging needs?

The Future Warfighter

The future warfighter will come from a home less threatened by the extreme prospect of nuclear war but still disconcerted by lack of certainty in a risk-filled and shrinking world. The warfighter's family and friends will be unlikely to have much direct knowledge and understanding of (or sympathy for) the profession of arms or the conduct of war; as a nation, we have a diminished tolerance for human casualties, particularly among our own sons and daughters. Because changes in social values and lifestyles have increased physical and psychological "softness" in many Americans, the warfighter will probably be less willing or able to endure traditional hardships of conflict without a great deal of training and preparation. Moreover, he or she will serve a society so comprehensively influenced by the media that the television camera has become a weapon of war, one that not only shapes public opinion and affects national morale, but is also capable of influencing operational and even strategic outcomes.

Despite changes in society and in the warfighter's disposition, the United States still expects military success at the lowest cost to the nation in money and manpower. Expectations for high-quality, low-cost military health care to support the warfighter are equally high. It is evident that the contemporary warfighter expects wartime health care to be equal or superior to peacetime care.

The Future Battlefield

The business of warfighting, the sharp end of the operational spectrum, is not going to get easier in the foreseeable future. Technology is increasing the lethality of weapons and changing the way we fight. More accurate and lethal weapons mean that fewer are needed—and that fewer personnel on the battlefield are needed to operate them. Although this means there are fewer people in harm's way, the increasing lethality places increasing demands on the smaller number of warfighters who have to remain on the battlefield. They will have to disperse more widely and move faster than ever to avoid detection, protect themselves, and outmaneuver the enemy. The result is that they have become increasingly difficult to find and recover when they are wounded. There was evidence in the Gulf War that despite the low casualty numbers and the wealth of medical support, some casualties took many hours to reach definitive care, the consequence of high-speed combat and long evacuation routes.

Technology has also negated the traditional limits of night and even weather on combat. The 24-hour battle, with all its physical and psychological demands, is now a reality. The land battle of the Gulf War lasted little more than 100 hours, but for the warfighter it was a 100-hour battle with no respite. During that period, the Coalition Forces covered hundreds of miles at high speed. Combat was more often encounter battles than deliberate, planned attacks. The weapons systems enabled fighting on the move: tanks engaged and killed targets in the dark at distances of over 2 miles, with first-time hits expected. The speed of maneuver and the complexity of the battlefield meant that fighting units and their supporting formations were often separated by many miles of hostile desert, filled with mines, unexploded ordnance, and surrendering enemy units. Many combatants became so physically and psychologically exhausted that one commander, Major General Rupert Smith, described his forces as being "stressed by their own success."

Importance of Conserving the Fighting Force

Our future warfighters will become increasingly difficult to find, expensive to train, and difficult to replace. There will also be so few that even the loss of small numbers will have a dramatic effect on combat power. For example, the modern B2 bomber is said to have the equivalent combat power of 70 aircraft from the Vietnam War era. However, if one member of the B2 crew becomes sick or injured, his replacement will be a specialist in very short supply. If a replacement cannot be found, the nonavailability of the aircraft could mean a significant loss of combat power and might even affect the tactical outcome. The same argument is true of the Army's Abrams Main Battle Tank, the Apache attack helicopter, and the Patriot Missile. Even the Navy is not immune. Major surface warships of the future will have crews of less than 100, but how many can be lost to disease and injury before the ship can no longer fight?

This modern phenomenon makes the traditional military medical role of conserving the fighting force ever more vital. Preventive medicine and health promotion should be reestablished as the major tasks of military health care; until recently, these tasks have been eclipsed by the preoccupation with treating and evacuating the wounded from battle. The need to conserve the fighting force also significantly raises the profile of Disease and Non-Battle Injury (DNBI) as a factor in medical planning.

Even if most future U.S. military operations are relatively low-intensity operations like those recently experienced in Somalia, Bosnia, and Kosovo, U.S. forces will still have to organize and train for high-intensity conflict, under the military dictum "Train for war, adjust for peace." Operations like peacekeeping are no less demanding than actual combat; they are merely different. Modern combat will be intense but of short duration, peacekeeping operations tend to be protracted, and although levels of violence are lower, there is always the risk of death and injury. Many of these operations take place in countries where the social infrastructure is destroyed and the risk of disease and injury is high. The frequency of this type of operation and its open-ended nature result in a marked increase in "operational tempo," or deployments for units and individuals. This in turn increases the physical and emotional stress on individuals and their dependents and contributes to the demand for very high levels of healthcare support.

Need for Transformation

Clearly, the warfighter's needs for tomorrow's conflict have so fundamentally changed that the MHS requires a comparable transformation in the provision of health care in both war and peace. The underpinning debate concerns how best to reconcile the needs of readiness with the often competing day-to-day demands of the peacetime mission. In the future, operational health support must be capable of providing the highest standards of care from the outset; it can no longer afford to adopt the traditional approach of getting better through experience as operations develop. The most pressing dilemma facing the Surgeons General is how best to obtain the necessary training in peace to prepare for war, given that peacetime hospitals and medical centers in the main are unable to provide vital experience like military-relevant trauma care. Even where such training is available, it cannot meet the needs of the three services' clinical specialists, particularly surgeons and OR staffs.

The problem of training the "First Responder" combat medic is much larger and far from being resolved. The First Responder is the vital first link in the chain, without whom the casualty will never get off the battlefield alive. History shows that even with highly sophisticated care at subsequent echelons, combat mortality and morbidity rates rise without well-trained First Responders. How this training can best be achieved (continuation training included) is a complex issue and the subject of contentious debate. Emerging technologies like telemedicine may provide some answers, but they must be focused on training and should not attempt to substitute for expertise. Current developments in the arena of medical simulation and virtual reality may provide the best option. The DoD is actively pursuing research and development in this area, under the aegis of Medical Research and Materiel Command.

We must face and solve these dilemmas to avoid repeating the lessons of history, poignantly described in a postconflict report of British medical efforts during the Crimean War: "How wide and various is the experience of the battlefield and how fertile the blood of warriors in raising good surgeons" (Allbutt 1898). Although this censure has been a common theme of postconflict medical reports, it should not (and need not) be an indictment of health support for future operations.

Other Considerations

Included in health care's future business is the question of how best to provide health care in peace and operations for dependents and retirees.

The latter in particular are the major consumer of peacetime military health care at the hospital level and, given current trends, they will dramatically increase in number. The result can only be substantial cost increases, even if the increase in retirees is accompanied by subvention of Medicare funding. However, the argument is far from simple. On one hand, retirees and dependents are a major limitation on readiness because much effort and many resources are required to ensure they are provided for when the MHS is deployed. On the other hand, without the broad clinical practice that retirees in particular provide, it would be impossible to render the breadth of patient care necessary to train, accredit, and retain in peace many vital specialist providers like surgeons and anesthesiologists. Resolving this dilemma will be vital to the future of operational healthcare support.

Principles and Precepts of Military Health Care

Even a cursory examination of our long-held operational healthcare principles and precepts raises some key questions that will have to be addressed. As already discussed, the traditional roles of maintaining health, preventing disease, and treating and evacuating sick and wounded from the battlefield are being carefully reexamined. Also pressing is the need to redefine the function of casualty rates, the basis of medical force planning. Traditionally, warfighting staffs, in concert with the medical staff, have predicted the expected rate of combat casualties expressed as a percentage of the force deployed over time. This calculation, often shown as a figure or casualty estimate, is used to determine the capabilities and size of the deployed healthcare support. It seems certain that future political and military imperatives will dictate minimum casualty rates in all but the most exceptional and dire military operations. The question is this: On what criteria will casualty rates be developed? Will a casualty rate be expressed as a realistic estimate or an optimistic, politically acceptable guess for an operation? Will these rates continue to be the tool used to dictate the shape and size of deployed healthcare support, even if the predicted rates are too small to be used to produce viable medical organizations?

Future Casualty Evacuation and Treatment Processes

Modern warfighting doctrine dictates that casualties require almost immediate replacement from reserves, and the drive to limit deployed logistic footprints severely constrains the shape and size of in-theater medical support. The result is a growing trend to evacuate all but those with the most minor sicknesses and injuries out of the theater as quickly as possible. The USAF medical services are currently developing a sophisticated intra-theater evacuation system known as "Care in the Air." As laudable as this might be, it is critically dependent on airframes. The approaching end of the operational life of such aircraft as the C9 and C141 will almost certainly produce constraints on USAF planning. There is also an urgent need to review traditional evacuation policies designed to treat in theater, hold, and return to duty the maximum number of combatants who could be "repaired" within a given time frame. Casualties treated and retained in an operational theater become a logistic and security liability until they return to duty; in addition to their medical treatment, they have to be housed, fed, watered, and protected from enemy attack.

There is also a pressing need to reexamine the current system for casualty notification, a vital element of the casualty treatment and evacuation process. The aim must be to provide faster, more accurate information about casualties from a theater of operation to dependents and the operational and administrative staff. Only by creating these higher standards of reporting and tracking will the military cope with the increasing demands of news media reporting and the "CNN Curve" and meet rising expectations of dependents and families.

Impact of DNBI

As the threat of large numbers of traditional combat casualties—i.e., the results of bullets and bombs—diminishes, the impact of DNBI has increased, particularly the effect of "unknown" hazards as exemplified by Gulf War Syndrome. The most effective means of combating such threats is gathering data and analyzing it in the classic epidemiological method. This, together with the development of specific preventive measures, is known in modern military healthcare parlance as "Force Protection."

In light of the perceived growing threat to U.S. Forces from terrorist attacks using chemical or biological agents as weapons of mass destruction, these Force Protection measures may well include vaccination against specific disease threats. The development of accurate, timely, and seamless data capture and information management for this purpose continues to test the MHS. The aim should be to develop a rugged and seamless system providing a Computerized Personal Medical Record that follows the warfighter from the moment of enlistment until retirement and beyond. Such a record would gather data on operations and record health status and treatment throughout a service career. Whatever approach is adopted, there is an urgent operational requirement to replace the current system of paper-based records and data capture, little changed since the Civil War.

Effect of Technology

Finally, there is a need to examine the overall effect of technology on deployed health support. Many questions will arise, such as the following:

- What will be the true impact of technology on the quality of care at every level, and how will it reshape the traditional structures?
- What medical capabilities are vital in deployed healthcare organizations?

- How valid are echelons of care on the seamless digital battlefield?
- Will there be a need in the future for such distinct Army and Marine organizations as Battalion Aid Posts and Medical Battalions?
- How valid is the concept of deployable hospitals for all three services?
- Is there a continuing role for hospital ships configured like the USS *Mercy* or *Comfort* in the electronic maritime combat environment?
- What functions are being made operationally redundant by new technology-driven processes like Telemedicine?
- What impact can simulation and modeling have on training in combat medical skills?

Answering these questions and others will be vital to mapping the future direction of military health care. We can only answer them by continuing to review the roles and mission of military health care in peace and war, and this review process will only be relevant if it is conducted in close concert with the warfighter. To paraphrase the great nineteenth-century French leader Clemenceau, "military health care is too important to be left to military healthcare professionals." The review process should be an evolving military medical doctrine shaped to meet the warfighter's needs, compatible with the requirements of all three medical services, and adaptable enough to be used in multinational operations across the spectrum of conflict. This doctrine should be the basis for the design of training, equipment, and logistic support of future military healthcare organizations.

Conclusion

The future of military health care is one of rapid and major change, which will bring with it great uncertainty and much opportunity. Transforming military health care to manage the "whitewater" of change in this new century will not be easy to achieve. As we steer toward the future, we must begin recognizing the needs of the new warfighter, managing the effects of technology and a diminishing fighting force, and restimulating the ongoing deliberations between the three military health services by including the military healthcare consumer at every level of the debate.

References

Allbutt, C. 1898. *British Medical Journal.*
Koop, C.E. 1994. Address to the Association of Military Surgeons of the United States, Orlando, FL.
Mazzar, M. 1994. The Revolution in Military Affairs. U.S. Army War College Strategic Studies Institute, Carlisle, PA.

3
Federal Support for Healthcare Information Systems

Morris F. Collen

Before the 1940s, medical research in the United States was supported primarily by private funding and by philanthropic foundations and endowments (Shyrock 1947). However, after the Hill-Burton Act of 1946, tens of millions of dollars went to hospital construction, opening the door for the introduction of new technologies into hospitals. After World War II, the early development of healthcare informatics was mainly supported by federal government grants and contracts.

In 1959, Senator Hubert Humphrey conducted hearings that concluded the time was appropriate for the federal government to support biomedical computing. The National Institutes of Health (NIH) promptly initiated funding to support research and development projects and establish regional and university-based biomedical computer centers. Throughout the 1960s, funds streamed from NIH and other federal agencies, encouraging the use of computers in medicine. In the 1970s, funding decreased and the NIH computer resources program was abruptly reduced. In a decade marked by economic recession and inflation, Medicare and Medicaid grew in size and costs. In the 1980s, as healthcare expenditures became a national concern, technology was often condemned as the primary reason for the phenomenon (Starr 1982).

In assessing the impact of federal funding on health care, we focus on two areas. The first is agency funding for research and development efforts in both the private and public sectors, and the second is information systems work in support of direct patient care provided by the Veterans Administration (VA) and the Department of Defense (DoD).

Federal funding supported much of the early research and development in medical informatics. It did so with minimal direction or coordination, resulting in a "bottom-up" approach. This stands in contrast to national "top-down" approaches taken in some other countries, notably Japan. This broad-based early work laid the foundation for the evolution and diffusion of healthcare informatics in this country. Medical and bioengineering organizations, commercial organizations, medical schools and universities, and federal agencies all played major roles (Collen 1986). In the 1990s, with the growth of the Internet and web technologies, the pace of cross-sector collaboration accelerated. We strongly believe it will continue to do so in this new millennium.

The VA and DoD are two of the largest healthcare systems in the world. Each has several hundred freestanding clinics, well over a hundred hospitals, hospital admissions of a million or more, and outpatient visits in the neighborhood of a quarter million per year. The VA and DoD have long histories with their multifacility healthcare systems and offer very different models. The VA took a decentralized "bottom-up" approach, relied predominantly on in-house development, and generally enjoyed high user satisfaction. The DoD took a centralized "top-down" approach, purchased vendor turnkey systems, and registered variable user satisfaction. Today, as discussed elsewhere in this book, the VA and DoD are looking to the private sector for approaches and solutions proven in diverse settings, leveraging what works, and benefiting from private sector experience with financial systems. These two federally funded systems can offer the private sector valuable lessons on providing care that crosses geographic boundaries, follows the patient across time, and shares the focus on wellness so critical to the DoD. We believe that, in the area of multifacility systems, technology transfer is just beginning. As it increases markedly, it will be valuable to both sectors.

In the pages that follow, we give a brief overview of the impact of federal funding for healthcare informatics, highlighting areas where technology transfer has occurred. We also relate the work done by the VA and DoD in providing information systems support for their multifacility systems, documenting past accomplishments in hopes of fostering technology transfer now and in the future.

Research and Development in Medical Informatics

National Library of Medicine

The National Library of Medicine (NLM) has long been an innovator in healthcare informatics. In 1879 its first director, John Shaw Billings, initiated the *Index Medicus*, a bibliographic listing of articles in biomedical journals. The NLM revolutionized this Index in 1964 by implementing the computer-based Medical Literature Analysis and Retrieval System known as MEDLARS. In 1971, the NLM introduced MEDLINE, an online version of MEDLARS, with files dating back to 1966. Under its current director, Donald A.B. Lindberg, the NLM has continued this tradition of innovation, extending free access to its resources via the web-based PubMed. By making biomedical information easily available in the United States and throughout the world, the NLM has helped to transform the information-intensive enterprises that make up health care.

The NLM assumed leadership in the critical area of medical nomenclature, an area beyond the reach of any single private entity. In the 1980s, the NLM launched the Unified Medical Language System (UMLS) project to facilitate access to machine-readable information located in various sources, including scientific literature, factual databases, knowledge-based expert systems, and computer-based patient records (Humphreys and Lindberg 1989). This work, of course, is critical to the full use of the literature indexed by the NLM. It is also critical to population-based health and outcomes research. The NLM continues to develop the UMLS, mapping terms across SNOMED, Read Code, and other terminologies and helping the biomedical community address the difficult problems posed by medical nomenclature.

The NLM has launched other initiatives, training professionals and encouraging institutional change. Pre- and postdoctoral training programs in medical informatics, first funded by NLM in the 1970s, produced many of the professionals now working in private and public settings. Programs like these continue today at Harvard, Minnesota, Stanford, and other academic health centers. Extramural programs funded by NLM in the 1980s, such as the Integrated Academic Information Management System (IAIMS) initiative, supported institutional change. Academic health centers designated as IAIMS sites—initially Columbia-Presbyterian Medical Center, Georgetown University, and the universities of Maryland and Utah—used computers and communication networks to link varied information bases, support diverse activities, and create integrated systems (NLM 1984, 1986). By developing new applications and approaches, and by defining the importance of human factors, these early leaders helped set the stage for innovations undertaken by hospitals that joined to form integrated delivery systems in the 1990s.

For the NLM, medical informatics was clearly a priority. By 1989, approximately 10% of its budget directly supported medical informatics.

National Institutes of Health (NIH)

The NLM's parent organization, the National Institutes of Health (NIH), also looked to academic institutions as change agents for medicine. Grant funding from the NIH supported many early biomedical computing centers, including those at Tulane, the University of California Los Angeles, Johns Hopkins, the University of Utah (home of the first U.S. department of medical informatics), and the Massachusetts Institute of Technology (a multicenter research resources program). By the end of 1966, NIH supported a total of 48 centers, with over $8 million in total annual support (Raub 1971).

The NIH also sponsored early work in artificial intelligence at academic centers under its biotechnology resources program. In 1973, the

Stanford University Medical Experimental Artificial Intelligence in Medicine (SUMEX-AIM) was launched, including a network of computers at Stanford, Rutgers, and the University of Pittsburgh, with collaboration from the University of Missouri-Columbia (Lindberg 1982). This evolved to a long-distance communications network for a user community involved in roughly 20 research projects spanning a broad range of applications.

The NIH also targeted profit-making organizations through negotiated contracts to help develop biomedical informatics (Lusted 1961). In 1964, NIH contracted with the Washington University Computer Laboratories in St. Louis, Missouri, to address the design and application of minicomputers in health care. In 1965, the NIH established a Division of Computer Research and Technology (DCRT). The DCRT contributed significantly to the computer processing of natural language text, and by 1970 it was the largest health computing facility in the nation (Gee 1970)—one more testament to the critical role federal funding played in the development of healthcare informatics.

Other Programs

Established by Congress under the Heart, Cancer, and Stroke Act of 1965, the Regional Medical Program (RMP) included 54 computer-based RMPs by 1967. Programs included clinical laboratory systems, clinical data collection studies, multiphasic screening systems, and tumor registries. During the 1960s, the U.S. Public Health Service, through its Chronic Disease Division, also supported computer applications for multiphasic screening systems and preventive medicine (Waxman 1961).

National Center for Health Services Research and Development

In 1968, the National Center for Health Services Research Development (NCHSR&D) was organized within the Health Services and Mental Health Administration. The Center supported computer-based information systems in 1969 and 1970, including medical records projects, hospital information systems, clinical laboratory systems, X-ray information systems, physiological monitoring systems, pharmacy information systems, a multiphasic screening system, and patient interviewing projects.

In addition, NCHSR&D funded two Health Services Research Centers with healthcare information systems as their principal focus. According to their estimates, more than $31 million was spent between 1962 and 1970 on projects using computers in healthcare delivery. During the 1970s, the

Center evaluated several hospital information systems and supported office information systems, clinical laboratory systems, radiology systems, automated interpretation of electrocardiograms, automated patient monitoring systems, and computer-based consulting systems.

Department of Defense

Other initiatives were funded by the Department of Defense (DoD). The Defense Advanced Research Project Agency (DARPA) contributed to academic computer science departments, notably at the University of California at Berkeley, Carnegie Mellon, Stanford, and the Massachusetts Institute of Technology. One far-reaching project began in 1966, when DARPA contracted with Bolt, Beranek, and Newman, in Cambridge, Massachusetts, to create a wide area network called ARPANET. Initiated in 1969 using packet switching, ARPANET became the first nationwide digital network and was used to connect academic computer centers conducting research for DoD. By 1972, ARPANET linked 29 computer centers, each with its own communications minicomputer, to a single terminal at the DoD.

The basic technology developed for ARPANET was soon released for commercial private development. Eventually, as the chapter on Enhancing Private Biomedical Technology (Chapter 4) describes in greater detail, ARPANET evolved into the global Internet in a truly remarkable instance of technology transfer.

Health Care Financing Agency

In the 1970s, the growth of Medicare and Medicaid and associated costs reshaped health care and the role of the Health Care Financing Agency (HCFA). According to Lindberg (1978, p. 346), "The most profound effect upon medical information systems certainly was the introduction of the Medicare system . . . These federal programs have created whole industries within the computer field . . . of health care services required for 'third party' reimbursement."

In 1983, HCFA instituted fixed Medicare payments for 468 diagnostic related groups (DRGs) based on International Classification of Diseases (ICD) codes. As a result, every hospital accepting Medicare patients could collect the data to satisfy Medicare billing requirements. With Medicare accounting for about 40% of all hospital beds in use in the United States, HCFA became a powerful force in the diffusion of hospital information systems in private sector institutions.

Federal agencies played a key role in the early development of healthcare informatics by initiating and supporting seminal activities. In the years ahead, we will see the continued influence of this federally funded innovation in both the private and public sectors.

Multifacility Healthcare Systems

The Veterans Administration

In the 1950s, the VA maintained a central computerized file of all VA patients, including identification data, claims, and Social Security numbers. A patient treatment file contained inpatient admission and discharge data, surgical procedures, diagnoses, and patient disposition data. Every month, VA hospitals submitted decks of punched cards to the central processing center, each card representing data for a completed hospital episode (Christianson 1964). Revised to include outpatient visits, the patient treatment file became a management tool used by the VA Central Office (Rosen 1968).

In the 1960s and 1970s, the VA began to explore the use of computers in its clinical program. The 710-bed VA hospital in Washington, D.C., piloted an automated hospital information system (AHIS) in 1965 and had several modules operational by 1969 (Christianson 1969). Judged inadequate for the VA's requirements, the system was terminated. Several other VA hospitals independently developed additional clinical applications, mostly using MUMPS for applications programming and File Manager for the database management system (Ivers et al. 1983). File Manager allowed the user to define new files, add new attributes to existing files, and list or search the files for any combination of data elements (Timson 1980).

Throughout the 1980s, the VA focused on decentralizing operations among the medical centers. Early in this process, a task force inventoried computer capabilities and developed plans to implement existing software developed in house. To carry out the work of the task force, the Medical Information Resources Management Office (MIRMO) was formed in 1982. Two years later, MIRMO published what was known as the Department of Medicine and Surgery Automated Data Processing Plan (DM&S ADP), including procurement and budget strategies. In the meantime, MIRMO had established six regional Verification and Development Centers (VDCs), whose directors were charged with overseeing and directing the central program—specifically, preventing duplicate efforts, ensuring system exportability, and developing a management information system supported by standard data dictionaries. In 1983, the VA established Special Interest User Groups (SIUGs) made up of experts in the field and the central office. The SIUGs were tasked with fostering computer literacy and supporting systems development throughout the VA. Members were involved in a wide range of activities, from developing functional requirements to helping the VDCs and serving as advocates for program area interests.

As stated in their plan, the VA's objective was "to decentralize to the field the responsibilities for ADP planning, budgeting, and operations to the maximum extent possible." To this end, the DM&S launched the Decentralized Hospital Computer Program (DHCP). Mostly written in MUMPS, DHCP included a basic set of software tools for database management, electronic communications, security, and software management. Known as the Kernel, this tool set allowed centrally developed software to coexist with locally adapted software and shared a common patient database with a system of applications known as the CORE system. Initially the CORE included patient identification and registration; admission, discharge, and transfer; ward census; clinic scheduling; and outpatient pharmacy. A full CORE system, planned for all VAMCs, added inpatient pharmacy, clinical laboratory, and radiology.

DHCP developers recognized the importance of standardization. Before any program was put to use at more than one location, it was verified by a VDC. A data dictionary established by the DM&S provided a common data structure for use in the various field-developed systems, ensuring standardization throughout the hospital network.

In 1983, Congress mandated the VA to procure, install, and assess three commercial hospital information systems and compare their effectiveness to the DHCP. It was generally acknowledged that the VA DHCP in the mid-1980s could not equal the capabilities of these commercial systems. The next year's DM&S ADP Plan reported that $48 million was being devoted to new computers and equipment as implementation of the full DHCP CORE system began. A mandatory training program for all DHCP users contributed to the successful implementation of its modules. Computer overview classes were held at least once a week, and physicians, nurses, and other functional user groups were taught together, allowing for diverse user-specific issues to be addressed in class (Catellier et al. 1987).

In 1987, at the direction of the U.S. Congress, the Office of Technology Assessment (OTA) conducted an independent review of the DHCP. According to its findings, "in the long term, DHCP may have limitations that could make it an unsuitable platform for the transition to the information system VA will need in the 1990s" (OTA 1987, p. 1). As the VA DHCP was not yet an integrated system but a series of interfaced applications, the OTA report focused on integrating patient data as a critical requirement.

By 1990, the DHCP contained clinical management modules for inpatient and outpatient pharmacy, clinical laboratory, radiology, anatomic pathology, blood bank, dietetics, medicine, surgery, oncology, nursing, mental health, dentistry, social work, quality assurance and utilization review, order entry, and results reporting. A health summary served as the beginning of a computer-based patient record that integrated clinical data from ancillary support packages and could be viewed by clinicians on displays or as printed reports. The admission, discharge, and transfer (ADT) module, the focal point in data collection for DHCP, included demographic, employment, insurance, and medical history information. ADT was used by other DHCP modules, including laboratory, pharmacy, radiology, and dietetics. The decentralized nature of the VA DHCP program was exhibited in its November 1989 report, which detailed the responsibilities of the

Verification and Development Centers (VDCs), now called Information Systems Centers (ISCs). Each ISC was responsible for a different set of modules.

Department of Defense

Like the VA, the DoD began its information systems work with a punched-card database, this one developed to help select candidates for the Air Force's Man in Space program (Schwichtenburg 1959). The 1960s saw independent development efforts within each of the three armed services, but it was not until 1973 that the DoD's Defense Systems Acquisition Review Council (DSARC) recommended combining the automated medical information systems efforts of the three military services into a single Tri-Service Program.

In 1974, the Deputy Secretary of Defense established TRIMIS, the Tri-Service Medical Information Systems Program (Bickel 1979) to improve the effectiveness and economy of healthcare delivery. TRIMIS was instructed to apply automated data processing techniques, centralize and coordinate application development, adapt advanced technology, and streamline and standardize the DoD's medical information systems.

In 1976, the TRIMIS Program Office (TPO) was established. Its direct management was transferred from the TRIMIS Steering Group to the Assistant Secretary of Defense for Health Affairs, with the Steering Group providing advice and guidance. The TPO focused on three major areas: functional work center applications to improve patient care, resources to improve management applications, and integration of functional and management applications into an overall replicable system, first for a single hospital and then for larger entities.

Guided by a master plan (Bickel 1978), TRIMIS addressed its objectives through three levels of automated data processing capabilities: in the work center, in the medical treatment facility (MTF), and in DoD higher commands. All were to be implemented in four incremental phases. In the beginning, commercially available applications were piloted (known as Initial Operational Capabilities or IOCs) in selected high-volume work centers. This work supported the next phase, the evolution of standardized systems with expanded functional support in additional work centers, the development of standards needed to integrate the initial modules, and the design of a Network Integrating System (NIS). The third phase involved designing a Composite Hospital System (CHS), culminating in specifications for integrating the standardized systems within the military treatment facilities (MTFs). The final phase called for implementation of a DoD Health Care Information System (HCIS) to manage both resource and patient-centered data on a systemwide basis.

In 1978, the TPO reported on support for Tri-Service Wards and Clinics Support at three different sites, comparing the automated pilot system to the traditional manual alternative. Total costs (11 years discounted) for the automated system were 0.5% less than for the manual system. Benefits included fewer redundant services, reduced requirements for clerical support, improved outpatient pharmaceutical management, reduced workload burden, and less patient time away from active duty (TRIMIS 1978).

By 1979, the TPO had put a number of IOCs in place. Without an integrating system, however, users had to access each module individually to retrieve data from their respective databases. Furthermore, Congressman Brooks issued a report that year criticizing TRIMIS for designing a system from scratch and disregarding the years of costly research, development, and testing that had preceded their efforts (Brooks 1979). The report also judged requirements for the computer-based patient record and the healthcare provider functional requirements as "gold-plated" enhancements. The TPO decided to move directly into the third phase and develop plans for a comprehensive, fully integrated system.

In 1980, as it had for the VA, Congress directed the DoD to install and assess two or three competing commercial hospital information systems. In addition, because of concerns about the possible duplication of effort between the DoD and the VA, Congress directed the DoD to test the feasibility of using the VA DHCP software. An external analysis conducted by the Mitre Corporation in 1984 found that the TRIMIS functionality demonstrated by the VA system was 30% adequate for CHCS.

In 1984, to integrate its military healthcare information systems more completely, the Assistant Secretary of Defense for Health Affairs established the Defense Medical Systems Support Center (DMSSC). The assessments completed earlier were used to formulate specific requirements for what was now called the Composite Health Care System (CHCS), and the TPO released a request for proposal (RFP) to the vendor community, excluding the requirements judged to be "gold-plated" in the Brooks report. A second RFP, also without these requirements, was released in March 1987.

In 1988, the DoD chose Science Applications International Corporation (SAIC) as its vendor. The selected CHCS architecture was to be decentralized at the hospital level, with a mainframe computer in each hospital linked to its associated clinics by a communications network. Independent clinics separate from hospitals were to receive their own mainframe computer. The system included a comprehensive data dictionary, a standard terminal display presentation and editing tool, and electronic mail for all users. CHCS would provide patient care data through integration with the functional work centers of clinical dietetics, laboratory, nursing, patient administration, patient appointment and scheduling, pharmacy, and radiology. CHCS would provide support to order entry and test results reporting (Mestrovich 1988).

In 1989, sites were selected for beta testing. Most of the IOC modules were to be replaced in the early 1990s by CHCS installations (Andreoni

1990). TPC prepared a test and evaluation master plan to review and monitor CHCS functional effectiveness (TRIMIS 1988), and the Arthur D. Little Group obtained a contract to provide a benefits assessment of CHCS.

Even at the end of the 1980s, CHCS had not yet planned to provide an integrated, computer-based patient record, nor did it satisfy such healthcare professional functional requirements as the inclusion of patients' medical histories, physicians' physical examination findings, or consultation reports. These functions awaited a later phase of enhancements in the 1990s, when the DoD, the VA, and the Indian Health Service joined to develop comprehensive, lifelong, computer-based patient record systems. By the late 1990s, CHCS was deployed in all major DoD facilities, and was one of the largest and most comprehensive multifacility healthcare information systems in the country.

As federal and private multifacility systems address issues of cost and outcomes in a managed care environment, technology transfer holds promise for both. Chapters elsewhere in this volume review current work in the federal sector that draws upon and contributes to private sector initiatives.

Technology Transfer

This chapter recognizes the major influence the federal government has had on the diffusion of healthcare information systems and on medical technology transfer. We applaud that influence and urge legislators to continue to support the use of healthcare information systems—primarily to improve the quality of patient care, and only secondarily to decrease its cost.

Acknowledgment. The author wishes to thank the American Medical Informatics Association for permission to draw from the work reported more fully in his book, *A History of Medical Informatics in the United States* (Bethesda, MD: American Medical Informatics Association, 1995) and refers the reader to that volume for archival information.

References

Andreoni, A.J. 1990. From the DMSCC Director's Desk. *CHCS Parameters* 1:1.

Bickel, R.G. 1978. The TRIMIS Planning Process: Decisions, Decisions, Decisions. In: Emlet, H.E., ed. *Challenges and Prospects for Advanced Medical Systems.* Miami: Symposia Specialists, pp. 175–181.

Bickel, R.G. 1979. The TRIMIS Concept. *SCAMC Proceedings*, pp. 839–842. Long Beach, CA: IEEE Computer Society Press.

Brooks, J. 1979. Memorandum re: Investigation of the TRIMIS Project, March 27.

Catellier, J., Bernway, P.K., Perez, K. 1987. Meeting the DHCP Challenge: A Model for Implementing a Decentralized Hospital Computer Program. *SCAMC Proceedings*, 595–598. Los Angeles, CA: IEEE Computer Society Press.

Christianson, L.G. 1964. Medical Data Automation in the VA. *Mil Med* 29:614–617.

Christianson, L.G. 1969. Toward an Automated Hospital Information System. *Ann NY Acad Sci* 161:694–706.

Collen, M.F. 1986. Origins of Medical Informatics. *West J Med* 145:778–785.

Gee, H.H. 1970. Organization and Influence in Biomedical Computing. *J Inform Med*, pp. 437–450.

Humphreys, B.L., Lindberg, D.A.B. 1989. Building the Unified Medical Language. *SCAMC Proceedings*, pp. 475–480. Washington, DC: IEEE Computer Society Press.

Ivers, M.T., Timson, G.F., Blankensee, H., Whitfield, G., Keltz, P., Pfeil, C. 1983. Large Scale Implementation of Compatible Hospital Computer Systems within the Veterans Administration. *SCAMC Proceedings*, pp. 53–56. Silver Spring, MD: IEEE Computer Society Press.

Lindberg, D.A.B. 1978. Computers in Health Care. Hearings before the Committee on Science and Technology, U.S. House of Representatives, May 1978.

Lindberg, D.A.B. 1982. Computer Networks Within Health Care: The State of the Art in the USA. In: Peterson, H.E., Isaksson, A.J., eds. *Communications Networks in Health Care*. Amsterdam: North Holland, pp. 109–120.

Lusted, L.B. 1961. Summary of Discussions on Medical Data Centers. In: *Proceedings of the Third IBM Medical Symposium*. Endicott, NY: IBM, pp. 203–213.

Mestrovich, M.J. 1988. *Defense Medical Systems Support Center (DMSSC) Fact Book*. Falls Church, VA: DMSSC.

NLM (National Library of Medicine). 1984. *Planning for Integrated Academic Information Systems*. Proceedings of the NLM Symposium. Bethesda, MD: NLM.

NLM. 1986. Second IAIMS Symposium Emphasizes Health Sciences Education. *NLM News* 41:1.

OTA (Office of Technology Assessment). 1987. *Special Report: Hospital Information Systems at the Veterans Administration*. Washington, DC: OTA.

Raub, W.F. 1971. The Life Sciences Computer Resources Program of the National Institutes of Health. In: *Proceedings of 1971 Annual Conference*. New York: ACM, pp. 693–700.

Rosen, D. 1968. Medical Care Information System of the Veterans Administration. *Public Health Rep* 83:363–371.

Schwichtenberg, A.H. 1959. The Development and Use of Medical Machine Record Cards in the Astronaut Selection Program. In: *Proceedings of the First IBM Medical Symposium*. Poughkeepsie, NY: IBM, pp. 185–204.

Shyrock, R.H. 1947. *American Medical Research, Past and Present*. New York: The Commonwealth Fund.

Starr, P. 1982. *The Social Transformation of American Medicine*. New York: Basic Books.

Timson, G. 1980. The File Manager System. *SCAMC Proceedings*, pp. 1645–1649. Long Beach, CA: IEEE Computer Society Press.

TRIMIS (Tri-Service Medical Information Systems). 1978. *A Study of Costs and Benefits*. Bethesda, MD: TRIMIS Program Office.

TRIMIS (Tri-Service Medical Information Systems). 1988. *TEMP: Trimis Composite Health Care System Test and Evaluation Plan.* Bethesda, MD: TRIMIS Program Office (TPO).

Waxman, B.D. 1961. Public Health Service Support of Biomedical Computing. In: *Proceedings of the Third IBM Medical Symposium.* Endicott, NY: IBM, pp. 199–202.

4
Enhancing Private Biomedical Technology: The Role of Federal Programs

Steven J. Phillips

During the early days of World War II, American soldiers fighting in the scorching sun of the Pacific Islands, working on the decks of ships, or stranded on the open ocean rapidly became victims of incapacitating sunburn. Recognizing the critical need for a skin agent to protect GIs, the government began experimenting with sun-protecting chemicals like red petrolatum, the inert residue that remains after crude oil is processed into gasoline and heating oil. Red petrolatum's natural red pigments proved to be effective in blocking the sun's ultraviolet rays, and the Army Air Corps issued it to pilots and crews in case they were downed in the tropics. Dr. Benjamin Green, who assisted the military in developing sunscreens, believed there was a vast, untapped commercial market for sunning products. After the war, he helped develop sunscreen into a creamy white lotion scented with the essence of jasmine, a product that became known as Coppertone.

As this account indicates, government-sponsored programs have enabled the multidisciplinary transfer of technology to the private sector, resulting in significant advances in health care for the American public and for all of humankind. Federal programs involved in the development of biomedical devices, biogenics, and information and communication technologies have a long history of profound impact on private health care. Nonprofit government programs play a significant role in initiating and sustaining a level of biomedical technology transfer that the industry is not likely to achieve by itself. These programs can assess the needs and evaluate alternative sources for cutting edge biomedical technologies. In addition, by viewing the "big picture," federal programs can evaluate merits, coordinate resources, and provide a minimum infrastructure to catalyze biomedical technology transfer to the private sector. We believe that *how* the transfer occurs is of little consequence, so long as it does occur on a regular basis.

Because space does not permit a detailed discussion of all the federal programs that promote technology transfer to the private sector, this chapter provides a broad overview of a selected subset of these programs. The programs can be separated into three basic categories: programs that are active, interactive, and passive in the transfer of biomedical technology to the private sector. These three are not mutually exclusive, as they often overlap and interact.

Active Programs

The National Institutes of Health (NIH) is the primary "active program" that encourages and enhances biomedical technology transfer into the private sector. The NIH, which has its origins in the last part of the nineteenth century, began as the Marine Hospital and slowly metamorphosed into its present premier status. During its evolution, the NIH played many roles. It is rumored that an interesting nonscientific role played by the NIH during the early days of World War II was as a cover for the Office of Information (OIC). The OIC became the Office of Strategic Services (OSS), the precursor to the Central Intelligence Agency (CIA). Supposedly, Colonel "Wild" Bill Donovan, director of the OSS, used the NIH as a cover for his clandestine operatives in the same way James Bond used "Universal Exports." (A detailed history of the NIH can be found on its website.)

The NIH—composed of 25 separate institutes and centers—underwent rapid growth and development following WWII (see Table 4.2 later in this chapter). Congress has had significant input into its positive evolution. Important NIH-enhancing legislation includes the 1944 Public Health Service (PHS) Act and the 1986 Technology Transfer Act. The PHS Act helped define the shape of future medical research, and the Technology Transfer Act codified and fostered partnerships between NIH and the private sector for the development of therapeutic products. In the late 1980s, for example, the NIH and the Department of Energy launched the Human Genome Project with the goal of mapping and sequencing the entire collection of human genes. This once secret project, centered at Los Alamos Laboratories in New Mexico, was transferred in the 1990s to the NIH's National Library of Medicine (NLM). This transfer was a significant step in allowing public access to the human genome map.

As one of eight agencies of the Department of Health and Human Services, with a congressional appropriated budget more than $13 billion, the NIH is the primary federal agency that provides competitive federal grants to nongovernment entities. The grants are given primarily to universities, hospitals, and private research and development (R&D) companies that are spinoffs from universities or government agencies.

All the Institutes at the NIH have active extramural grant programs. These meritorious grants can include large multiple year renewable project grants in the multimillion dollar range. For example, meritorious grants were given to support telemedicine initiatives, the National Library of Medicine's Visible Human project at the University of Colorado, and the Virtual Hospital at the University of Iowa. The National Heart, Lung, and Blood

Institute (NHLBI), which played a primary role in developing the Artificial Heart, is now partnering with the NLM on a National Heart Attack Alert Project.

Another highly successful program for grants provided by the NIH's Institutes is called the Small Business Innovative Research program (SBIR). The SBIR provides meritorious grants in the $50,000 range to private sector companies, mostly research and development organizations, for product development research. Often, an SBIR grant will progress into a large project grant. There are many "success stories" of SBIR grant programs. An example is a company called Nimbus, Inc., located in Ranchero Cordova, California. Nimbus, through the SBIR grant program and private investments, enabled its founder, Dr. Richard Wampler, to develop and commercialize a heart assist device called the Hemopump (discussed in detail in the next section).

Another federal agency devoted to technology transfer is the National Science Foundation (NSF). Although not specifically devoted to biomedical technology transfer to the private sector, the NSF deserves mention because of its indirect but strong influence on that process. The mission of the NSF is far more broad based than that of the NIH. Created by Congress in 1950, the NSF invests more than $3.3 billion per year in nearly 20,000 research and education projects in science and engineering.

Passive Programs

Unintentional, "passive" technology transfer occurs when information released to the public from federal programs is translated into biomedical products. These technologies contribute to the disciplines of communication and information, transportation, and device development. An example of device development is the Hemopump, mentioned in the previous section.

The Hemopump

When a portion of U.S. satellite technology was declassified in the 1980s, Dr. Richard Wampler explored the information and was attracted to the description of a miniaturized engine used to turn satellites in orbit. The "guts" of this satellite motor were based on the principle of the Archimedes screw, invented by the ancient Greek scientist to lift water from wells. This technology, in its original form and with modern variations, is still in active use today.

Dr. Wampler's creativity translated this information, obtained "passively" from declassified satellite technology, into lifesaving biomedical technology. His Hemopump is a temporary axial flow pump that can support the circulation of a patient in acute heart failure or even cardiac arrest. The device, which is about the size of a pencil eraser, is mounted approximately 10 inches from the end of a hollow silastic tube that is the same diameter as the pump. An insulated cable and lubrication system connects the Hemopump to its external electric motor encased in a bedside console. Through surgical techniques similar to cardiac catherization, the Hemopump is inserted into the femoral artery and passed retrograde into the left ventricle, where the end of this strawlike tube remains while the body of the Hemopump is in the aorta. When the Hemopump spins via its long cable, it gently but rapidly aspirates stagnant blood from the left ventricle and pumps it into the aorta, thus taking over most of the workload of the heart. This action not only keeps the patient alive but also allows the heart to rest and potentially recover. Alternatively, if cardiac recovery is not possible because of irreversible damage, this temporary pump can support the patient until an alternative therapy like bypass surgery or a heart transplant can be performed. Many surgeons around the world have successfully used the Hemopump in patients.

Another example of "passive" biomedical technology transfer is in the realm of magnetohydrodynamics. Roughly translated into English, magnetohydrodynamics uses magnetic forces to propel fluids. A form of magnetohydrodynamics is used to cool nuclear power plants. The very high temperatures developed in the reactor would melt a conventional pump/cooling system. Generally, nuclear reactors are cooled by using a magnetic force (which does not melt) to propel a coolant, usually liquid sodium, around the core. The positively charged liquid sodium is propelled through large-bore pipes by appropriately spaced electromagnets. Thus, magnetohydrodynamics provides the technology for moving liquid sodium, which can absorb the heat generated by the reactor, thereby preventing a meltdown. This information is public, and technical details can be obtained in most libraries.

Other uses of magnetohydrodynamics are not so public. Remember Tom Clancy's *Hunt for Red October*? The Red October was a Russian nuclear submarine propelled by a stealth engine. Submarines are identifiable, in part, by the sonar sounds their engines make, but this Russian stealth engine consisted of a magnetic pumping system that had no moving parts, which rendered it essentially noiseless. In principle, this magnetohydrodynamic engine sucks in seawater (which is mostly sodium chloride) and silently jets it out the rear of the submarine with enough force to move it rapidly through the ocean. Since the mid-1970s, research on this "fictional" Red October magnetohydrodynamic pump has in fact been a high-priority, classified U.S. government collaboration with Russia. Much of this research has been performed under a Department of Defense (DoD) contract with Argone Laboratories, located near Chicago. The project at Argone involves a 25-ton electromagnet and a miniature artificial ocean where research on this stealth submarine engine is being performed. The Russians have a similar laboratory outside Moscow.

The author's research group was able to use the available information on magnetohydrodynamics to build a miniature magnetohydrodynamic engine that would propel blood. The early prototype engine or pump is the size of a shoe box, has no moving parts to wear out, and can pump blood at 6 to 8 liters per minute at 120 mmHg pressure.

The Hemopump and the magnetohydrodynamics pump are prime examples of how formerly secret federal programs, unrelated to and unintended for medical science use, have had significant benefits for health care once declassified. Another example is the unlimited battery life nuclear technology provides for heart pacemakers. Nuclear energy, initially developed for destructive purposes, is "passively" evolving into biomedical uses.

Many federal programs, such as the Human Genome Project, fall under the category of "passive" but have components that evolve into the "active" category. Our successful civilian air ambulance system, for instance, evolved from military transport helicopters of WWII into the Medic helicopters of the Korea and Vietnam conflicts. Another good example is the Internet.

The Internet

The sentiments that sparked the development of the Internet can be traced back as far as 1957, when the Soviet Union launched the first orbital, artificial satellite. Sputnik, a technological feat that rattled the post-WWII self-assurance of the United States, fueled the creation of the Advanced Research Projects Agency (ARPA) and increased funding for U.S. space programs and missile research. In the midst of this heightened awareness of U.S. vulnerability to nuclear attack, the spotlight soon fell on improving and safeguarding communication. Military strategists turned their attention to the need for a communication network capable of surviving nuclear assault. An ideal network would lack central authority; rather, every computer on the network would be equally capable of originating, transmitting, and receiving messages. This way, even if portions of the network were destroyed, messages could still be transmitted to the remaining computers.

In the early 1960s, ARPA funded experiments that linked computers through telephone hookups. Through the innovation known as packet switching, computers in different locations could be linked and several users could share a single communications line. ARPA's experiments led to the creation of ARPANET, a system that was used to facilitate communication among many government agencies in the 1970s. Through the system, computers could share data and researchers could exchange e-mail and conduct online conferences. Once these basic functionalities were in place, ARPA supported the development of internetworking (or "internet") protocols for transferring data between different types of computers around the world, enabling ARPANET to erase national boundaries and establish a global network. By the late 1970s other computer networks began linking to ARPANET, a feat that became much easier after 1983, when the military segments of ARPANET broke off to form MILNET. The world was

TABLE 4.1. Internet timeline.

1969—ARPANET was conceived to survive nuclear attack. Project begins with four "supercomputers" linked together at military and educational institutions

1970s—Independent networks thrive

1973—First international connections to ARPANET (Norway and England)

Early 1980s—Transmission Control Protocol/Internet Protocol (TCP/IP) was adopted as the official communications protocol by the Department of Defense. TCP/IP had become the new standard in internetworking, was ported to PCs and mainframes, and remains the backbone of the Internet today

1982—The term "Internet" is used for the first time

1984—National Science Foundation forms NSFnet, which will connect researchers and educators across America

Mid- to late 1980s—Universities worldwide go online

1987—Number of Internet hosts exceeds 10,000

1989—Number of Internet hosts exceeds 100,000

Early 1990s—Large corporations flock to the Internet

1991—Tim Berners-Lee creates the multimedia World Wide Web

1991—Paul Lidner and Mark McCahill write the first point-and-click system, Gopher, which achieves widespread popularity within a year

1991—Commercial network service providers make their debut

1992—Beginnings of hypertext and hypertext links; Hyper Text Markup Language (HTML) is the backbone of the today's web, allowing graphics and text to be formatted for viewing by web browsers

Number of Internet sites exceeds 1,000,000

1993—Mosaic desktop browser for WWW introduced by *NCSA*. WWW expands at a 341,634% growth rate of service traffic

Clinton and Gore become first U.S. President and Vice President to receive e-mail addresses

1994—The Internet achieves widespread commercialization and popularization

First virtual bank is created

"Welcome to the White House" site goes online

1995—Entry of Microsoft

Internet stocks skyrocket on Wall Street

1996—Concept of intranets developed

Number of Internet sites exceeds 12 million

1998—60 million Americans go online during the year to search for health information

In the United States, Internet advertising generates $1.92 billion

U.S. companies spend an estimated $10.9 billion on intranet development

The U.S. Internet economy is worth $301 billion, creating jobs for $1.2 million people

1999—Internet users number an estimated 195 million worldwide

The e-commerce industry records a 150% revenue growth rate, generating $95 billion in revenue by the end of the year

2003—Global e-commerce revenues will top $1.3 trillion

2005—Internet users will number an estimated 717 million worldwide

---

connected in a worldwide computer net that would see exponential growth in the decades to follow. (For further information on Internet history, see Table 4.1.)

Beginning in the mid-1980s, the Internet attracted hundreds, then thousands, of universities, research companies, and government agencies, many of which offered free access to the public. In the mid- to late 1980s, the

National Science Foundation Network (NSFNET) began connecting the academic networks that connected universities and research consortiums, expanding the Internet's scope and influence. When commercial Internet traffic was migrated to commercial network providers in 1995, 5 years after ARPANET was retired, millions of new users began flocking to the Internet for government, health business, computer, educational, medical, religious, political, and scientific information.

Throughout the 1990s, the Internet has grown at astonishing rates, and this expansion will no doubt continue in this new century. At the time of this writing, Internet users numbered an estimated 131.1 million in North America and 248.6 million worldwide, and the Computer Industry Almanac estimates that by 2005 those numbers will rise to 230 million and 717 million, respectively. More than just a novelty or diversion, the net has become an integral part of its users' lives. A survey of more than 1,000 Internet users in the United States reported that that two-thirds would rather give up their phone and TV access than their Internet connection, and close to 50% of the users considered the Internet a necessity.

Grown apart from its military roots, the Internet now has the potential to touch or transform nearly every facet of life for every demographic. A glance at statistics for the United States alone indicates how users benefit from this technology: 31% of Internet users in the United States are now purchasing regularly online, including 92% of senior citizens with Internet access; an estimated 20.3 million households will perform financial trading online by 2003, up from 4.3 million in 1998; two of three children with access to a home computer use it to help them do their homework; approximately 24.2 million U.S. households will bank online by 2004, up from 7 million in 1998; and over half the total online banking population—13.7 million households—are expected to pay bills online by 2004 (statistics from Nua Internet Surveys, *www.nua.ie*).

Although crucial issues like privacy, security, confidentiality, and validity need to be fully addressed, the Internet's implications for both public and private sector health care are particularly dramatic. Web-savvy patients can pursue self-education through approved medical websites and literature and seek support and advice through specially tailored mailing lists, newsgroups, and bulletin boards. Physicians comfortable with the technology can supplement doctor–patient communication through e-mail and their own web pages. Healthcare professionals can fulfill their commitment to lifelong learning through continuing education courses and online medical literature. Both healthcare professionals and patients can save time and frustration through online scheduling and billing, referral and health insurance management, and online drugstores.

The Internet continues to evolve into online programs and databases like those created by the largest medical library in the world, the National Library of Medicine. MEDLINE, the NLM's online database, houses over 10 million references to journal articles in the health sciences, including nursing, dentistry, pharmacy, and allied health. The database includes 4,300 journals in more than 30 languages, dating back to 1966; 7,300 references are added weekly. For consumers, the NLM offers MEDLINE*plus*, with dictionaries, databases, links to organizations, directories, clearinghouses, and information on health topics. These offerings continue to mature and expand to benefit biomedical science.

The overwhelming success of the Internet is a prime example of military technology transfer to private sector health care. Initially developed for the military and for rapid communication between physicists, the Internet is not only altering the way healthcare professionals interact, it is transforming the way care itself is managed and delivered.

Interactive Programs

The National Aeronautic Space Administration (NASA) states on its website that it is "deeply committed to spreading the unique knowledge that flows from its aeronautic and space research." NASA actively involves clinicians, the medical device industry, and government health agencies in the technology transfer process. To ensure the availability of NASA technology to the medical community, NASA's methodology emphasizes projects that lead to the development of commercially available medical products incorporating NASA technology. The development of an improved artificial sphincter is one of many examples of the successful transfer of aerospace technology to medicine. Early collaboration between the medical device industry and NASA was critical to the success of this effort to reduce patient risk and healthcare costs by incorporating high-reliability aerospace components in a new prosthesis.

The successful transfer and commercialization of NASA-sponsored research and technology occurs in many ways—information dissemination, technical assistance, technology licensing, cooperative research and development, and other forms of collaboration and partnerships. Examples abound, from spacesuit technology to protect patients with porphyria from harmful ultraviolet rays to software that displays breast tumors in three dimensions. NASA has interactive programs with the National Institutes of Health, the Department of Health and Human Services, and a variety of researchers, universities, and private companies.

The American space program has helped revolutionize the practice of medicine. A few of today's space-derived improvements include blood pressure monitors, exercise and rehabilitation equipment, ultrasound images, surgical lasers, self-adjusting pacemakers, and advanced EKG monitoring systems. A recent example of NASA's interactive technology transfer program is the DeBakey–NASA artificial heart pump. In the mid-1980s, world renowned heart surgeon Dr. Michael DeBakey and his pioneering cardiac surgical team at the Baylor Medical Center performed a heart transplant on a NASA engineer. This relationship evolved into a collaborative effort between Dr. DeBakey and NASA that resulted in the DeBakey–NASA heart assist pump. The combination of NASA's computer and engineering expertise with Dr. DeBakey's medical knowledge created a cutting edge heart assist pump the size of a battery. To date, this pump, after nearly 10 years of collaborative effort, has been successfully implanted in the chests of 10 patients with end-stage heart disease.

Along with biomedical technology transfer efforts, NASA held a 1993 competition to select six Regional Technology Transfer Centers that would implement the Technology Access for Product Innovation (TAP-IN) program. This project helps companies access DoD, Department of Energy (DOE), and NASA technologies. During the past 3 years of operation, TAP-IN assisted more than 6,000 industry and federal laboratory clients, helping firms enter new markets and introduce commercial products.

Federal Regulatory Agencies

This chapter has not yet covered the federal regulatory agencies, like the Food and Drug Administration, that influence biomedical technology. As stated in the introduction, it is virtually impossible to cite all the federal agencies that participate in technology transfer to the private biomedical sector. Federal agencies like the National Institutes of Health, the National Science Foundation, the National Aeronautic Space Administration, the Department of Energy, the Veterans Administration, and many others all partner with the private sector, supported by Congress. These agencies deserve the credit for many of the unprecedented and dramatic advances in medical care and research of this century (Table 4.2).

All these agencies have promoted biomedical technology that has touched every aspect of medicine, from dentistry to sophisticated diagnosis and treatment modalities. Virtual reality research has permitted blind persons to use audio and visual virtual realities to navigate. The contribution of the Veterans Administration made notable contributions to the area of rehabilitation medicine. Not only have VA programs developed rehabilitation training strategies, the VA has contributed significantly to the development of a spectrum of devices, from ultrasonic head controllers for powered wheelchairs to neuroprosthetic devices.

Conclusion

As this chapter has illustrated, federal programs have played an important role in supporting and promoting the development of private sector biomedical technology. Humankind has reaped significant benefits from this multidisciplinary transfer of technology, whether through active programs like the NIH grant process, passive venues like declassified information

TABLE 4.2. Institutes and Centers of the National Institutes of Health.

The National Institutes of Health (NIH) is one of eight health agencies that are part of the U.S. Department of Health and Human Services. It is composed of 25 separate Institutes and Centers:

National Cancer Institute (NCI)
National Eye Institute (NEI)
National Heart, Lung, and Blood Institute (NHLBI)
National Human Genome Research Institute (NHGRI)
National Institute on Aging (NIA)
National Institute on Alcohol Abuse and Alcoholism (NIAAA)
National Institute of Allergy and Infectious Diseases (NIAID)
National Institute of Arthritis and Musculoskeletal and Skin Diseases (NIAMS)
National Institute of Child Health and Human Development (NICHD)
National Institute on Deafness and Other Communication Disorders (NIDCD)
National Institute of Dental and Craniofacial Research (NIDCR)
National Institute of Diabetes and Digestive and Kidney Diseases (NIDDK)
National Institute on Drug Abuse (NIDA)
National Institute of Environmental Health Sciences (NIEHS)
National Institute of General Medical Sciences (NIGMS)
National Institute of Mental Health (NIMH)
National Institute of Neurological Disorders and Stroke (NINDS)
National Institute of Nursing Research (NINR)
National Library of Medicine (NLM)
Warren Grant Magnuson Clinical Center (CC)
Center for Information Technology (CIT)
National Center for Complementary and Alternative Medicine (NCCAM)
National Center for Research Resources (NCRR)
John E. Fogarty International Center (FIC)
Center for Scientific Review (CSR)

from the DoD and DOE, or interactive programs like NASA and the Veterans Administration.

In many ways, the United States enjoys the best healthcare system in the world. We believe the primary reason for this is that our extensive federal and private programs have allowed us the unique opportunity to build on past medical advances that have made enormous contributions to improving health care. At the beginning of this new millennium, health researchers are unveiling the fundamental properties of cells and genes, the structure of proteins, and the circuitry of the human brain, advances built upon discoveries in physics, chemistry, and computer science that were supported by federal agencies. As we make new discoveries and forge breakthroughs, federal support will help revolutionize the practice of medicine.

Readings

Brienaz, D., Angelo, J., Henry, K. 1995. Consumer Participation in Identifying Research and Development Priorities for Power Wheelchair Input Devices and Controllers. *Assist Technol* 7(1):55–62.
Brown, J.N. Jr., Wooten, F.T., Fischer, W.A. 1979. Technology Transfer in Medicine. *CRC Crit Rev Bioeng* 4(1):45–79.

Citron, P. 1995. The Effects of Regulation, Reimbursement, and Product Liability on U.S. Medical Technology Innovation. *J ASAIO* 41(3):M242–244.

Coleman, C. 1997. Aerospace Technology Comes Home. *Caring* 16(7):40–41.

Ford, J., Sheredos, S.J. 1995. Ultrasonic Head Controller for Powered Wheelchairs. *J Rehabil Res Dev* 32(2):280–284.

Friedman, D.S. 1991. Biomedical Applications of NASA Technology. *Med Des Mater* 1(2):54–57.

Goodwin, C.D. 1996. Technology Transfer at US Universities: Seeking Public Benefit from the Results of Basic Research (review). *Technol Health Care* 4(3):323–330.

Griffin, W.E.B. 1998. *The Secret Warriors*. New York: Putnam.

Jeffcoat, M., Clark, W.B. 1995. Research, Technology Transfer and Dentistry. *J Dent Educ* 59(1):169–184.

Langbein, W.E., Fehr, L. 1993. Research Device to Production Prototype: a Chronology. *J Rehabil Res Dev* 30(4):436–442.

Lindberg, D.A., et al. 1995. The High-Performance Computing and Communications Program, the National Information Infrastructure and Health Care. *J Am Med Inform Assoc* 2(3):156–159.

Max, M.L., Gonzalez, J.R. Blind Persons Navigate in Virtual Reality (VR); Hearing and Feeling Communicates "Reality." *Stud Health Technol Inform* 39:54–59.

Murphy, E.F. 1978. Technology Transfer. *Bull Prosthet Res* Spring:1–7.

Neumann, P.G. 1995. Telemedicine—the Diagnostic Tool of the Future. *Health Care Law Newsl* 10(8):7–9.

Nua Internet Surveys. "How Many Online?" *www.nua.ie*, last accessed 3/00.

Panati, C. 1987. *Panati's Extraordinary Orgins of Everyday Things*. New York: Harper & Row.

Peckham, P.H., Thrope, G., Woloszko, J., Habasevich, R., Scherer, M., Kantor, C. 1996. Technology Transfer of Neuroprosthetic Devices. *J Rehabil Res Dev* 33(2):173–183.

Perry, S. 1984. Diffusion of New Technologies: Rational and Irrational. *J Health Care Technol* 1(2):73–88.

Perry, S., et al. 1997. Health Technology Assessment: Decentralized and Fragmented in the US Compared to Other Countries. *Health Policy* 40(3):177–198.

Phillips, S.J., Barker, L., Balentine, B., VandeHaar, J., Slonine, D., Core, M., Zeff, R.H., Kongtahworn, C., Skinner, J.R., Grignon, A., Toon, R.S., Wickemeyer, W., Spector, M., Wampler, R. 1990. Hemopump Support for the Failing Heart. *ASAIO Trans* 36(3):629–632.

Phillips, S.J., Zeff, R.H., Thornton, K., Barker, L. 1993. A Disposable Heart Lung Machine—Results of Animal Testing. *ASAIO J* 39(3):M204.

Phillips, S.J. 1998. Statement on Implementation of the Food and Drug Administration Modernization Act of 1997 before Subcommittee on Full Committee on Commerce. Proccedinsg of /Hearings.nsf The House Committee on Commerce. *http://www.com-notes.gov/cchea*.

Rouse, D.J., Brown, J.N. Jr., Whitten, R.P. 1981. Methodology for NASA Technology Transfer in Medicine. *Med Instrum* 15(4):234–236.

Stout, C. 1999. Negotiating the Technology Maze. *Behav Healthcare Tomorrow* 8(1):58–59, 62–64.

Satava, R.M. 1998. Accelerating Technology Transfer: New Relationships for Academia, Industry and Government. *Stud Health Technol Inform* 50:1–6.

Russell, L.B. 1982. Appropriate Health Care Technology Transfer to Developing Countries. *Health Affairs* (Millwood) 1(3):133–141.

Vernardakis, N., Stephanidis, C., Akoumianakis, D. 1997. Transfering Technology Toward the European Assistive Technology Industry: Mechanisms and Implications. *Assist Technol* 9(1):34–46.

Wadman, M. 1999. NIH Strives to Keep Resource Sharing Alive. *Nature* (Lond) 399(6734):291.

Wampler, R.K., Frazier, O., Howard, L., Allan, M., Smalling, R.W., Nicklas, J.M., Phillips, S.J., Guyton, R.A., Golding, L.A.R. 1991. Treatment of Cardiogenic Shock with the Hemopump Left Ventricular Assist Device. *Ann Thorac Surg* 52:506–513.

Wasuna, A.E., Wyper, D.Y. 1998. Technology for Health in the Future. *World Health Stat Q* 51(1):33–43.

Selected Websites

http//:www.nasa.gov
http//:www.micromedtech.com
http//: www.nhlbi.nih.gov
http//: www.nlm.nih.gov
http//:www.nih.gov
http//:www.nsf.gov
http//:www.doe.gov

5
The Parthenon Strategy in Military Medicine

LT. GEN. (RET.) CHARLES H. ROADMAN II

> *America spends more on health care than any other nation. And*
> *we get what we pay for. The problem is that it isn't what we*
> *want, or need, or could be getting.*
> —*George C. Halvorsen*, Strong Medicine (*1993*)

Health care in the United States is being driven by rapidly increasing technical capability, escalating cost, and the perception that the healthcare system is not adding value to the individual or to the society that is funding it. These facts and perceptions produce conflict, currently unresolved, between the patients, providers, and payors of health care. This conflict hinges on issues like what level of health care individuals are entitled to, what care should be provided, and who will pay for the benefit. Currently, the general sentiment is that health care should be perfect, immediate, and free.

The existing healthcare system has grown over time without the end in mind; that is, those responsible for its evolution have tended not to focus on what the entire system needs to look like and how it should function. Rather, the healthcare system is as follows:

- Organized around a cottage industry mindset (Berwick et al. 1999), with built-in inefficiencies based on nonintegrated healthcare organizations for medical practice, information transfer and analysis, and identification of best clinical practices
- Oriented on a disease "piecework" approach to care delivery focused on the patient and organ system currently exhibiting signs or symptoms; this approach ignores the context of the patient and the surrounding community as the core cause of the health problems
- Driven by cost and financial rewards that motivate overuse by patients, excessive treatment by providers, and cost containment strategies that fail because they conflict with the patient's concept of entitlement or are antithetical to the good practice of medicine

Because the organizational construct of the current system is not conducive to centrally directed change, the convergence of major external forces will demand that the entire medical system seek a new equilibrium through a self-organizing trial and error process. Clearly, however, there is a growing mandate that medicine as an industry change the way services are conceptualized, funded, and delivered.

Coping with Change

Healthcare planners faced with the dilemma of unconstrained demand, crisis of quality, and constrained budgets have three choices: to do nothing, to do more of the same, or to do something different. The clear mandate is for medicine to do something different. That quest is fraught with hazard, as the real issue of how health care is delivered in the United States is cultural. Therefore, much of the attention of leadership must be focused on the culture of medicine and of the organizations that deliver healthcare services. The difficulty of change in culture is well documented. As the work of Stacey demonstrates, change often breeds lack of agreement on what to do and lack of certainty in the outcomes (Zimmerman et al. 1998). When there is scarce agreement and low certainty of outcome, the organization descends into chaos. Leadership must work to lift the organization out of that chaos and into a zone where constructive growth and change can occur.

To do this, different approaches and techniques must be employed, depending on the specific changes desired and the region inhabited by the organization. To increase the level of agreement, a leader must concentrate on fostering a common view of the situation and nurturing alliances. To increase the perception of certainty, the leader must concentrate on strategy, doctrine, and demonstrated victories. In the final analysis, the responsibility of leaders is to pull organizations into moderate ranges of agreement and certainty.

The pace and amount of change in the post-Cold War world has resulted in tremendous discomfort because it is hard to distinguish the important issues from the unimportant ones. Essentially, the signal to noise ratio is unfavorable; with so much static, it becomes difficult to pick out the real message. This problem impedes communication and hinders the development of an agreement–certainty plot that is conducive to positive change. To overcome this obstacle, the U.S. Military Academy at West Point offers a successful construct for identifying major issues and forces. For many years, West Point has used a historical teaching tool called the "threads of continuity" to explain why one commander succeeds in a military campaign while the losing commander fails. The object is to demonstrate that the major factors preceding conflict shape outcomes just as much as do tactics used on the actual battlefield.

Understanding Healthcare Pressures

Although many of the major forces are external to the commander and not controlled by that individual, they must be understood and adapted to the strategy and tactics. In the same way, medical leaders who wish to cultivate agreement must explain the major forces exerting pressure on the system and develop strategies to deal with them.

The major forces pressuring the healthcare system are as follows.

- Economics: The United States is currently spending 12% to 16% of its gross domestic product (GDP) on health care. Unfortunately, the outcomes we generate are no better epidemiologically than those in nations spending half as much. Consumers have clear expectations of increased efficiency, effectiveness, best practices, and outcome report cards. Also, the utilization of health care is disconnected from market forces because of private and federal third party payment. Health care is a job-related benefit.
- Societal expectations: Simply put, members of our society want the best health care that others will buy for them. Although the majority of disease is caused by lifestyle, most want a treatment, a pill, or some potion to restore health. Consumers will balk at a personal lifestyle change and do not wish to accept accountability for their current health condition. Additionally, there are no existing financial incentives to engage market forces to encourage modified consumption.
- Technology: The digital age and the concurrent explosion of innovation in medical appliances have worked to increase the cost of practicing "state of the art" medicine. The Congressional Budget Office has estimated that 62% of the healthcare cost increases from 1996 to 2000 were driven by technology integration—not increased services, patient load, or increased quality of outcomes. The task of the medical community is to employ information technology with the same zeal that it does clinical applications, but with prudence and an eye on cost management.
- Politics: The United States is struggling with the concept of health care. Is it a right or is it a privilege? A great debate currently is being argued by three major constituents: the providers, the payors, and the patients. A fourth "P," the politicians, will become increasingly involved as we realize that future fiscal issues with medicine will center on financing health care for the aging population.
- Doctrine: The most obvious doctrinal issues are the change from inpatient to outpatient care, which brings infrastructure changes from hospital-based to ambulatory-centered medicine, and the change from fee-for-service medicine to managed care, which tightens the focus on utilization management, case management, and clinical practice guidelines. The less obvious doctrinal shift from interventional care to preventive care is also an important issue.

- Leadership: Leadership in the healthcare industry has migrated, during the past 50 years, from the physician to the nonphysician. This business focus has resulted in pursuing efficiencies, which often conflict with the concept of best patient care "at whatever cost."

In response to these unrelenting external forces, medical leaders can respond with the tools of strategy, tactics, logistics, professionals, and leadership. By systematically stepping back and looking at the big picture, leaders can get a broader view of the task at hand and calm the desire to "just do *something*," which leads to hasty decisions and invites further difficulty.

Case Study: The Parthenon Strategy

In 1992, using a technique developed by Eliyahu Goldratt (1992), the author evaluated the Air Force Medical System (AFMS), an interventive closed staff model Health Maintenance Organization. The goal was to determine the source of the system's dysfunction and to develop a strategic plan to correct the core causes.

The assessment of the AFMS revealed seven critical structural/behavioral areas that needed improvement. The goals were these:

- Improve the concept of enterprise: At every level in the organization (individual provider to clinic to hospital to Major Command), members needed to sharpen their awareness of being part of a larger system.
- Clarify enterprise goals: Each individual or subunit needed to move beyond isolated decision making and strengthen focus on the larger goals of the organization.
- Expand the practice of strategic planning: Once larger goals were explicitly defined, the organization needed to generate principles around which to plan.
- Encourage better use of business skills: Once an all-encompassing strategic focus was developed, the organization would have to focus on guiding crucial business skills like resource allocation planning and return-on-investment calculations.
- Improve coordination of process decisions: The organization needed to counter the ill effects of processes being "stovepiped" by clinical specialty or professional training. Often, individuals and teams spent time and resources minimizing the impact of decisions made by others.
- Move away from "management to the local optimum": Rather than deeming the default decision process "the best," everyone needed to understand the impacts of individual actions on the system at large.
- Ensure that all work added value to the organization: After the overall vision of the system had been strengthened, the organization needed to examine current programs and projects and discontinue those that did not advance its strategic viability.

In 1992, the AFMS began to develop strategies to minimize the effect of these seven conditions. The initial challenge was describing an overarching theory about how the system might work and assess whether we were successful at implementing the "ought-to-be" system (Builder 1994; Hock 1999).

The theory the AFMS developed was this: health care could be efficient and effective if it was organized as an integrated system with a unifying strategy and was focused on quality (in all venues) with good business practices. The developed strategy identified five critical success factors for the AFMS:

- Medical readiness
- Use of TRICARE
- Use of rightsizing
- Development of healthy communities
- Customer satisfaction

These critical success factors were assembled into a focusing strategy that would enable all 52,000 AFMS medics to understand how their work directly contributed to the success of the system. There was one clear question all individuals had to ask themselves: *Are my actions contributing to the strategy?* If the answer was "no," they needed to discontinue those actions. If the answer was "yes," they needed to continue and expand their efforts.

An icon was deployed to give the AFMS a visual image or brand identity. That icon, the Parthenon Strategy (Figure 5.1), was to be the focus of

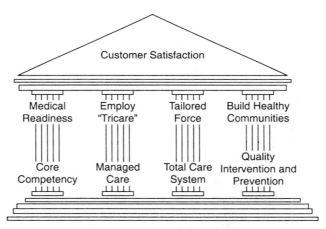

The pillars each represent areas of performance that must be integrated to lead to organizational success.

FIGURE 5.1. The AFMS Parthenon Strategy icon.

change within the AFMS. The purpose of the architectural depiction of the strategy was to visually demonstrate the dependent nature of the components, the real synergy of an integrated approach, and the potential to solve rather than "band-aid" problems if everyone works together toward a common goal. A brief description of the components of the Parthenon strategy follows.

Parthenon Pillar 1: Medical Readiness

The AFMS is a part of the Department of Defense (DoD) healthcare system that has as its primary mission the medical support of contingency and combat operations. Consequently, the medical system should be conceptualized as the "HMO that goes to war." In 1994, the AFMS medical equipment and the manpower assigned to it were still Cold War oriented. The Chief of Medical Readiness was assigned the task of reengineering medical readiness to be lighter (requiring less strategic airlift) and more clinically capable. She undertook the task and within 4 years had completely redesigned the doctrine, the equipment packages, and the manpower assigned to our two major programs: Air Transportable Hospitals and Aeromedical Evacuation. The readiness community recognized and resisted change in their old programs, as did line commanders of the USAF who saw that the format of deployable assets was changing.

Parthenon Pillar 2: Use of TRICARE

By definition, integration of the healthcare system implied managed care with an active focus that would ensure the "right care for the right patient at the right cost every time." TRICARE, the DoD medical system for the military clinics and hospitals, also provides contracted care in the civilian medical community. The program was developed in 1991 and has been in transition up to the present. The DoD system has the potential to be the model managed care system for the nation, with a central focus on patients and their health. Implementation of TRICARE has been very difficult because of resistance to change by providers and patients due to funding mechanisms and the requirement to enroll and schedule patients.

Parthenon Pillar 3: Use of Rightsizing

This pillar is an active resource allocation plan to ensure that there is efficiency/effectiveness in the size and capability of the medical system based on the patient populations served. Striving for a critical balance of fixed and variable costs, the program depends upon a successful transition to enrollment-based resource management (EBRM). Resources are allocated against population requirements determined epidemiologically. At many Air Force bases, this has required a change in the pattern of care delivery from hospitals to ambulatory care units. The patient population determines the site of treatment and the age/sex/race adjusted case mix expected. Great resistance was encountered from patients, providers, and congressional staffs, all of whom perceived change for their constituents and decreasing benefits.

Parthenon Pillar 4: Development of Healthy Communities

A shift in focus to population medicine implemented a transition from intervention to prevention. It has long been documented that 70% of premature death is due to lifestyle (poor nutrition, alcohol consumption, smoking, unsafe sex, lack of activity). This understanding clearly drives the point that although the causative agents of disease, morbidity, and mortality are primarily community issues, the medical response was to provide more and more care at an accelerating cost. The shift from this "fix the body" approach to the goal of population health (a "Fit Fighting Force") was a critical change. Great resistance to the transition was encountered from providers, who had trained in intervention and not prevention; from patients, who did not accept responsibility for their own balance of mind, body, and spirit (Dalai Lama 1999) and from politicians, who saw commodities like cigarettes as a benefit rather than a clear health hazard.

Parthenon Capstone: Customer Satisfaction

The *sine qua non* of any service industry is the satisfaction of its customers. Organizations must recognize that the product of the system adds value to the recipient, or the payors of the service. The military system must concentrate on a series of customers, beginning with the patient and family and ending with the wing commander and the combatant Commander in Chief (CINC). Each must see how value is added to their lives and mission by the USAF Medical Service.

Success of the Parthenon Strategy

Despite resistance from patients, providers, and staff who feared change, the Parthenon Strategy engendered impressive success stories. One example of the Parthenon (enterprise) model at work is the USAF community's suicide prevention program, implemented from 1996 to the present. From 1990 to 1994, suicide accounted for 23% of all active duty Air Force deaths and was the second leading cause of death. Although the suicide rate in the USAF community in 1994 was approximately 40% lower than the rate in a comparable civilian population of the United States, the Air Force had documented a disturbing increase in the number of suicides. It had been assumed that the rate should be low, since the USAF population had completed secondary education, were fully employed, and had housing and comprehensive healthcare benefits. Members also have been screened for mental illness before entry into military service since 1974, and the organizational structure of military units is designed to provide support. Each member has a commander and a first sergeant whose primary task is genuine interest in the health and well-being of their troops.

In 1996, leadership at the highest levels expressed growing concern over the increasing suicide rate. This prompted an in-depth study of the problem by a cross-functional team of civilian and military experts, both medical and nonmedical.

The team goals were as follows:

- Prevent suicides in the United States Air Force
- Identify risk and protective factors thought to impact a wide spectrum of social, behavioral, and health problems (not only suicides and suicide attempts) to establish at-risk populations
- Implement a systemwide comprehensive database to allow for analysis of risk populations and risk factors
- Evaluate every facet of the Air Force community, attempting to change institutions (e.g., investigative agencies, military justice, prevention and treatment services) within the Air Force as well as the culture of its global community
- Demedicalize the issue of suicide, transferring responsibility for community issues to the community leaders

The overall approach was to produce a comprehensive, community-wide prevention strategy to reduce predisposing factors (emphasizing early interventions) and strengthen protective factors. Initiatives fell into three primary areas of need:

- Preventive services: Services were reengineered to tighten the weave in the safety net under each member of the USAF community. A limited psychotherapist/patient privilege was established to protect members charged under the Uniform Code Military Justice. Mental health providers were mandated to initiate community-based primary prevention. Services of the six major agencies involved in preventive services (Mental Health, Family Support Centers, Child and Youth Development, Health and Wellness Centers, Chaplains, and Family Advocacy) were integrated at the base level to assess risks and tailor a community action plan with outcome metrics.
- Surveillance database: Gathering suicide data from the Air Force population was facilitated by standardized data systems that accurately track each member. The Air Force Office of Special Investigations investigated each member death. After the first year of extensive data collection, there

were three primary risk factors for suicide: financial management problems, troubled personal relationships, or trouble with the law.
- Mandatory Air Force annual suicide prevention and awareness training: This training was designed to place a safety net under Air Force personnel who had the three predisposing factors for suicide or demonstrated signs of stress. The emphasis was on "buddy care" as a suicide prevention technique. The training was provided to more than 80% of USAF members in each of calendar years 1997 and 1998. Supervisors and leaders within each military unit, medical providers, attorneys, and chaplains received more intensive training as "gatekeepers."

Every senior line of the Air Force sent frequent messages to the field "recognizing the strength of individuals who confront issues in their lives and seek professional help" (e.g., marital, family, legal, or financial counseling; mental health care; spiritual guidance). These messages mandated that military leaders ensure that members facing significant stress be identified and receive the care and support of their military unit and their local community. Again, suicide was seen as a community issue, not just a medical one.

The suicide rate among USAF members fell significantly from 16.4 per 100,000 in 1994 to 9.4 in 1998 (p for trend, <0.002; see Figure 5.2). This downward trend continued into 1999, with the estimated annual rate only 2.2 suicides per 100,000 persons—nearly 80% lower than the lowest annual rate in the previous 19 years (Figure 5.2).

The lack of controls precludes making definitive assessments of causal relationships with any part or even the totality of the program. However, suicide rates in the other military services do not demonstrate similar trends over the same period (Figure 5.3).

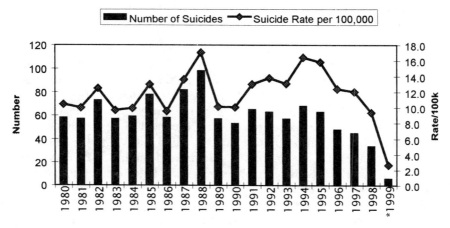

FIGURE 5.2. Annual count and rate of suicides among Air Force members from 1980 to 1999.

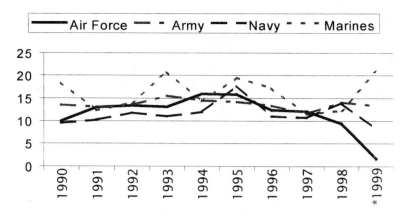

FIGURE 5.3. Suicide rates by branch of military service, 1990–1999. Data are annu-alized rates based on suicides occurring through the end of June 1999.

The Air Force's approach to suicide prevention emphasized the role of the entire community (not only health care) in reducing and preventing factors thought to predispose many to social, behavioral, and health problems, including the focal problem of suicide. A comprehensive program of education and awareness training for all personnel, combined with integrated preventive services in every community, set out to fundamentally change the culture of the Air Force community and the structure and function of its institutions.

Conclusion

The fundamental task of leadership is to develop a consistent and compelling vision of what could be possible if the dreams, resources, and actions of all people are aligned. Problems that are chronic and viewed as intractable can be evaluated and converted to opportunities, but several crucial pieces must be in place. The organization must be viewed as a complex and adaptive system, synergy between all "parts" must be demanded, and action must be initiated to accomplish the dream. We strongly believe that our resources are not constrained because we provide excellence in service and products—rather, we constrain ourselves when we fail to nurture dreams and visions and neglect our mission to lead and change.

References

Berwick, D.M., Godfrey, A.B., Roessner, J. 1999. *Curing Health Care.* San Francisco: Jossey-Bass.

Builder, C.H. 1994. *The Icarus Syndrome.* New Brunswick: Transaction Publishers.
Dalai Lama. 1999. *Ethics for the New Millennium.* New York: Riverhead Books.
Goldratt, E. 1992. *The Goal: A Process of Ongoing Improvement.* Great Barrington, MA: North River Press.
Halvorsen, G.C. 1993. *Strong Medicine.* New York: Random House.
Hock, D. 1999. *The Birth of the Chaordic Age.* San Francisco: Berrett-Kohler.
Zimmerman, B., Lindberg, C., Plsek, P. 1998. *Edge Ware.* Irving, TX: VHA, Inc, pp 136–143.

6
Alignment in a Large Enterprise: Department of Defense Military Health System

BRIG. GEN. KLAUS SCHAFER, CAPT C. FORREST FAISON III,
COL. LEO COUSINEAU, LT. COL. (RET.) HARRY YOUNG, AND
PETER RAMSAROOP

The Military Health System (MHS) of the Department of Defense (DoD), currently responsible for the health care of approximately 8.2 million beneficiaries worldwide, is one of the largest healthcare delivery systems in the world. The vision of the MHS, as stated in the 1999 MHS Optimization Plan (Military Health System Reengineering Coordination Team 1999), is to be "responsive and accountable to DoD, line leadership, and our beneficiaries to ensure force health protection and optimize the health of MHS beneficiaries by providing best value health services using best clinical and business practices." The two cardinal missions of the MHS are to ensure the readiness of the fighting force and to maintain the medical capability to respond to contingency operations.

To support the vision and missions, the MHS invests more than 1 billion dollars ($1.2B) annually for technology development, acquisition, and maintenance. Most of this investment is uncoordinated at the enterprise level. This lack has often resulted in the procurement and attempted integration of technologies that are not aligned with the enterprise vision and mission. Furthermore, a lack of overarching prioritization for most pressing technology requirements has hindered targeted resourcing of investments. When purchases were made, many resulted from "techno-seduction" and gave little consideration to objective benefits or alternatives.

Overall, these efforts were far from cost-efficient. The disparity of the technologies precluded cost savings through bulk purchases, standardized maintenance contracting, and other economies of scale. Cost avoidance was not realized through standardized consideration of technology alternatives or resource sharing opportunities with non-DoD healthcare partners.

This pattern, if continued, will yield a mushrooming technology resource burden with nebulous links to the MHS mission and poor return on investment. This scenario will ultimately increase variation while inhibiting the standardization of healthcare practice and impeding benefits to the MHS.

Telemedicine: The Impact of Misalignment

One example of the impact of misalignment on the enterprise is the MHS experience with telemedicine. The MHS has invested in telemedicine technologies since at least 1992, and by 1997, telemedicine represented a cumulative investment of more than $300 million. Of this, all but $15 million had been executed at the local level and lacked coordination either within the services or between the services. A review by the General Accounting Office in 1997 found that these disparate investments had created multiple enterprise challenges:

- Applications were mostly proprietary with little concern given for contribution to an electronic patient record or data standardization/sharing.
- Telemedicine deployments were overlays on existing processes with little consideration given to successful clinical process redesign or integration.
- Most applications were automations of existing physician–patient interactions. As such, they relied on synchronous, high bandwidth communications. Support was expensive, and without valid business case analyses, it was not justifiable or sustainable over the long term. Because of this, most early telemedicine applications were terminated within 1 year of start-up.

Despite these early results, there continued to be a high level of interest in the potential benefits of telemedicine. In 1994, the Assistant Secretary of Defense for Health Affairs convened a Telemedicine Board of Directors, composed of the Principal Deputy, the three service Surgeons General, and the Commanding General, U.S. Army Medical Research and Materiel Command (USAMRMC). The purpose of this board was to oversee the DoD Telemedicine Testbed at the Medical Advanced Technology Management Office (MATMO) at Fort Detrick, Maryland. MATMO was an Army organization created to perform telemedicine research and prototype deployments, the latter of which garnered limited funding or support from the other services.

Chairmanship of this board rotated among the three Surgeons General. Although the board met quarterly to explore new and emerging telemedicine technologies, it was never officially chartered and held no decision-making or funding authority. Emerging telemedicine technology information was shared, but lacking a charter or other official mandate, the board's ability to achieve alignment through strategic oversight and guidance was unsuccessful.

Arguably, information sharing without mandated leadership oversight or guidance contributed to the mushrooming telemedicine proliferation. Anecdotal information sharing further fueled investment in unproven technologies without defined mission contribution, as opposed to a systematic, planned investment in mature technologies with defined, quantified mission contribution demonstrated by valid business case analysis. Also, these early deployments involved little analysis of alternatives. In Bosnia alone, from 1995 to 1997 the MHS spent nearly 20 million dollars ($20M) to demonstrate the potential of telemedicine in an operational setting, only to find they could have achieved similar results through less costly, nontechnological means.

In summary, early efforts were marked by uncontrolled proliferation and underutilized leadership power and influence in effectively aligning the investment for telemedicine to the goals of the enterprise.

Enemies of Progress: Why Achieving Alignment Is Difficult

In December 1996, the Chair passed to the Surgeon General of the Navy. Recognizing that most of the challenges and lessons learned from the telemedicine experience were shared by other emerging technologies, the Chair recommended a plan to expand the focus of the board. The members approved, and it became the Technology Insertion Board of Directors (TIBOD) to continue information sharing on other emerging technologies beyond telemedicine.

Even with this change in place, the role of the board continued to be information sharing, not decision making. Because the board had no authority to ensure alignment of the technology investment with MHS vision/missions, technology proliferation continued unfettered. Many technologies could not be objectively or demonstrably aligned with the strategic goals of the enterprise, and those that were aligned were frequently behind schedule or over budget. This lack of alignment also included widespread lack of functional input from the end users. Thus, technologies were frequently designed and deployed without business process redesign or objective requirements analysis. This practice led to widespread dissatisfaction among the healthcare providers, hobbling integration and suboptimizing return on investment.

The historical paradigm had allowed program managers wide latitude in product development/deployment with limited functional input and little need to map their products to objective, prioritized mission requirements. In part, this was facilitated by DoD funding practices, in which individual program managers developed their budgets independently and budget approval was performed by various groups at various levels within the enterprise. For example, information technology (IT) was reviewed and prioritized by the Deputy Surgeons General in the Information Management Proponent Committee. This group did not prioritize non-IT medical technologies, research technologies, or other technology investments, and there was no review of any technology costing less than $100,000. As such, lack of overarching coordination facilitated stovepipe efforts and created several potential resource drains.

The Technology Insertion Board of Directors recognized this problem and its potential threat to MHS viability. It became evident to the board that a CEO-level leadership forum was needed to successfully align the enterprise technology investment and plug resource drains. In April 1998, the Chair recommended a reinvention of the Technology Insertion Board. The new goals would be to champion technology "integration," become a decision-making body, and use the leadership power and influence of its members to successfully align technology investment with the goals of the MHS and its healthcare partners. This reinvention was approved by the board members at the June 1998 meeting.

The reinvention involved a complete change in the way the MHS identified, reviewed, cross-functionally related, funded, and deployed technology investments. This approach was a dramatic departure from the previously isolated activities of relatively independent program managers. As such, middle management was reluctant to include these program managers in their activities. Parochialism, protection of narrowly focused territory, and overall resistance to change dominated early efforts to effect this reinvention. The power of the middle manager and the informal communications network became evident.

At first glance, one might assume that if a board of Flag and General Officers like the Surgeons General of the services wished to have some executive level decision-making authority over an issue, they would have it—particularly if the issue impacted the delivery of health care. However, it is their duty to provide the vision and then let the middle managers execute that vision. The pace and intensity of that execution determines the success or failure of the leadership's vision. Accountability must be in place to ensure that middle managers are held responsible for executing the vision and contributing to overall enterprise progress and efficiency. Without accountability, nothing changes. Collective synergy and unity of purpose are lacking and are subjugated to the most common "enemies of progress" within the MHS.

The first of these enemies of progress is parochialism. Within the military complex, activities are organized and funded to accomplish specific missions. In today's environment of rightsizing, protection of narrowly focused territory has become a constant issue. Public statements of support for the concept of "jointness" are frequently followed by actions behind closed doors that bar any long-term realization of joint operations. To most, the concept of joint operations translates to further downsizing of people and dollars, coupled with a sharp increase in mission requirements. The military culture is not aligned with the need for joint efforts; without a reinvention to address this fact, such efforts are frequently doomed.

The second enemy of progress is comfort with the status quo. Concern over the loss of power and influence will cause certain elements within an organization to resist any form of change, regardless of the long-term benefit to the enterprise. This should not be surprising in the military culture because program managers and others are often promoted according to the size of the budget they control and the resources they direct. Placing those resources at risk for review and realignment potentially dilutes the impact of their duties and places individual careers at risk. For this reason and others, middle management resisted change.

If anything, these enemies of progress reinforced the need for the functions proposed by a Chair of the board. The current state of technology integration was recently described in a memorandum to the ASD (HA), which identified the following systems issues facing the MHS:

- Technology represents a multibillion dollar annual investment for the Military Health System (MHS). Goals of that investment should be to improve efficiency, quality, and cost savings.
- Multiple committees, workgroups, and organizations manage portions of the investment. However, none are positioned to strategically guide it, and none exert senior executive level influence on the identification, integration, and evaluation of technology solutions to ensure that goals are met.
- Nowhere do we collectively or methodically examine technology investment prioritization or mission contribution across the entire system of beneficiary health care. This frequently results in competing, duplicative, delayed, or suboptimized technology investments.

At the June 1998 meeting, the board members unanimously recognized these problems and endorsed the need for change. The reinvented board would provide a unique forum for collaboration, use its power and influence to defeat the enemies of progress, and accelerate successful technology integration in support of MHS efforts to achieve population health. Their strategy would align diverse efforts and use technology to power and inform their doctrine.

Creating a Strategy to Achieve Alignment: Technology Integration Board of Directors

In June 1998, the Chair of the board passed to the Surgeon General of the Air Force. Immediately, the Chair sponsored a full-day fact finding offsite (Technology Day) to identify the scope of technology deployment and contribution in the MHS. In August 1998, he sponsored a strategic offsite at the Uniformed Services University of the Health Sciences to define the role of the board and create the concept of operations. Attendance at that offsite represented the DoD healthcare corporation and its major subsidiaries and partners: the services, the Joint Staff, the R&D commands, the Veterans Administration, and others.

In preparation for this offsite, the Chair defined his vision for the board, now known as the Technology Integration Board of Directors (TIBOD).

Ideally, technology would enable the MHS to accomplish the specific capabilities inherent in its mission. Capabilities consist merely of *people*, trained to do *processes*, using *tools* (of which technology is one), supported by *policies*. The work of the TIBOD would be a systematic, objective evaluation of these five variables to ascertain the best solution for each capability. Cross-functional relationships, critical dependencies, gaps, and other issues would be identified and quickly brought to leadership attention for resolution. In this regard, technology would become directly traceable to mission capabilities.

The TIBOD aimed to create an objective, repeatable methodology to assess technology for its mission contribution as well as any constraints impeding its use. The goal, as indicated in the previous section, was to use the board to "create the strategy to align disparate efforts and use technology to drive and enable doctrine," all based on objective evaluation of the five variables just mentioned. The board would function as both a champion of change management and a cross-functional integrator of disparate efforts. In addition, the board would be a resource sponsor to identify and recommend support for mission-critical efforts to the Assistant Secretary of Defense for Health Affairs, allowing completion and deployment on time and within budget.

A TIBOD forum was chosen based on the benchmarking of similar best industry practices in which integrated delivery networks used CEO forums to set strategy and guide technology decisions. Because the medical marketplace was rapidly evolving and had multiple destabilizing factors, a CEO-level technology board was essential to success. The board would provide an executive level forum to coordinate and collaborate on the assessment, integration, and evaluation of technology across the healthcare continuum and to identify and overcome system constraints in using technology. The goals would be to use technology to

- Improve readiness
- Increase access and improve quality
- Move from interventive to preventive health care
- Improve efficiency
- Provide cost savings

A comprehensive overview of existing MHS efforts was done to ensure there was no overlap with current efforts. The board discovered that no other group possessed the membership, methodology, or influence to accomplish what they needed to accomplish. As such, it became clear that the board existed not so much to insert technology as to ensure successful integration of technology.

At the conclusion of the offsite, an initial version of the Technology Integration Board of Directors (TIBOD) charter was completed and circulated. In developing that charter, the group adopted the following guiding principles:

- Technology is an enabling tool to accomplish the mission. Process drives the technology, not the reverse.
- The focus of any technology action should be mission contribution, not techno-fascination or techno-seduction.
- Nontechnical critical success factors (training, processes, policy revisions, etc.) will determine the success or failure of any technology investment: the technical performance of the equipment is secondary. These nontechnical factors need to be worked out up front and should guide technology decisions.
- To optimize standardization and opportunities for resource sharing, planning should occur across the entire spectrum of DoD healthcare delivery. The board membership should be representative of that spectrum.
- Planning should allow the leadership to develop a technology portfolio, which could be used to assist in resource decisions, planning, and advocacy by mapping technology investments directly to the mission.
- CEO-level leadership is essential to set strategy for the organization, identify how technology contributed to accomplishing the mission, advocate technology actions in times of resource constraints, champion change management, and foster sharing and cooperation to improve resource use.

To support the TIBOD, the Chair directed that an Executive Work Group (EWG) be formed and chaired by a flag officer. The EWG would implement the methodology and provide a clear linkage between technology investments and enterprise vision and mission, both current and future; this is graphically illustrated in Figure 6.1 in the later section on Operationalizing the Strategy. The Air Combat Command (ACC) Surgeon, a Brigadier General, was appointed as the first EWG chair as direct representative of the end user. Workgroup membership consisted of senior officer representatives from each of the TIBOD principals.

Based on the fact that no other group was positioned for success in this area, the EWG began to develop a process model, analytical methodology, and concept of operations.

Process Model

To operationalize the TIBOD concept, the MHS mission was laid out as a series of dependent capabilities. The MHS vision of population health was also mapped out as a series of dependent capabilities—i.e., what must be done, and in what order, to achieve population health.

Analytical Methodology

Based on best industry and Service practices, and in close consultation with industry experts, the EWG developed a systematic, objective methodology to sequentially evaluate all five variables for each capability. This methodology was based on the *Theory of Constraints*, developed by Eliyahu Goldratt (1992). The goal of this methodology was to assess technology and ensure successful technology integration in meeting the capabilities outlined in the process model. Following initial development, the methodology was verified and validated by industry experts at First Consulting Group for completeness. The methodology uses a series of fact-based questions to identify the best combination of people, training, processes, tools, and policies necessary to accomplish a given capability. The product of the methodology is an integrated decision package that includes recommendations for these points:

- Staffing
- Process redesign
- Technology solutions
- Required process and policy implementation or revision
- Metrics plan
- Resource requirements for initial implementation and long-term sustainment

Not every emerging technology produces a financial return on investment. Mission-specific requirements and DoD-unique circumstances would preclude a financial return on investment in many cases but could provide a significant nonfinancial return on investment as far as mission contribution or other measures were concerned. The Balanced Scorecard, developed by Kaplan and Norton (1996), was adopted for the metrics portion of the process. This is the methodology used by the GAO and other Federal agencies in its surveys, and it is the most comprehensive view available of both financial and nonfinancial measures of success.

Concept of Operations

Once the methodology was finalized and validated by industry experts, the EWG developed the concept of operations for the TIBOD. Clearly, the TIBOD could not constrain organizational progress, but the EWG realized that it did not possess the knowledge or experience to work all necessary issues. The group decided that most work would be done by TIBOD-sponsored workgroups of 10 to 12 subject matter experts, depending on subject under consideration. The TIBOD would augment these groups with industry consultants, technology experts, business analysts, and futurists.

Workgroups would have 3 months to develop an integrated decision package for presentation to TIBOD, with the elements listed. Each workgroup would be responsible for identifying long-term oversight and coordination so that after the TIBOD approved the integrated decision package for submission to ASD(HA), the TIBOD would hand off the workgroup to a long-term oversight and coordinating organization. Guiding the entire process was a firm belief that all enterprise actions, including technology decisions, should map directly to the enterprise vision and mission. To help fulfill this objective, TIBOD-sponsored workgroups would be chartered and directed toward specific mission capabilities.

The role of the EWG was to map the recommendations provided by TIBOD-sponsored workgroups to the process model to clearly illustrate how they will help the MHS accomplish its mission. In addition, the EWG would demonstrate how the resource requirements identified would affect other current or planned technology investments. Using the model to identify the cross-functional relationships between capabilities, the EWG could clearly demonstrate how people, process, tool, or policy decisions for one capability might affect other capabilities, thereby increasing leadership awareness of critical dependencies during the decision-making process.

Daily support for the TIBOD, EWG, and sponsored workgroups would be provided by a TIBOD Support Office.

Operationalizing the Strategy: Capability-Focused Workgroups

On January 29, 1999, the current state of technology integration in the MHS, the role of the TIBOD, the process model, the methodology, and the concept of operations were briefed to the TIBOD. The recommendations to continue TIBOD efforts and to adopt and test the methodology were unanimously approved by the members. There was, however, one major constraint. In December 1998, a comprehensive review of all MHS strategic plans had been completed by the MHS Healthcare Reengineering Office, Directorate of Information Management, Technology and Reengineering. These plans were compared, first with each other to identify alignment within the MHS, and then against overarching National and DoD level Strategic Plans to identify alignment of the MHS within the DoD. Documents reviewed included the following:

- National Military Strategy
- Defense Security Planning Guidance 00-05
- Joint Vision 2010
- Quadrennial Defense Review 97
- Joint Warfighter Science and Technology Plan 98
- Joint Strategic Capabilities Plan
- Joint Health Service Support Planning Guidance
- Force Health Protection Capstone Document
- Military Health System Strategic Plan 98-03
- Medical Programming Guidance 00-05
- Medical Readiness Strategic Plan 98-04

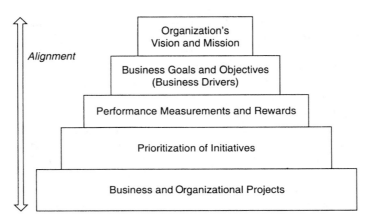

FIGURE 6.1. Business planning model.

A review of the Military Health System Information Management and Information Technology Strategic Plan was not completed, as it was under revision.

Results of this side-by-side gap analysis revealed multiple discrepancies between MHS strategic plans with no clear overarching prioritization of goals and objectives. Further, there was marked discrepancy between MHS strategic plans and DoD strategic plans, giving the impression that MHS strategy and direction were at odds with the warfighters. In keeping with the business planning model illustrated in Figure 6.1, the first task for the EWG was to reconcile the disparate strategic documents and propose an aligned MHS Strategic Plan.

The EWG developed a strawman MHS Strategic Plan, which addressed the gaps among the many MHS plans and between MHS and DoD plans. Upon completion and endorsement by the EWG in March 1999, the strawman Strategic Plan was forwarded to the MHS Strategic Planning Committee (SPC) for review and discussion. This strawman would serve as the basis for revising the existing MHS Strategic Plan to reconcile noted differences.

While awaiting MHS SPC action, the EWG took the opportunity to map the goals and objectives of the strawman against current MHS activities/priorities, as contained in the Reengineering Coordination Team's (RCT) MHS Optimization Plan. The MHS Optimization Plan represents a series of 29 initiatives as part of an overarching strategy for implementing the "High Performance MHS." These represent the current focus/thrust of MHS leadership. The focus of the plan is to shift from providing primarily interventional services to better serve MHS beneficiaries by preventing injuries and illness. According to the plan, MHS optimization has three underlying tenets:

- Effectively use readiness-required personnel and equipment to support the peacetime health service delivery mission.
- Equitably align resources to provide as much health service delivery as possible in the most cost-effective manner within the MTF.
- Use the best evidence-based clinical practices and a population health approach to ensure consistently superior quality of services.

Results of the mapping revealed several interesting findings:

- Several of the goals and objectives contained in the strawman strategic plan were not included in the optimization plan. That is, current MHS priorities would miss several line-DoD goals and objectives.
- Many of the goals and objectives in the strawman were also published as CINC requirements and were missing from the Optimization Plan. Current MHS priorities would miss several important priorities for the CINCs, our primary warfighting customer.
- Many of the goals and objectives in the strawman were published goals or objectives of the Department of Veterans Affairs, but were absent from the Optimization Plan. Resource sharing with the VA might be limited if goals and objectives were not shared.
- There were multiple critical factors on which the strawman depended for completion. These dependencies had a track record of being late or over budget. Without a change in business practices, it was doubtful that the goals and objectives of the strawman (and concurrently, the goals and objectives of MHS support to line-DoD, the CINCs, and others) could be accomplished.

These discrepancies were briefed to the TIBOD and RCT. Both committees agreed that a detailed Plan of Action and Milestones (POA&M) to address the gaps was needed to achieve the overarching goals of population health.

At the end of the June 1999 TIBOD meeting, the EWG was tasked to develop the roadmap that would bring the MHS to population health and achieve both the CINC requirements and the requirements necessary to optimally support line-DoD. The roadmap should make use of collaborative opportunities with the VA and others by aligning goals and objectives where it made good business sense for the MHS.

Concurrent with these activities, the TIBOD, while endorsing the concept of the process model and methodology, agreed that there were some significant technology investment challenges and potential resource drains that required immediate attention. The members also agreed that the methodology should be tested on these challenges before wide application elsewhere. The EWG recommended two investments for TIBOD involvement: telehealth and digital imaging, both approved for action at the January 1999 TIBOD meeting. Reasons for these recommendations were these:

- Extremely high political visibility
- Magnitude of current and projected investments
- Number of process and policy constraints
- Previous technocentric focus
- High potential payoff

In March 1999, the Telehealth Work Group held its initial meeting. The group's members included Telehealth leaders from Veterans Affairs, academia, industry, the Joint Staff, and Army, Navy, and Air Force Medical, Logistics, and Research and Development communities. Members agreed that any discussion of technology must be based on a required capability and what combination of the five variables of people, training, process, tools, and policy could best meet that capability. From the capabilities identified in the process model, the workgroup identified remote access to care as most relevant to the role of telehealth.

Based on the industry planning model described earlier, the EWG developed a series of questions designed to help the workgroup systematically review the five variables; this would help determine how best to achieve remote access to care and what role, if any, telehealth played in that area. Using the methodology and the Balanced Scorecard to develop measures of success, the workgroup reviewed more than 100 current telehealth initiatives to determine which of the projects had a valid business case for using telehealth as the best way to achieve remote access to care. None of the known DoD telehealth projects had sufficient data to complete a valid business case. The inability to develop significant amounts of hard, non-anecdotal data has been cited in numerous studies as one of the leading barriers to large-scale, cost-effective telemedicine use. Based on this, the workgroup identified a need for training and a standardized planning methodology for future telemedicine projects; this was modeled after the TIBOD methodology. At the end of its efforts, the Telehealth Workgroup made the following recommendations:

- Adopt the Telehealth Program Planning Methodology to execute process design opportunities and to achieve the preferred environment. The TIBOD should immediately adopt and promulgate the Telehealth Program Planning Methodology.
- Continue with three current telehealth initiatives, guided by the Telehealth Program Planning Methodology. These initiatives, which all showed promise for a valid business case analysis, included the teledermatology efforts being conducted by the Army and Region 10, the CBA/Innovation Fund Healthcare Consortium Home Health Initiative in Region 9, and the Joint Medical Operations Advanced Concept Technology Demonstration in support of Pacific Command. Independent evaluations of these initiatives would be conducted for 9 to 12 months and then reassessed.
- Apply the Telehealth Program Planning Methodology to all other current and new start-up initiatives. The project sponsor/manager for each

remaining current project and any new start-up effort must complete the Telehealth Program Planning Methodology with the goal of developing a comprehensive Telehealth Program Plan for each project. P8 funding should stop for projects unable to complete the program planning methodology and alternate funding sources (grants, for example) should be pursued. All projects, regardless of funding, should collect metrics data specified in the program planning methodology, and there should be no new starts without fully completing the business case questions of the program planning methodology. Any telehealth projects with valid business cases should be forwarded for technical integration, standardization, and promulgation.

- Establish a DoD Joint Telehealth Coordinating Committee to assess the benefit and viability of telehealth initiatives through monitoring conformity to the program planning methodology. This Joint Telehealth Coordinating Committee should act as POC for any subsequent telehealth projects with a valid business case, and TIBOD should retain oversight pending results of independent evaluations (not to exceed 12 months).

Concurrently, in March 1999, a Radiology Work Group was formed to begin to address the issues surrounding digital imaging. Like the Telehealth Work Group, the membership included recognized radiology leaders from the armed services, Veterans Affairs, and from the radiological industry. Other members included representatives from the Joint Staff, Service logistics, and the research and development communities. In this case, the question was what combination of people, processes, and tools would best support radiological diagnosis and treatment.

The need for immediate action by the Radiology Work Group was even more significant because the MHS was facing several major constraints in its effort to provide radiology services to its beneficiary population. These were identified by the workgroup as the following:

- Looming radiologist staffing shortfalls in the Air Force and Navy
- Lack of an overall corporate plan
- Numerous unaddressed process issues
- Unexplored interim alternatives and collaborative efforts
- Unexplored yet rapidly evolving PACS market
- Critical data such as workload, inventory status, and analysis of alternatives was unavailable for evaluation

Despite these findings, multiple efforts worth tens of millions of dollars were currently under way.

The workgroup developed an action plan to address the issues of data collection, deployment prioritization, the development of objective analysis of alternatives to address staffing shortfalls, and the development of a long-term oversight and coordination plan. The action plan was presented to the TIBOD at the June 7, 1999, meeting. The TIBOD recommended that the workgroup begin by developing the long-term oversight and coordination plan that would provide a mechanism to develop solutions to the constraints noted earlier.

Moving to the Future: Using Alignment to Achieve Population Health

According to the Draft Population Health Improvement Guide by the MHS Reengineering Coordination Team (RCT), the two cardinal missions of the MHS are to ensure the readiness of the fighting force and to maintain a medical capability to respond to contingency operations. The goal is to optimize the health of the eligible population, active duty, retirees, and their families. Using the TIBOD process model as a baseline, the TSO developed a roadmap and critical path (Figure 6.2) by comparing the capabilities identified in the process model with the those identified in the RCT Population Health Improvement Guide, the Air Force Medical Service (AFMS) Population-Based Health Plan, and the Army and Navy Strategic Plans for Preventive Medicine.

Although each of the documents varied slightly in their description of capabilities required to achieve population health, the following critical success factors were identified:

- Remember that identification, enrollment, and assessment of the health status of a population is the foundation of any population health program.
- Develop, based on the assessment, a comprehensive demand forecast and demand management plan to provide comprehensive preventive services to the enrolled population.
- Provide condition management.
- Identify and evaluate key clinical and process outcomes.
- Continually measure the improvement in the population's health status and in the delivery system's effectiveness and efficiency.
- Base population health on a total community approach.

The TIBOD can assume three major roles to help the MHS achieve population health. First, it can serve as a catalyst for collaboration, coordination, and action among organizations responsible for the planning and execution of population health, such as the MHS 2025 Work Group, RCT, Department of Veterans Affairs, industry, academia, and others. Second, it will establish the TIBOD process methodology as the gold standard for identifying capabilities required to achieve population health, developing service delivery alternatives, and making investment recommendations based on best clinical and business practices. Finally, the TIBOD will use the power and influence of its collective membership to provide oversight for the man-

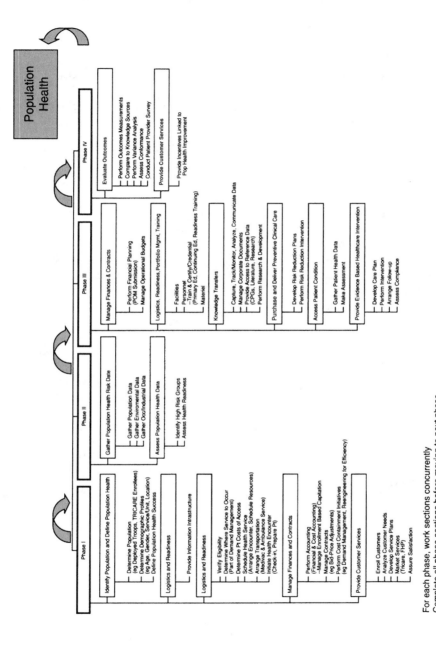

FIGURE 6.2. Population health roadmap and critical path.

agement of the technology portfolio and evaluation of population health outcomes. Based on these outcomes, the TIBOD will "create the strategy to align disparate efforts and use technology to drive and enable" population health.

Successful Alignment: Difficult But Not Impossible

In the previous sections, we have described the importance of alignment to the long-term success of a large enterprise. We have identified some of the major constraints to achieving successful alignment and provided a few ideas on how to use best industry practices to reach this goal. Although we used the MHS as an example, the lessons learned—both positive and negative—can be applied to any organization undergoing significant change.

Change is difficult but essential. The paradigm shift from curative to preventive medicine carries with it enormous medical, financial, and moral implications. Despite numerous challenges from the "enemies of progress," it is absolutely imperative to achieve the ultimate goal of population health. Although achieving successful alignment through best industry practices is difficult, it is not impossible if senior leadership exerts its power and influence to articulate the vision, effect coordination, increase the pace of execution, and provide incentives to reward success.

References

Goldratt, E.M. 1992. *The Goal*, 2nd Ed. Great Barrington, MA: North River Press.

Kaplan, R.S., Norton, D.P. 1996. *The Balanced Scorecard*. Boston: Harvard Business School Press.

Military Health System Reengineering Coordination Team. 1999. *MHS Optimization Plan*. Available on www.tricare.osd.mil; last accessed July 2000.

United States General Accounting Office Report. 1997. *Telemedicine: Federal Strategy Is Needed to Guide Investments*. Available on www.gao.gov; last accessed July 2000.

7
Reengineering the Veterans Healthcare System

KENNETH W. KIZER

The Veterans Health Administration (VHA) in the U.S. Department of Veterans Affairs (VA) manages the largest fully integrated healthcare system in the United States. In 1995, the VHA initiated the most radical redesign of the veterans healthcare system to occur since the system was formally established in 1946. This chapter provides an overview of the veterans healthcare system, and it describes selected aspects of the system's re-engineering. While still a work in progress, the first 5 years of this re-engineering effort have produced dramatic improvements in quality of care, access, and service satisfaction, while simultaneously documenting a 25% reduction in per patient costs.

A Brief History of the Veterans Healthcare System

The United States has always provided special benefits to veterans of its armed forces. The first American law specifically providing benefits for veterans was passed by the Plymouth Colony in 1636; this law provided lifetime support for any soldier who was maimed while defending the colony against the Pequot Indians. In 1789, one of the first laws passed by the new U.S. Congress provided pensions for soldiers who fought in the American Revolution.

Since these early times, the nation's interest in issues regarding veterans has waxed and waned, generally in accordance with the interval since the last armed conflict. In 1862, President Abraham Lincoln signed legislation authorizing the National Cemeteries, and 3 years later, he signed legislation creating the National Home for Volunteer Soldiers in Togus, Maine. Homes for disabled Civil War veterans were subsequently opened at numerous sites throughout the country. In 1917, the United States Government Life Insurance program was established, and in 1930, President Herbert Hoover signed legislation consolidating the many disparate veterans programs into an independent federal agency known as the Veterans Administration (VA). The most far-reaching expansion of veterans benefits resulted from the Servicemen's Readjustment Act of 1944, which became known as the "GI Bill of Rights." This landmark legislation offered low interest loans for veterans to purchase homes, farms, or small businesses; unemployment benefits; financial assistance for education; and healthcare and rehabilitation services.

Veterans benefits have always included some health care, but such benefits were limited to infirmary-type services and were provided by the U.S. Public Health Service (USPHS) until after World War I, when Congress authorized hospital inpatient care as a veterans benefit and transferred several USPHS hospitals to the Veterans Bureau. Subsequently, the beginnings of a veterans healthcare system began to form within the Veterans Administration. However, the VA's nascent healthcare capabilities were rapidly overwhelmed by the massive numbers of World War II veterans needing medical care, leading Congress to authorize the creation of a new VA Department of Medicine and Surgery and a formal veterans healthcare system in 1946.

Since World War II, the veterans healthcare system and other veterans programs have grown markedly. In recognition of this and other factors, President Ronald Reagan established the Department of Veterans Affairs in 1989 as the 14th cabinet-level department in the executive branch of the federal government. (Because of its familiarity, the Department was still abbreviated as "VA.") The new Department of Veterans Affairs was charged with coordinating the full range of services for veterans, and the VA is now the second largest agency in the federal government, next to the Department of Defense.

The principal operating units of the Department of Veterans Affairs are these:

- The Veterans Health Administration, which manages the veterans healthcare system and accounts for more than 80% of the Department's staff and about half of its budget
- The Veterans Benefits Administration, which provides disability compensation and pensions for about 3.3 million veterans and administers a number of education, home loan, and insurance programs for veterans
- The Memorial Affairs Administration, which manages 115 national cemeteries located throughout the United States and Puerto Rico
- The Board of Veterans Appeals, which adjudicates disputes about VA benefits

Assets and Missions of the Veterans Healthcare System

Today's veterans healthcare system is one of the largest and oldest formally organized healthcare systems in the world. In federal fiscal year (FY) 1999, the VA provided "hands-on" health care to more than 3.6 million persons at more than 1,100 sites of care, located in all 50 states and the District of Columbia, Puerto Rico, the U.S. Virgin Islands, Guam, Samoa, and the Philippine Islands. It operates with a medical care budget of about $18 billion and approximately 182,000 staff. In FY 1999, the VA's principal physical assets included 172 hospitals, more than 600 ambulatory and community-based clinics, 132 nursing homes, 206 counseling centers, 40 domiciliaries (residential care facilities), 73 home healthcare programs, and various contract care programs. Among the VHA's staff in FY 1999 were approximately 13,000 physicians, 53,000 nurses and 3,500 pharmacists, among thousands of other healthcare professionals.

Originally created to treat combat-related injuries and to help rehabilitate veterans with service-connected disabilities, the veterans healthcare system has expanded in both size and responsibility over the years. The VHA now has five principal missions:

- Medical Care: The primary mission of the veterans healthcare system is to provide medical care to improve the health and functionality of America's veterans and reduce the burden of disability from conditions occurring during their service in the armed forces—especially those conditions related to combat. Although all veterans were originally eligible for VA health care, such eligibility was limited by Congress over the years. By the late 1980s, VA health care had essentially become a "safety net" system (Wilson and Kizer 1997). Unlike Medicare and Medicaid, VA health care is not an entitlement program; the number of persons the VA is able to serve each year is limited primarily by the amount of funding provided by Congress. Of note, in FY 1999, VA health care was opened to all veterans, according to a new enrollment system required by the 1996 landmark eligibility reform legislation.
- Education and Training: The VHA's second statutorily mandated mission is to conduct education and training programs that will enhance the quality of care provided to veterans. In FY 1999, the VHA provided clinical training to more than 110,000 students and trainees in 47 healthcare disciplines through affiliations with over 1,200 universities, colleges, and other institutions of higher education. Almost two-thirds of physicians in the United States have received at least some of their training through the VA. The veterans healthcare system has become an integral part of healthcare higher education in the United States.
- Research: The VHA's third statutory mission is to conduct research that will enhance health care for veterans. Over the years, the VHA's research program has been exceptionally productive, and its investigative portfolio has become diverse, encompassing a wide array of projects ranging from basic science studies and multiinstitutional clinical trials to health services delivery and clinical outcomes projects. Indeed, being nested in a fully integrated healthcare delivery system and having a stable patient population with a high prevalence of chronic conditions provides VA

investigators with unparalleled opportunities to translate research questions into studies and research findings into clinical action. Currently, the VHA has combined intramural and extramural research funding of about $1.1 billion per year.

- Contingency Support and Emergency Management: The VHA is mandated by law to be the primary backup to the Department of Defense (DoD) medical care system in times of war and to help the U.S. Public Health Service (PHS) and National Disaster Medical System provide emergency care to victims of natural and other disasters (Kizer et al. 2000). Because of the devolution of the DoD and PHS healthcare systems in recent years, the veterans healthcare system has become the federal government's primary asset to actualize disaster plans requiring a medical care response.
- Homelessness: About 35% of homeless adults are veterans, and the VA has become the nation's largest direct provider of services for homeless persons, providing medical care to more than 65,000 a year and providing other services to many more (Rosenheck and Kizer 1998). The VA is the only federal agency providing substantial assistance directly to homeless persons.

Prologue to Change

Powerful societal, demographic, and industry-wide forces have markedly transformed American health care in the past two decades. Most prominent among these forces of change have been the market-based restructuring of health care and the rise of managed care; the explosion of scientific and biomedical knowledge; the concomitant technological advances that have dramatically expanded the ability to treat illness and injury; unprecedented developments in information management; and the changing demographics of the aging U.S. population. While buffeted by these same forces of change, the VHA was slow to respond to them.

When it was created, and as it developed in the 1950s and 1960s, the veterans healthcare system was patterned after the best of American health care. It emphasized hospital inpatient care, medical specialization, and innovative technology. During its early years, the VA established a distinguished record of educating physicians, conducting cutting edge research, and providing veterans with specialized medical care that was often unavailable in the community (e.g., blind rehabilitation, psychiatric care, prosthetics, and care for spinal cord injuries). Unfortunately, the system's accomplishments often were overshadowed by untoward incidents involving individual VA medical centers. Considerable evidence supports the belief that quality of care problems have been no more prevalent in VA hospitals than in private hospitals, but because of the VA's extreme amount of oversight and its public nature, such occurrences at VA facilities have typically drawn marked media attention. Indeed, various situations have been dramatized and memorialized in such films as *Born on the Fourth of July*.

In addition to its public image problem, the VA as a system did not embrace needed change as soon as it should have. This deficiency is not surprising in light of the system's political nature, its many special interest groups, its highly centralized and hierarchical management structure, its changing leadership, and the inertia inherent to large organizations. All these factors combined to suppress innovation, slow decision making, and make change very difficult to achieve. The VHA was especially tardy in changing its patterns of hospital utilization.

By the early 1990s, a number of internal and external reports identified serious operational and managerial problems in the veterans healthcare system (Booth et al. 1991; Smith et al. 1996; General Accounting Office reports; VHA Task Force reports). Veterans health care was criticized for being too hospital focused and specialist based, resulting in uncoordinated, fragmented, and episodic treatment of illness in which patients too often "fell through the cracks." Instead of functioning as a healthcare *system* that provided a coordinated continuum of care, the VA operated as a collage of independent and competing medical centers, much as its private sector counterparts did.

VA health care was also too difficult to access, both geographically and temporally, with patients sometimes traveling hundreds of miles for routine care and enduring a months-long backlog for a routine appointment. There was marked, unexplainable interfacility and interphysician variation in how care was provided, and Congressionally appropriated medical care funds were distributed to facilities by a highly complex and poorly understood process that perpetuated unnecessary inpatient care and other inefficiencies. Likewise, the rules governing veteran eligibility for care had become anachronistic, often requiring hospitalization for simple procedures done routinely on an outpatient basis in the private sector. Because these rules were encoded in statute, an act of Congress was required to change them. Key Congressional leaders had resisted doing so for many years from fear that rationalizing the eligibility rules would result in increased utilization and expenditures. However, major systemic change clearly was needed.

The VHA Transformation

In late 1994, after a short period of preparatory work and consensus building, a plan was proposed to fundamentally transform VA health care. This approach would use population health and managed care principles tailored to the complex needs of the VA's service population of older, sicker, and socioeconomically disadvantaged persons (Kizer 1995). Space here allows for only a brief description of the major changes undertaken and some of the results achieved during the 5-year period FY 1995–FY 1999.

The reader is referred to the original documents and other publications for a more detailed discussion of the transformation plan and principles upon which it was based (see Suggested Readings at the end of this chapter).

One of the greatest threats to the quality of health care is fragmented service delivery (Berwick 1996), and in 1995, fragmentation of care was probably the single biggest problem that needed fixing in veterans health care. The VHA transformation sought to correct the fragmentation of service delivery by a set of initiatives that aimed to structurally and procedurally coordinate healthcare services. We explore these initiatives in the following subsections, beginning with the two most visible steps: implementation of universal primary care and creation of integrated service networks.

Implementation of Primary Care

Although a number of VA medical centers had implemented primary care pilot projects in the late 1980s and early 1990s, only about 10% of VA patients had been enrolled in primary care by the end of FY 1994, and most VA medical centers had no primary care program. One of the first major initiatives in the VHA's transformation was the decision to implement systemwide universal primary care. The VHA approach to primary care was largely patterned after the British firm model, as this model of primary care was judged better able to serve the VA patient population of primarily older males with a high prevalence of chronic illness than the family practitioner model prevalent in the United States.

By the end of FY 1998, less than 4 years after launching its primary care initiative, essentially all patients in the VA healthcare system had been assigned to a primary care team, and more than 80% of patients queried could name their primary caregiver.

Implementation of Integrated Service Networks

In the fall of 1995, the VHA's myriad sites of service delivery were organized into 22 Veterans Integrated Service Networks, or VISNs (pronounced "visions"), according to the then prevailing patient referral patterns. Clinical care assets and beneficiaries were aggregated into each VISN so that they could provide a continuum of primary to tertiary care. To some extent, the VISNs follow political jurisdictional boundaries like state and county lines. A typical VISN encompasses 7 to 10 VA medical centers, 25 to 30 ambulatory care clinics, 4 to 7 nursing homes, 1 to 2 domiciliaries, and 10 to 15 counseling centers, and provides "hands-on" care to about 150,000 to 200,000 persons each year.

The VISN has become the veteran healthcare system's basic budgetary and management unit. Designed to promote both vertical and "virtual" integration, it provides an imperative for pooling and aligning resources to meet the needs of a defined population. It provides a structural template for coordinating services, for ensuring the continuity of care, for reducing service duplication and administrative redundancies, for improving the consistency and predictability of service, and, overall, for optimizing healthcare value.

Other Strategies

Concomitant with the implementation of primary care and the VISNs, a number of other initiatives were launched to better coordinate and integrate care. For example, in an effort to promote better locally integrated service delivery, 52 VA medical centers were merged into 25 local integrated care networks between September 1995 and September 1999, stressing improved access, service, and quality in each case (Kizer 1998). Similarly, both single and multiinstitutional service lines (e.g., primary care, mental health) were implemented in several VISNs, multidisciplinary Strategic Healthcare Groups were organized at VHA Headquarters, and a standardized National Formulary of prescription and nonprescription drugs, dietary supplements, and medical supplies was created (Kizer et al. 1997).

Eligibility Reform

The major cause of the fragmentation of service delivery in the veterans healthcare system was the set of statutes governing eligibility for care; these eligibility rules focused VA healthcare primarily on a veteran's service-connected disability, which did not always coincide with the veteran's greatest healthcare needs. Therefore, a key strategy of VHA transformation was gaining authority to treat the entire patient, instead of just his or her service-connected disability, and to be able to do so in the most appropriate medical setting.

Although attempts to change the eligibility rules governing veterans health care had been made for many years, such proposals had been unsuccessful. The new proposal employed a different line of reasoning than had been used before; it focused more on accountability and system management needs than on expanding access to care, and it promoted the concept of formal enrollment as a way to control growth of the system, should this be necessary. The combination of the concepts of enrollment and greater system accountability appeared to sway the opinion of certain historically resistant senators and seemingly helped secure passage of the landmark Veterans Eligibility Reform Act of 1996.

This new law substantially revised the statutes governing veterans care, putting inpatient and ambulatory care on the same statutory footing so that the VA could provide whatever care a patient needed in whatever were the most medically appropriate settings. The law also gave the VA broad authority to contract with private practitioners, health plans, or other entities to provide care for VA patients (i.e., to integrate "virtually"). Previously, this had not been permitted.

Capitation-Based Resource Allocation

Another major problem with veterans health care in 1995 was the manner in which the VHA distributed Congressionally appropriated medical care funds. The resource allocation methodology used at that time, as well as various earlier models, was neither predictable nor widely understood, and it perpetuated inefficiencies. A key strategy of the transformation effort was to create a predictable, fair, and easy-to-understand methodology for allocating funds, which also took into account the national demographic shifts of the 1970s and 1980s and the high degree of illness and disability prevalent in the VA's service population. To this end, a new capitation-based resource allocation system known as the Veterans Equitable Resource Allocation (VERA) methodology was implemented in 1997 (Veterans Health Administration 1997, 1998) after gaining the requisite statutory support needed to sustain such an effort (Khuri et al. 1995). We recognized how politically unpopular such a change would be, because of the resultant shift in funds from northeastern and northern midwestern states to southeastern and southwestern states.

In brief, under VERA, patients are divided into two categories based on the types of services they required in the preceding 3 years, and each category is given a national price based on an averaging of the expenditures for the services provided. These national prices are then adjusted for each VISN according to the cost of labor and five other variables.

For fiscal years 1997 through 1999, 96% of VA patients, accounting for 62% of expenditures, fell into the VERA "Basic Care" category, while the remaining 4% of patients (38% of expenditures) fell into what is considered "Complex Care." Basic Care provides a scope of benefits slightly broader than what is offered by Medicare managed care plans, while Complex Care includes services largely covered by non-Medicare funds (e.g., long-term care and advanced HIV disease).

Interestingly, while the VA's Basic Care benefit package is slightly more generous than what is offered under Medicare managed care plans, its annual capitation rate is between a third and a half of what Medicare pays HMOs to care for Medicare beneficiaries. The systemwide average annual expenditure per patient (combining both Basic and Complex Care patients post-VERA to allow comparison with expenditures pre-VERA) decreased from $5,479 in FY 1994 to $4,105 in FY 1999, a 25.1% decrease in constant dollars.

VERA simplified the VHA budgetary and resource allocation process while ensuring that resources were allocated equitably. VERA also provides strong incentives for system managers to ensure that care is coordinated, continuous, and provided in the most appropriate setting. It promotes multidisciplinary cooperative approaches to care, and it supports innovative approaches to care by permitting or facilitating the transfer of resources among providers so that the costs of innovation in one setting can be offset by gains in another area. Overall, VERA introduced unprecedented financial discipline into the veterans healthcare system while it facilitated coordination and continuity of care. (For further discussion of VERA, see Chapter 16, Resource Allocation Dilemmas in Large Federal Healthcare Systems, this volume.)

Expanding Access by Shifting to Ambulatory Care

A further critical problem with veterans healthcare in 1995 was its overreliance on inpatient care. Thus, another key strategy of VHA transformation was to reduce unnecessary inpatient care while expanding access by emphasizing ambulatory care *whenever medically appropriate*. This approach was visibly manifested by the institution of preadmission screening, rigorous admission and discharge planning, universal primary care, and systemwide telephone-linked care, as well as the creation in all facilities of "hoptel" beds for patients needing lodging but not hospital care.

As tangible evidence of the shift to ambulatory care, VHA closed 28,886 of its 52,315 (55%) acute care hospital beds between September 1994 and September 1999. Bed days of care per 1,000 patients dropped from 3,530 to 1,136 (68% decrease), while ambulatory care visits per year increased by more than 11 million, i.e., from 25 to 37 million per year (35% increase). In comparison, the number of VA nursing home beds decreased less than 3% during this 5-year period, and the number of domiciliary beds decreased about 15%.

Compared to FY 1994, inpatient admissions to VA hospitals in FY 1999 had fallen by almost 350,000 (36%), even though the number of patients being cared for by the system during this time had increased 24%. Likewise, the percentage of surgeries performed on an ambulatory basis increased from 35% of all VA surgeries in FY 1996 to more than 75% in FY 1999. Total surgical productivity increased nearly 5% with the shift to more ambulatory procedures, even though surgical staffing decreased about 10% (356,546 surgical procedures were performed in FY 1998 compared with 344,791 in FY 1996).

Similarly dramatic changes in inpatient capacity were made in substance abuse, posttraumatic stress disorder (PTSD), and other mental health programs—areas widely viewed as being too dependent on inpatient care. For example, during the 4-year interval FY 1995 through FY 1998, 59% (112 of 190) of substance abuse treatment programs shifted from inpatient to outpatient. During this same time, inpatient PTSD units decreased by 52% (21 of 40 closed), while outpatient PTSD programs increased by 13% (rising from 87 to 98) and PTSD Residential Rehabilitation Programs increased by 90% (from 10 to 19). In FY 1998, about 8% more psychiatric or substance abuse patients were being treated than in FY 1995, and there was no evidence that treatment was less successful than before the shift to outpatient care.

To make care more accessible and to increase coordination and continuity of care, 302 new community-based outpatient clinics were established during the 5-year period FY 1995 through FY 1999. No new funds were appropriated for these clinics; they were all established from savings achieved in other programs. For example, the VA's Pharmacy Benefits Management Group with its National Formulary documented more than $654 million in savings on the cost of drug purchases alone from FY 1995 to FY 1999. (While it may be obvious, it is worth pointing out that this type of redirection of funds is only possible in a fully integrated and capitated healthcare system. This achievement would never have been possible in the private sector, with its fragmented approach to reimbursement.)

Associated with the VHA's new approaches to providing care, systemwide staffing decreased by 25,867 full time equivalent (FTE) employees (12%) between September 1995 and September 1999 (from 207,940 FTE to 182,073 FTE), even though approximately 700,000 more patients were provided with "hands-on" care in FY 1999 than in FY 1994.

New Performance Management Program

The two paramount strategic goals of the VHA's transformation were ensuring that high-quality care was provided predictably and consistently everywhere in the system and that the *value* of veterans health care was optimal. (Value was operationally defined as being the sum of the performance metrics for access, technical quality, patient functionality, and service satisfaction divided by cost or price.) To achieve these goals, the VHA instituted a new performance management program in 1995. Under this approach, organizational vision and mission were aligned with quantifiable strategic goals; measures to track progress toward these goals were defined; and managers were held accountable for results achieved through prospective performance agreements.

Because accountability was key to the new performance management program, explicit performance contracts were used to hold managers specifically accountable for achieving challenging but realistic performance targets within defined timeframes. To date, these performance contracts are unique to the VHA in the federal government.

The VHA's new Performance Management Program was premised on quality improvement and quality innovation as key strategic goals. Toward this end, a 10-dimension accountability framework focused on process and outcomes of care was detailed. Within this framework:

- Performance measures were identified for a broad range of clinical and administrative processes

- Clinical performance measures were designed to support systemization of best research and best practices in the provision of healthcare services
- Numerous new quality management tactics were implemented (e.g., marked expansion of the use of clinical guidelines and care management, establishment of "Clinical Programs of Excellence," and development of new indices of best practices of care)
- A new performance measurement system for mental health was instituted
- The VA's National Surgical Quality Improvement Program was fully implemented (Khuri et al. 1995, 1998)
- The most comprehensive longitudinal and cross-sectional assessment of patient functional status ever performed anywhere was implemented
- Benchmark initiatives were launched in end-of-life care, pain management, HIV/AIDS care, cancer treatment, care management, and patient safety

Since initiating these efforts, substantial improvement in the quality of VA care has been documented by multiple methods. For example, the risk-adjusted 1-year survival rate of some of the VA's most vulnerable patient cohorts notably improved (Table 7.1); in other cohorts already having risk-adjusted 1-year survival rates greater than 95%, there was either no change or slight improvement despite the tumult in the system. Similarly, from FY 1994 through FY 1997, 30-day postsurgical morbidity and mortality decreased 30% and 9%, respectively, and the VHA surgical morbidity and mortality rates were the lowest reported for several high-volume procedures, including those for colectomy, cholecystectomy, abdominal aortic aneurysm repair, carotid endarterectomy, and total hip arthroplasty (Khuri et al. 1998).

The VHA's newly implemented prevention index (PI) and chronic disease care index (CDCI) documented marked improvement in adherence

TABLE 7.1. One-year risk-adjusted systemwide survival rates for nine VA patient cohorts.

Patient cohort	FY 1992	FY 1998	Percent change
Chronic renal failure	74.4%	81.4%	9.4%
Congestive heart failure	76.7%	83.1%	8.3%
COPD*	85.0%	88.5%	4.1%
Pneumonia	82.6%	89.3%	8.1%
Diabetes mellitus	94.7%	94.8%	<0.1%
Angina pectoris	96.0%	96.8%	<0.01%
Major depressive disorder	98.1%	98.3%	<0.1%
Schizophrenia	98.2%	98.2%	0.0%
Bipolar disorder	98.0%	98.5%	<0.01%

* COPD: chronic obstructive pulmonary disease.

to established clinical best practices (Tables 7.2 and 7.3). The VHA PI consists of nine clinical interventions that measure how well VHA practitioners follow nationally recognized primary prevention and early detection recommendations for eight diseases with major social consequences. These diseases are influenza and pneumococcal diseases; tobacco consumption; alcohol abuse; and cancer of the breast, cervix, colon, and prostate. (Many of the measures are the same as those in HEDIS.) In the aggregate, from FY 1995 through FY 1999, the PI rose from 34% to 81% (a 138% increase; see Table 7.2). To illustrate these changes, the percentage of at-risk patients documented as current on their influenza and pneumococcal vaccination increased from 28% to 76% (a 171% increase) and from 26% to 77% (a 196% increase), respectively. The number of at-risk veterans appropriately screened for colorectal and breast cancer increased from 34% to 74% (a 131% increase) and from 68% to 91% (a 34% increase), respectively.

The VHA's CDCI consists of 14 clinical interventions that assess how well VA practitioners follow nationally recognized guidelines for five high-volume diagnoses: ischemic heart disease, hypertension, COPD (chronic obstructive pulmonary disease), diabetes mellitus, and obesity. (Again, many of these measures are the same as those in HEDIS.) In the aggregate, this index increased from 44% to 89% (a 102% increase; see Table 7.3) from FY 1995 to FY 1999. The number of postmyocardial infarction patients on beta blockers increased from 77% to 94% (a 22% increase); the percent of diabetics having at least one annual hemoglobin A1c measurement and a retinal eye exam increased from 51% to 93% (an 82% increase) and from 47% to 67% (a 43% increase); and the percent of hypertensive patients

TABLE 7.2. The VHA's Prevention Index (PI) results for FY 1996–1999.

Indicator	VA FY 95/96[a,b]	VA FY 97[a]	VA FY 98[a]	VA FY 99[a]
Immunizations				
Pneumococcal	26%	61%	73%	77%
Influenza	28%	61%	71%	76%
Cancer (CA) screening				
Colorectal CA	34%	62%	72%	74%
Breast CA	68%	87%	89%	91%
Cervical CA	64%	90%	93%	94%
Prostate CA discussion	1%	37%	63%	66%
Tobacco consumption				
Screening	49%	86%	95%	95%
Counseling	35%	79%	93%	93%
Alcohol consumption				
Screening with standard instrument	2%	40%	65%	69%

[a] Average percentage of VA patients receiving the preventive or treatment intervention.
[b] Some of the baseline data were obtained in late FY 1995, but most were obtained in FY 1996.

TABLE 7.3. The VHA's Chronic Disease Care Index (CDCI) results for FY 1996–1999.

Indicator	VA FY 95/96[a,b]	VA FY 97[a]	VA FY 98[a]	VA FY 99[a]
Ischemic heart disease				
Aspirin therapy	91%	92%	95%	97%
Beta Blocker therapy	71%	83%	93%	94%
Cholesterol management	74%	98%	99%	99%
Hypertension				
Nutrition counseling	37%	78%	88%	91%
Exercise counseling	26%	76%	89%	91%
COPD				
Inhaler use (outpatient)	19%	44%	75%	80%
Inhaler use (inpatient)	16%	61%	61%	—
Diabetes mellitus				
Foot inspection	73%	90%	95%	96%
Foot pulses checked	46%	74%	84%	84%
Foot sensation checked	35%	69%	78%	78%
Retinal eye exam	47%	69%	73%	67%
Hemoglobin A1c	51%	85%	91%	93%
Obesity				
Nutrition counseling	44%	85%	92%	94%
Exercise counseling	26%	78%	89%	92%

[a] Average percentage of VA patients receiving the preventive or treatment intervention.
[b] Some of the baseline data were obtained in late FY 1995, but most were obtained in FY 1996.

with documented blood pressure control of lower than 140/90 increased from 25% to 45% (an 80% increase).

Improved quality of care also was demonstrated by use of a new palliative care index. In accreditation scores from the Joint Commission on Accreditation of Healthcare Organizations, and by various other methods, it rose from 54% in FY 1997 (the year it was implemented) to 96% in FY 1999.

While the VHA's experience in implementing and institutionalizing quality improvement is similar to that of the private sector, its experience is also unique in some ways. For example, the VHA's extensive involvement with health professional training and research provides unique opportunities for increasing the knowledge base about and encouraging innovation in quality improvement. With this in mind, the VA National Quality Scholars Fellowship Program was launched in collaboration with the Center for Evaluative Clinical Sciences at Dartmouth Medical School in 1998. The VA Faculty Fellows Program for Improved Care for Patients at the End of Life (funded by the Robert Wood Johnson Foundation) was initiated in the same year. Similarly, the Quality Enhancement Research Initiative (QUERI) was implemented in 1998 in an effort to capitalize on the VHA's unique portfolio of providing patient care, teaching, conducting research, and continuously measuring outcomes. QUERI attempts to purposely link research activities to clinical care so that new scientific knowledge is adopted in as close to real time as possible.

To accomplish its goals for systemwide quality improvement, the VHA has employed an operational strategy that combines central direction or "regulation" (e.g., directives that define and set standards or expectations for quality or efficiency) with close monitoring of performance to determine if expectations are being met. Competition and rewards build upon the professionalism and passion of healthcare workers to do what is best for patients. Conceptually, this blended strategy is similar to the approach used to improve cardiac surgery outcomes in New York State (Chassin 1996; Chassin et al. 1996; Hannan et al. 1994), although the nature of the regulation and competition in this case are primarily internal to the organization.

Service Satisfaction

The VHA improvements in technical quality have been accompanied by improvements in service satisfaction, although the changes in this regard have not been as dramatic. In FY 1995, customer service standards were implemented in the veterans healthcare system, and management was held accountable for making improvement. Using the patient service satisfaction instrument promulgated by the Picker Institute for Patient Centered Care in Boston, statistically significant improvements in patient satisfaction and reductions in the number of complaints were observed between FY 1995 and FY 1999 in essentially all areas.

Similarly, in May 1999, a national survey of veterans commissioned by the National Partnership for Re-inventing Government (NPRG) using the American Customer Satisfaction Index (ACSI) found that veterans who used VA health care were increasingly satisfied with their service. The ACSI is a rating produced quarterly for private sector firms by the University of Michigan Business School, the American Society for Quality, and the consulting firm of Arthur Andersen. In this study, 80% of veterans said care had improved in the previous 2 years, and they gave an overall satisfaction rating of 79 (on a scale of 0 to 100). The latter was significantly higher than the score of 72 recorded by the general public for all industry sectors or the score of 70 for private hospitals.

Improving Information Management and Data Integrity

Managing large amounts of information is integral to providing health care, and the success of any healthcare organization today is highly dependent on its ability to manage information. Improving the VHA's information management capabilities was a further key transforming strategy. Fortunately, the VHA had several historical information technology-related conditions that facilitated its ability to respond to the new direction given in FY 1995.

Because the VHA's primary healthcare information management system was implemented at a time when VA medical centers did little or no billing, the primary emphasis in many of its core applications was to improve operational efficiency and support clinical care delivery, rather than provide support for billing or fiscal purposes. Although this caused some problems when these financial functions were later needed, the benefit was that the system captured a great deal more clinical information than the vast majority of other existing healthcare information systems. This information provided a strong foundation when performance measures and other quality care monitors would draw on this clinical information base.

Similarly, the primary information system at the VA medical centers was both integrated in its databases (i.e., all data were kept in a central database) and designed to be decentralized, as evidenced by its original name, the Decentralized Hospital Computer Program (DHCP). This system was designed to allow each facility to write its own local applications, and even to exchange these with other facilities, without causing conflicts among the local applications. The data were made available to other programs on the system without having to connect to different computers. The DHCP architecture also provided an infrastructure to serve as the primary data feed for national databases; in fact, over 120 national databases were populated by data initially captured and stored in DHCP.

The VHA also had a long tradition of local innovation in IT, particularly in clinical computing. The experience gained from many local projects initiated to meet diverse local needs proved to be important because these projects often served as prototypes for solutions to national problems. This historical factor increased the VHA's ability to use automation to support some of the changes in management structure and clinical business processes that were integral to the transformation effort. Beginning in 1996, the VHA took a major step toward improving its information management by investing significant resources in several initiatives that established a communications platform robust enough to support the VISN concept. These initiatives included:

- Improving the telecommunications infrastructure within every facility and VISN office from one that could support only a dumb terminal-based (CRT-based) system to one designed for networking PCs throughout the buildings
- Standardizing the use of the Microsoft Office suite across VHA
- Agreeing on the use of Microsoft Exchange as the e-mail system for VISNs
- Developing a common VHA intranet
- Developing a method to consolidate databases

These initiatives guaranteed at least a minimum level of connectivity and response across the VHA, and in some cases imposed a de facto standard for exchanging and collaborating on work products.

As a result of the various initiatives related to upgrading the IT infrastructure, the VHA was able to quickly move forward with nationwide implementation of a VA Computerized Patient Record System (CPRS). Implementation of CPRS at "key sites" in each VISN began in February 1997. Once each VISN had implemented CPRS at their key site, they then moved forward with bringing up CPRS at all the other sites within the VISN. The last site in the system to bring up CPRS did so in December 1999, less than 3 years after this initiative was launched. The VHA is now one of the few healthcare systems to have fully implemented an electronic medical record.

In addition to enabling the VHA to implement CPRS, the IT infrastructure upgrade was key to the deployment of the VistA Imaging System, which interfaces with the VA Computerized Patient Record System. Other additions to the repertoire of clinical systems in the VHA are now possible as a result of the investment in the infrastructure.

One other major information management initiative that should be mentioned was the effort to implement a uniform, systemwide validated cost accounting and decision support system. A product from Transition Systems, Inc. was chosen and is now up and running at every VHA facility. However, from the beginning of this effort there has been considerable resistance to using the system, and it is only now beginning to be used for management purposes.

In this same vein, a number of other initiatives were launched to standardize data collection, increase the reliability and consistency of data acquisition, and otherwise improve the integrity of data management. Space does not allow a discussion of either these efforts or other transformation strategies like increasing partnerships and other external relationships; restructuring the research and education programs; decentralizing decision making; and diversifying the sources of funding. However, the results achieved in these areas have been substantial, and some of these strategies are discussed in more detail in this chapter's list of suggested readings and in other chapters of this volume.

Conclusion

Although linked exclusively to veterans in the minds of most Americans, today's veterans healthcare system provides many services that benefit the entire U.S. population. The VHA offers the potential to serve as a national laboratory for addressing many important healthcare questions now confronting the nation. This potential has greatly increased in the aftermath of the system reengineering that took place during the 5-year period of FY 1995 to FY 1999. The transformation of the VHA is still a work in progress, but the results thus far have demonstrated a 25% reduction in per patient costs, improved access to healthcare services, greater service satisfaction, and unequivocally higher quality of care.

Acknowledgment. Portions of this chapter appear in modified form in other publications, including: Kizer, K.W. 2000. Re-Inventing VA Healthcare—Systematizing Quality Management and Quality Innovation. *Medical Care* (in press); Kizer, K.W. 2000. Promoting Innovative Nursing Practice During Radical Health System Change. *Nursing Clinics of North America* (in press); and Kizer, K.W. 1999. The "New VA": A National Laboratory for Health Care Quality Management. *American Journal of Medical Quality* 14: 3–20.

References

Berwick, D.M. 1996. Payment by Capitation and the Quality of Care. *N Engl J Med* 335:1227–1231.

Booth, B.M., Ludke, R.L., Wakefield, D.S., et al. 1991. Non-Acute Days of Care Within Department of Veterans Affairs Medical Centers. *Med Care* 29S:AS51–AS63.

Chassin, M.R. 1996. Improving the Quality of Health Care: What Strategy Works? *Bull NY Acad Med* 73:81–91.

Hannan, E.L., Kilburn, H., Racz, M., et al. 1994. Improving the Outcomes of Coronary Artery Bypass Surgery in New York State. *JAMA* 271:271–276.

Khuri, S.F., Daley, J., Henderson, W., et al. 1995. "The National Veterans Administration Surgical Risk Study: Risk Adjustment for the Comparative Assessment of the Quality of Surgical Care." *J Am Coll Surg* 180:519-531.

Khuri, S.F., Daley, J., Henderson, W., et al. 1998. The Department of Veterans Affairs NSQIP: the First National, Validated, Outcome-Based, Risk-Adjusted and Peer-Controlled Program for the Measurement and Enhancement of the Quality of Surgical Care. *Ann Surg* 228:491–507.

Kizer, K.W., ed. 1995. *Vision for Change: A Plan to Restructure the Veterans Health Administration.* Washington, DC: Department of Veterans Affairs.

Kizer, K.W. 1998. *A Guidebook for VHA Medical Facility Integration.* Washington, D.C.: Veterans Health Administration.

Kizer, K.W., Ogden, J.E., Ray, J.E., 1997. Establishing a PBM: Pharmacy Benefits Management in the Veterans Health Care System. *Drug Benefit Trends* 9(8):24–27,47.

Kizer, K.W., Cushing, T.S., Nishimi, R.Y. 2000. The VA's Role in Federal Emergency Management. *Ann Emerg Med* (in press).

Rosenheck, R., Kizer, K.W. 1998. Hospitalizations and the Homeless. *N Engl J Med* 339:1166.

Smith, C.B., Goldman, R.L., Martin, D.C., et al. 1996. Overutilization of Acute-Care Beds in Veterans Affairs Hospitals. *Med Care* 34:85–96.

Veterans Health Administration. 1997. *VERA—Veterans Equitable Resource Allocation.* Washington, DC: Department of Veterans Affairs.

Veterans Health Administration. 1998. *VERA—Veterans Equitable Resource Allocation.* Washington, DC: Department of Veterans Affairs.

Wilson, N.J., Kizer, K.W. 1997. The VA Health Care System: An Unrecognized National Health Care Safety Net. *Health Aff* 16:200–204.

8
Shaping Future Healthcare Professionals

VICE ADM. (RET.) JAMES A. ZIMBLE AND MARION J. BALL

As change revolutionizes health care in the twenty-first century, medical education must keep pace with an unprecedented wave of innovation and demand. Faculty and curricula of medical schools will need to address an expanding roster of challenges: significant advances in technology, shifts in patient populations, new disease entities, and organizational and industry-wide changes.

In this time of transition and transformation, the military offers the best model for both private and public sector medical education. Long before the private sector, with its state-by-state requirements, could begin to address factors like increasing globalization of patient populations and the need for fast, remote access to information, the military was already devising solutions. This chapter will serve as a testament, demonstrating how the Uniformed Services University of the Health Sciences (USU) in Bethesda, Maryland, has enhanced and updated its curricula to prepare for the future of medicine. As the medical school uniquely focused on the training of United States uniformed services medical personnel, USU is in an ideal position to address military medicine's requirements: keeping large and dispersed populations healthy, training students for disaster and combat trauma, accessing data and expertise from remote locations, and delivering "good medicine in bad places." Many of USU's technological and curricular innovations are equally applicable to the private and public sectors. All represent the progressive thinking medical schools must consider when updating their educational goals.

USU: An Overview

As a federal health sciences educational university, USU was established by Congress in 1972 to train healthcare professionals for the Department of Defense (DoD) and the United States Public Health Service. Organized under the DoD, USU is governed by an Executive Committee of the three military Surgeons General. A 14-member Board of Regents, 9 of whom are prominent figures in U.S. health care appointed by the President, provide guidance regarding academic issues.

The F. Edward Hébert School of Medicine

The School of Medicine, named for Congressman F. Edward Hébert, admitted its first class of 32 students in 1976, and the number of enrollees has grown steadily since then, admitting 165 annually since 1992. Its graduate degree programs in anatomy, biochemistry, emerging infectious diseases, medical and clinical psychology, neuroscience, medical history, microbiology, molecular and cellular biology, pathology, pharmacy, physiology, public health, and tropical medicine and hygiene have experienced similar growth.

The School of Medicine is committed to remaining at the forefront of the healthcare industry's changes. Its curricula emphasize the unique aspects of military medicine, such as preventive medicine, disaster medicine, tropical medicine, survival in harsh climates, epidemiology, combat casualty care, and traumatic stress.

The Graduate School of Nursing

USU's Graduate School of Nursing (GSN) was established in 1993 and approved by the Assistant Secretary of Defense (Health Affairs) on February 26, 1996. The GSN's mission is to prepare Active Duty uniformed services nurses in masters level advanced nursing practice programs to deliver primary care, including anesthesia services, to Active Duty members of the uniformed services, their families, and other eligible beneficiaries. Through the GSN's two programs, Family Nurse Practice and Nurse Anesthesia, the school addresses two areas of current and future shortages in health care—primary care and anesthesia.

The GSN emphasizes health promotion and disease prevention from the nursing perspective, within the context of primary care and in a wide variety of national and international settings and communities. Besides contributing to the uniformed services peacetime healthcare delivery systems, graduates are prepared to aid military medicine and the Public Health Service by supporting combat operations and civil disaster and humanitarian missions.

Commitment to Progress

USU's mixture of civilian and military faculty help students prepare for the opportunities and challenges of current and future medical practice. In the past few years, a number of facilities, programs, and technological innovations have been introduced or expanded to meet the changing needs of medical students. Here, we examine five such facilities:

- The new Medical Simulation Center and Patient Simulation Laboratory
- The new Department of Biomedical Informatics
- The Learning Resource Center (LRC)
- Telehealth and Distance Learning
- The new interdisciplinary graduate program, Emerging Infectious Diseases (EID)

The New Simulation Center and Patient Simulation Laboratory (PSL)

As technology advances and the inpatient teaching base grows thinner, medical schools have both the impetus and the tools to respond to new challenges. Today's medical curricula must address:

- The fact that managed care practices and the dramatic increase in ambulatory care have led to fewer inpatients being available for teaching medical students, interns, residents, and other healthcare professionals
- The need to teach high-risk procedures without endangering lives
- The need to assess patient physical exams and patient history-taking
- Enhancement of medical readiness training (disaster training, sustainment of surgical skills, combat trauma, and stress management training)

To address these issues, USU launched two recent initiatives. The first is the National Capital Area Medical Simulation Center, expected to be fully operational by the start of the year 2000. The second is the new Patient Simulation Laboratory, which employs an anesthesia mannequin as a human patient simulator. Simulation techniques are not new—medical curricula across the United States are taking steps to incorporate them—but only USU has brought otherwise dispersed technologies together in a single facility.

The Military Medical Simulation Center

The groundwork for the military medical simulation center was established in July 1995, when the Dean of the USU School of Medicine and the Commander of the Walter Reed Army Medical Center (WRAMC) assembled a planning committee to create a model and establish objectives. The goal was to forge a cutting edge medical education laboratory that uses modern technologies (like medical simulation and information and telecommunication technology) to enhance teaching and training approaches. Four initial goals for the center were articulated:

- Develop and use military medicine databases for education and training
- Employ simulation techniques to enhance teaching and assessment of students' clinical interviewing, examining, and diagnostic skills

- Enhance the teaching, assessment, and documentation of medical readiness skills by using medical simulation capabilities
- Use medical simulations to enhance medical predeployment training

The center, used by both the medical and nursing schools and accessible to the faculty, staff, and students assigned to USU, WRAMC, the National Naval Medical Center (NNMC), and the Air Force's Malcolm Grow Medical Center (MGMC), would house three areas specially tailored to fulfill the committee's set goals. First, a Simulated Clinical Exam (SCE) would support standardized examination scenarios with actors portraying patients. The SCE consists of 12 clinical examination rooms, each equipped with two pan-tilt color cameras linked to specified VCRs. Interactions between the trainee and standardized patient are recorded on separate videos for subsequent analysis and teaching. Each training scenario or objective standardized clinical examination (OSCE) is scripted by an Educational Program Manager, who assists a Standardized Patient Trainer in managing the overall training exercise. Faculty and staff monitors, under the guidance of the Medical Director, observe the OSCE interaction via two-way mirrors or video monitors and provide the trainees with feedback.

The second area is the Computer Laboratory, where interactive computer-based tests would be given. Two types of computer-based tests would be used in the laboratory. The first would be interactive software on medical readiness decision making that would provide prospective medical leaders with complex decision-making problems often encountered during contingency missions. The second would be computer tests designed to prepare medical officers to take examinations such as the U.S. Medical Licensing Examination (USMLE).

Optimally, if selected and certified, this laboratory, which has been designed to meet the criteria of the National Board of Medical Examiners (NBME), could be authorized to conduct USMLE testing. Given that vision, the computer laboratory would also have color, pan-tilt cameras used to record events during high-stakes testing and allow for overall assessment of the testing process. The entire testing process thus would be managed by faculty and staff located in the adjacent Control Room, equipped with a two-way mirror and video monitors that would allow for easy observation. For USMLE testing, the site would be able to transmit real-time video, audio, and digital data back to the NBME.

Even more complex clinical scenarios would run in the Surgical Simulation Laboratory area. This area includes a fully equipped Deployable Medical Systems (DEPMEDS) Operating Room. DEPMEDS is the system of medical assemblage building blocks developed and used by the military to set up medical facilities in contingency operations. On one of the two DEPMEDS operating room tables, a human patient simulator would be used to provide simulated surgical training opportunities. The patient simulator planned for this area would allow for trauma, surgical, endoscopy, broncoscopy, intravenous catheterization, ultrasound, and anesthesiology training. The surgical simulation laboratory will also house a "Reach In," 3D-display Surgical Table that would be used to provide no-risk simulated surgical experiences to both students and residents. All operating room educational experiences would be recorded by remote controlled video cameras and monitored by the Surgical Director, the Operating Room Coordinator, and other faculty and staff members. The simulation center would also include equipment for teleconferencing and distance learning, two topics explored later in this chapter.

The simulation center concept was approved by the Defense Medical Readiness Training and Education Council in 1997, and the building renovation design was completed in 1998. Building renovation staffing, operational plans, and technology installation and testing continued throughout late 1999. Although the completed center was scheduled to open in early 2000, the center experienced its first student encounter in late September 1999, when a group of 24 students and 4 faculty members arrived to practice physical examination techniques.

The Clinical Simulator and Patient Simulator Laboratory (PSL)

The laboratory in the Department of Anesthesiology began in 1998 as a collaborative project between the National Naval Medical Center's Department of Anesthesiology and USU's Departments of Anesthesiology, Anatomy and Cell Biology, and Physiology. It has evolved into a fully interactive clinical training laboratory, equipped as an operating room with standard monitoring equipment, instruments, life support system, defibrillator, and complete audio/video recording equipment. Instead of flesh-and-blood patients, however, students practice both routine and high-risk procedures on a lifelike, computer-controlled mannequin.

Since the aviation industry discovered the positive effects of flight simulations on training, performance, and safety, other industries have worked to adopt these high-fidelity, low-risk training methods. USU's patient simulator includes more than 20 patient profiles, each with unique characteristics and more than 35 customizable "events," including cardiovascular conditions, allergic reactions, equipment failures, and anesthesia complications. The simulator is also equipped with an automatic drug recognition system, activated by syringes with computer chips that represent specific drugs. The mannequin responds realistically to the administered drug, whether it be a cardiovascular agent, an anesthetic, a neuromuscular blocker, or an infusion pharmaceutical.

Eight different groups of students/medical personnel make regular use of the PSL both as a training facility and as a research resource:

1. **USU Medical Students, first year, cardiovascular physiology**: For these students, the simulator is used to complement a teaching animal lab that demonstrates the basic interactions of heart rate, blood pressure, cardiac output, stroke volume, and circulatory resistance.

2. **USU Medical Students, third year, two-week anesthesiology rotation**: The simulator helps these students learn the fundamentals of anesthesia and practice connecting a patient to external life support. It also helps ensure that all the students are presented with a core learning experience.

3. **USU Graduate Students in Nurse Anesthesia (NA) in MSN degree program**: Students undergo basic and advanced simulator training, during which they must handle unique cases with unexpected complications. Some NA students use the simulator as a laboratory instrument for their required masters' degree thesis project.

4. **WRAMC Nurses in ICU certificate program**: These patients are exposed to advanced patient care scenarios that include extensive equipment use and critical medical situation training.

5. **Uniformed Anesthesia Residents from nearby military hospitals (NNMC, WRAMC, and Naval Medical Center Portsmouth [NMCP])**: These resident physicians are challenged with complex, specifically tailored medical scenarios, designed to prepare them for dealing with critical, time-sensitive situations. The most recent incoming class of anesthesia residents to WRAMC was given an extensive trauma training/evaluation with the simulator.

6. **Residents from the R. Adams Cowley Shock Trauma Center (in Baltimore, Maryland)**: These residents from the shock/trauma center use the simulator as the anesthesia residents do, for advanced and severe situations that have a high acuity but a low frequency.

7. **Collaborative Researchers with R. Adams Cowley Shock Trauma Center**: Here, the simulator is a test device that evaluates how experienced ER personnel make use of alarms during critical medical emergencies.

8. **MGMC's USAF Critical Care Air Transport Teams (CCATT)**: Once a month the school hosts a CCATT session, during which the three-person team treats the simulator as a real case. Practicing nurses, physicians, and respiratory therapists are involved in the CCATT training scenarios. They receive a call that their services are needed, gather their packs of gear, leave their hospital (MGMC), travel to the site of the patient (USU), evaluate the patient's condition, and provide sufficient treatment to ensure successful transport of the patient back to a hospital. Once they leave the hospital, they can use only equipment and supplies that they can carry.

The patient simulator offers many benefits to students and instructors. Without putting a life at risk, students can experience handling rare conditions such as malignant hyperthermia, learn to recognize a wide variety of problems, practice using instruments and equipment, hone decision-making skills, and accumulate first-hand experience with military-specific problems like combat trauma. Instructors can tailor each case to individual students, selecting the type, level of speed, and degree of severity according to the student's level of competence. If the instructor wants to give feedback or additional directions, the lesson can be paused and repeated as many times as necessary. Sessions are recorded and played back, thus enabling the students, with the guidance of their instructors, to analyze their performance and recognize their strengths and weaknesses.

Just as immunity is derived from infection, knowledge and wisdom are derived from experience. The patient simulator provides an ideal opportunity to nurture knowledge and wisdom in a risk-free environment. Because no life is at stake, instructors can purposely push students beyond their competency levels so they can learn and retain critical lessons the most effective way: by making mistakes.

The patient simulator is a valuable addition to the USU curricula, one that will play an expanded role in the years to come. Patient simulators have been gradually finding a place in medical schools across the United States, as well as all over the world. There are currently two commercial vendors of computer-controlled mannequin patient simulators; they share the market about equally. By the time this book goes to press, one vendor, Medsim, will have implemented 11 simulators in the United States: 7 in medical schools, 3 in nursing schools, and 1 in a podiatry school. If we assume that the other vendor has about the same number of devices in the United States, then we can conclude that about 10% of U.S. medical schools have patient simulators.

None of these schools, however, use their simulators for a wider range of students and classes than does USU, an institution that has become a focal point of many different medical education groups. The PSL at USU is successful because so many different instructors have taken the initiative to explore how it can support their educational missions. To date, every instructor who has tried the PSL has returned to use it for additional classes, and the Graduate School of Nursing program in Nurse Anesthesia has gone so far as to completely revamp its curriculum. Initially, the GSN used the simulator only a few times before sending students out for their clinical phase. Now the simulator plays an integral role from the very beginning of the academic phase, and it continues to be used about 1 day a week for the entire year.

The School of Medicine will begin including patient simulators in basic science curricula during the first and second years of the medical program, thus lending a clinical context to classes in physiology and pharmacology. Offering the single simulator in the PSL to teach a class size of more than 165 students, as was done for cardiovascular physiology, requires extraordinary juggling of schedules. This school year, collaboration between the PSL, the new Simulation Center, and the patient simulation facility at the Naval School of Health Sciences (located in the NNMC) will make three simulators available to better accommodate large class sizes. USU is also considering other preclinical medical school classes that may benefit from using the simulator as a demonstration device.

The New Department of Biomedical Informatics

The body of biomedical data and the field of informatics are both expanding rapidly. In response, healthcare experts are beginning to place more emphasis on the processes of knowledge retrieval and decision making, ranking it just as important as the knowledge itself. The drive to implement the most effective processes is fueling the move away from paper-based records and the increased recognition of the importance of computers.

Given this heightened awareness of technology's role in knowledge development, biomedical informatics has become an increasingly essential component of medical education. Graduating medical students must be able to use biomedical information to define, study, and solve problems and communicate their methodologies and results. Since January 1997, the Center for Informatics in Medicine (CIM) has enhanced USU informatics research and education through introductory computer courses, a workshop on Internet applications in diagnostic pathology, and development of such diverse areas as websites on educational technology, military graduate education, and HIV in the military.

For the last three entering classes since 1997, a coalition of CIM, the LRC, and appropriate Dean's Office has begun to prepare incoming USU students for the expanded role of informatics in their studies and professional careers. However, USU's School of Medicine and Graduate School of Nursing have recognized that if students are to fulfill the five key roles of physicians and nurses—lifelong learner, clinician, educator/communicator, researcher, and manager—they must have the benefits of a dedicated biomedical informatics program. USU's Department of Biomedical Informatics, proposed in June 1999, is conceived as a resource center to extend the medical and nursing curricula, serve as a clearinghouse for USU informatics applications, and provide a testing facility bed for informatics research. The new department will help USU fulfill its mission by these roles:

- Supporting the curricula through educational technology
- Extending the curricula through biomedical informatics
- Identifying and researching innovative informatics applications for military health care
- Providing consultants to military healthcare providers

The Department of Biomedical Informatics, recognized as a basic science department, will have three areas of specialization: bioinformatics, medical and nursing informatics, and education. It will extend and enhance an already strong curriculum through both departmental and interdisciplinary courses that will integrate basic sciences with clinical experiences, offer simulated clinical training experiences, continue current teaching efforts in introductory computing, and focus on student-centered learning with case-based, small-group sessions.

USU expects the Department of Biomedical Informatics to be more service focused than the traditional academic department. The current CIM will be retained as the department's service-based component. Research computing will be reassigned to this department and will no longer be a part of University Information Systems (UIS). The new department will be the heart of USU's academic computing support, propelling such activities as sequence analysis, statistical computing, and the student web page pilot project.

The new department will also solve problems associated with the university's widely dispersed informatics initiatives. In the past, attempts to incorporate informatics into USU curricula have been handled by individual departments, leaving the efforts vulnerable to collapse if a key member of the department left or was reassigned. The Department of Biomedical Informatics is conceived as a central resource into which all departmental informatics endeavors can be incorporated; this will be accomplished through collaborative arrangements offering joint faculty appointments in the department.

According to plans set forth by an ad hoc committee responding to the needs of the Surgeons General, resources for the new department will be phased in over the next 5 years. USU's ultimate goal for the department is to have a degree granting program in place. If the university can identify additional faculty and space, an interested student population, and an appropriate funding source before then, the degree granting program may become a high priority even sooner. USU's new Department of Biomedical Informatics is one more example of the university's commitment to anticipating and addressing changes in health care and providing models that can be transferred to the private sector.

The Learning Resource Center (LRC)

As new ways of collecting and disseminating information develop, medical schools have the incentive to reinvent their libraries, enhancing and supplementing elements of traditional paper-based resources with multimedia and computer-based resources. The complex information requirements of USU students, staff, alumni, and faculty have motivated the university to create an advanced model. By supplementing its print books and journals with a diverse collection of slides, videotapes, videodiscs, and CD-ROM products like Micromedix and Medline, the LRC at USU is quickly becoming *the* medical reference center for the Military Health Services System. Its microcomputers support word processing, graphics, desktop publishing, desktop presentation software, and a wide variety of medical education programs. For preservation and transmission of images, the LRC has also implemented a full-color imaging system for color copying and printing and flat-bed scanner fax machine.

By constantly updating and diversifying its resources, the LRC ensures fast access to crucial information. If students cannot locate a particular resource within the center, the LRC's mediated database and interlibrary loan services can link to local, national, and international resources. The surrounding area also offers such supplementary information sources as the National Library of Medicine (NLM), the National Agricultural Library, and the Library of Congress.

The "Library That Never Closes"

Because USU students, faculty, and alumni are dispersed across the globe, the university had to make provisions for quick retrieval of information from remote locations. Since January 1997, implementation of the Internet has expanded access to the LRC, making it globally accessible online 24 hours a day, every day of the year. This feature is ideal for alumni in remote sites—in fact, the registered number of users for the LRC's remote Internet services has grown to approximately 3,000. All information resources are tested for reliability and user-friendly access before they are moved to the Internet server, and revisions are made as necessary.

In 1998, the LRC expanded the scope of its Internet services with many new online resources that now equal those of a major medical library. The added resources can be divided into eight modules:

- Books: In addition to more than 120,000 traditional volumes (including a valuable collection of medical military history), the LRC offers more than 40 online books, from standard textbooks like *Harrison's Principles of Internal Medicine* and *Sabiston's Textbook of Surgery* to books covering all the major medical specialties. The volumes are constantly updated to reflect the most current thought and practice.
- Journals: In 1998, the LRC added more than 300 full-text titles to its Internet server, one of the largest in the country. These include all the 130 Academic Press titles, 50 Highwire Press titles, the Ovid Journals collections, and the MD Consult's 48 titles. Yearbooks on medical specialties are also available.
- Practice Guidelines: The LRC's Internet server contains more than 500 clinical practice guidelines contributed by more than 50 medical societies and government agencies.
- Patient Education: More than 2,500 patient education handouts are available through this module and can be personalized with special instructions from the attending physician or staff.
- Continuing Medical Education: The collection of more than 300 Continuing Medical Education (CME) modules provides topical updates

across 11 medical specialties and offers credits that can be applied toward the American Medical Association Physician's Recognition Award. All CME tests provide links to related information found in online literature and websites.

- Clinical Topic Tours: These online tours lead users through a focused collection of information from medical literature, establishing familiarity with current and accepted wisdom on a variety of significant topics. A new tour is provided each week.
- Today in Medicine: To keep users informed about the newest developments in medicine and nursing, this module includes clinical summaries, links to additional web sources, and current events from major journals, conferences, and government agencies.
- In This Week's Journals: This module allows users to scan key contents of the major weekly healthcare journals, from the *New England Journal of Medicine* to the *Journal of the American Medical Association* and other health professional journals. Concise article summaries are included.

The special needs of USU's dispersed populations made global access to the LRC's resources a necessity. However, as the practice of telehealth expands and more healthcare professionals must obtain crucial information where, when, and how it is needed, USU's Learning Resource Center can serve as a model for private sector medical libraries.

Telehealth and Distance Learning

With the development of Internet technologies and the globalization of patient populations, advancing telehealth and distance learning has become a major focus for private sector health care. As the nature of the Learning Resource Center demonstrates, the military already has been experimenting with these initiatives out of necessity—servicemen and women in remote populations cannot afford long absences from duty, and the healthcare professionals that serve them must be able to retrieve images and information from any location. Over the past decade, USU has rolled out several successful telehealth and distance learning initiatives, many of which can be adapted for the private sector.

Telehealth

With its time- and cost-conscious goal of moving information rather than people, telehealth became a crucial component of Army medicine more than 2 years ago. The DoD has become a champion of telehealth, recognizing its potential to meet the challenges associated with administering care to patients in far-flung environments. Telehealth, which includes techniques like digitized videoteleconferencing (VTC) and store and forward applications for image transmission, minimizes transportation time and expense by extending the care site, which optimizes staff workload and allows crucial service members to return to duty faster.

CCRC

The School of Medicine's Casualty Care Research Center (CCRC) has made much progress in the field of telehealth, training more than 400 personnel, providing 11 deployed telehealth courses to four countries, and taking the technology to Belize, Germany, Croatia, Macedonia, Bosnia, Saudi Arabia, and Ethiopia. For example, several years ago CCRC worked in conjunction with personnel from Fort Dietrick, Maryland, to develop methods of deployable telehealth for United Nations missions in Macedonia. This effort expanded when Fort Dietrick soldiers went into Bosnia with NATO forces to establish a foundation for communication between the 212th MASH, the primary medical treatment facility for the American sector in Bosnia, and the combat support hospital in Hungary. Meanwhile, the CCRC staff went to USU to give instructions on clinical applications, techniques, and medicolegal issues to units that would be deployed to Bosnia and Macedonia.

CCRC also provides clinical and technical telehealth training within the DoD by offering a 4-day course geared toward currently deployed telehealth users. Through such methods as hands-on training and case studies, this course teaches system design, clinical applications and techniques, tissue labs, and equipment options. Besides current telehealth system users, the course will be valuable for the telehealth industry, fixed-site consultants, and Army Surgeon General-mandated Medical Center Special Response Teams.

Another CCRC achievement has been the implementation of telehealth aboard the USS *George Washington*, an initiative that led the Navy to increase its use of telehealth equipment by 100%. More than 90 teledermatology cases have come from the USS *George Washington*; during 1998, CCRC staff were able to diagnose 4 cases of melanoma using telehealth techniques, and in 1 case, recommended a simple surgical procedure that could be performed on board. Not only did this approach save the patient from prolonged waiting and unnecessary testing, it also saved the Navy the expenses associated with the patient's travel and with losing a crucial member of their team.

Telegenetics Website

In response to the recognized need for genetic services, USU designed an Internet solution to assist with genetics education and services for the DoD. A Telegenetics website was initially developed in 1996 with the assistance of the U.S. Navy Telemedicine department and the Applied Physics Laboratory (APL) at Johns Hopkins University under the MIDN project. The Telegenetics site was moved to USU (www.usuhs.mil/genetics) in 1997 to focus on educational goals and to provide consultations in genetics to the DoD's deployed forces.

The mission of the Telegenetics website is to provide information and education about genetics to DoD primary care providers, specialist physicians, Uniformed Services University medical students, graduate students and researchers, and interns, residents, and fellows within DoD Graduate Medical Education programs. The website acts as an invaluable centralized knowledge resource, providing these recipients with online genetics lectures, written information, instructional aids like On-line Mendelian Inheritance in Man (OMIM), and links to articles, laboratory services, and patient support groups.

Through store and forward technology, the Telegenetics website also enables consultations about genetic disorders. Healthcare providers have accessed this site from within the continental United States as well as from international locations, including Yokota, Misawa, and Okinawa in Japan. Costs for transporting patients to consultants in genetics may be decreased by providing information about genetics to patients and healthcare providers in remote locations via the World Wide Web.

In the future, the USU team responsible for maintaining the Telegenetics website will aim to fulfill these tasks:

- Incorporate video-teleconferencing capability to allow real-time consultations
- Integrate online Family Pedigree drawing program to improve genetic history intake
- Integrate Tele-Maternal Fetal Medicine (Tele-MFM) capability to allow store and forward examination of ultrasound, MRI, and CT images from remote locations and to enhance diagnostic capabilities in all DoD medical facilities
- Develop continuing medical education (CME) on the Web to enhance ongoing learning in genetics
- Use the Simulation Center to provide computer-assisted education for USU medical students in genetics, including cases, dysmorphology, cancer genetics, and adult genetics
- Use the Simulation Center to enhance learning in Obstetrical Ultrasound
- Assist in the development of Critical Pathways for clinical services in genetics

All fourth-year medical students at USU have been fully trained in deployable telehealth since the fall 1998 field training exercise "Bushmaster" was held. Now an integral part of the university's curriculum, telehealth will continue to fulfill one of USU's core missions: providing "good medicine in bad places."

Distance Learning

Web-based distance learning is advantageous for the same reasons tele-health is: it conserves expenses associated with travel, and it eliminates the necessity for excessive time away from work. It has proven to be cost-effective and highly satisfactory to both students and employers. To reap these benefits, the School of Medicine and the Graduate School of Nursing have collaborated and continue to collaborate with various departments on ambitious distance learning projects.

The Department of Pathology

The Department of Pathology was an early pioneer in the use of computer technology at USU. Today, computers are an integral part of the department's educational activities. For instance, computers are used to archive the department's varied collection of photographic images into a retriev-able database that can be searched by teaching faculty preparing for lectures, labs, and small group exercises. These images are used in the education of medical students, housestaff, and practicing physicians. A crucial component of this pathology database is the image source, because knowing the image source precludes the use of copyrighted material in its teaching exercises.

The department has developed a compact disc of approximately 1,000 photographic images of pathological specimens, an innovative way to help students prepare for their pathology labs and examinations. Directed to second-year medical students, the disc provides a comprehensive collection of images covering all major organ systems. The department finds that this compact disc increases the accessibility of images to students and results in significant financial savings for the department because duplication costs for lost or damaged 2×2 slides are eliminated.

Computers are also used in testing. Each year, USU students can access 14 online quizzes that use photographic images, answer the quiz questions in an open book format, and submit their answers electronically to the department. A databank of questions written by USU faculty are archived by computers and used in testing medical students. The use of archived questions allows the department to compare class performance from year to year and evaluate the quality of the questions, which has reduced ambiguity in examinations.

The Department of Pathology also uses Internet technology to provide a web page independent of the University's website. This page enables students to access information regarding pathology educational activities, links them with other medical schools and pathology websites, informs the public of departmental personnel and research activities, and advertises the department's Ph.D. program in pathology.

Finally, in recognition of the need for the deployed military physician to have access to CME credit, the department has used computer technology to provide CME credit to this group. Through the web page, physicians can review cases written by the pathology faculty, answer a series of questions based on the case, and receive CME credit. More than 300 CME certificates have been issued by USU for this activity.

Below are some other examples of USU's significant advances in distance learning.

The Department of Obstetrics and Gynecology

USU uses interactive, real-time video teleconferencing to link five different sites for its 6-week clerkship in obstetrics and gynecology. In sessions that last 60 to 150 minutes, site coordinators meet with the clerkship director and administrative personnel to discuss such crucial issues as curricula, student problems and evaluations, and faculty development. Since the sessions began in May 1998, USU has found that they enable the standardization of curricula, facilitate the sharing of ideas, reduce administrative tasks through centralized support, and improve the meaning, consistency, and level of detail in student evaluations.

The Graduate School of Nursing (GSN)

In 1997, USU's Graduate School of Nursing (GSN) initiated development of the Adult Nurse Practitioner Post-Master's Program. The 9-month multidisciplinary program, which aims to build a strong foundation of knowledge in adult primary care, advanced nursing practice, nursing research, and nursing theory, includes didactic coursework delivered with the aid of state-of-the-art distance learning technology. Interactive video teleconferencing and Internet technologies help prepare clinical nurse specialists to diagnose and manage adult primary care problems, all from remote sites that eliminate the costs of travel, tuition, and staff replacement.

Late in 1997, USU linked its Board of Regents conference room with 8 teaching sites and 35 advanced practice nurses across the country. Sites included were Atlanta, Georgia; Baltimore, Maryland; Los Angeles, California; Bronx, New York; Fayetteville, North Carolina; Charleston, South Carolina; Fort Leavenworth, Kansas; and San Diego, California. USU first reached Martinsburg, West Virginia, with a network of high-speed digital telephone lines from the compressed-video classroom, a method more cost-effective than satellite broadcasting. This site served as the hub that facilitated links to the other sites. As second class of 43 students began in June of 1999 with 10 teaching sites, including Puerto Rico.

To ensure that the distance learning courses meet the quality requirements of the accrediting bodies, the Offices of the Surgeons General and Federal Nursing Chiefs, and the Military Health Services System, the GSN has procured funding for research and evaluation protocols. Preceptors located at each site help verify the effectiveness of USU's distance learning classrooms; they ensure that the material is being understood and that questions are resolved immediately. All graduates from the class of 1999 have passed national certification exams in the upper percentile.

A recent distance learning initiative was formed to support pharmacology classes. Pharmacology is taught by live instructors, but students can access syllabi, lectures, and assignments via the Internet. These materials are available to students 2 to 3 days before classroom lectures.

The Medical Executive Skills Training Program

This program, which has been in existence for almost 5 years in traditional classrooms, is another recent distance learning initiative. The Department of Defense has defined 40 competencies that medical department executives must master before assuming leadership and command positions. For the 9 of these competencies that involve the use of data for clinical and management decision making, the Division of Health Services Administration is developing training modules. In one calendar year, USU hosts three 1-week courses for approximately 100 commanders and prospective commanders of medical treatment facilities. These programs also deliver continuing medical education credits.

The need to make this course available to a larger audience has prompted USU to develop a Distance Learning Course on the Internet. Beginning in the summer of 1999, USU began developing the Medical Executive Skills Training Course online. Within 6 months, five beta-test modules were online. These modules can be found at *http://medexec.usuhs.mil*. Future expansion efforts are ongoing.

Eventually, through its proliferation of annually reviewed online information, USU aims to provide "one-stop shopping" for medical education. In the near future, distance learning will provide the following benefits:

- For medical students, the USU website now includes a module on chest film interpretation, a complete set of images for radiographic anatomy, a child abuse module, and minilectures on brain and posterior fossa tumors. Eventually, all teaching handouts (including interactive materials) will be available online.
- For MHSS graduate medical education, resident-level handouts, including interactive lecture/tutorials and access to remote teaching files, will be offered online.
- For MHSS continuing medical education, online materials will resemble those offered for graduate medical education: interactive tutorials and web-based teaching files.
- For military telehealth, consults via e-mail attachments of images will enhance telehealth initiatives.

The New Interdisciplinary Graduate Program, Emerging Infectious Diseases (EID)

One of the primary concerns of military medicine is, quite naturally, ensuring that deployed military personnel are able to preserve their health and complete their job assignments. For this reason, USU is placing special emphasis on advancing clinical care, epidemiological services, preventive medicine planning, public health, and biomedical research, particularly in the area of infectious diseases. Many of the research programs at USU are directed toward understanding the molecular and cellular bases of current and emerging infectious diseases. These include studies on parasitic, bacterial, viral, and fungal pathogens. Research areas devoted to understanding these pathogens and the diseases they cause include studies on the pathogenesis, epidemiology, immunology, genetics, and physiology of these diseases.

USU's basic science and clinical faculty has been assembled to instruct students, conduct research, serve as consultants, and conduct projects relating to important areas that affect active duty military personnel. The depth and breadth of their studies are suggested by the active research protocols managed by the Research Administration Department at USU. As the sampling of grant titles in Table 8.1 demonstrates, USU faculty exhibits skills in clinical microbiology, laboratory microbiology, pathology, pharmacological management, parasitology, bacterial diseases, sexually transmitted diseases, immunology, vaccinology, pathogenesis of infectious diseases, epidemiology, virology, and tropical medicine.

TABLE 8.1. Sampling of Uniformed Services University of the Health Sciences (USU) grant titles.

Development of optical methods for new bioagent detection instrument
Molecular analysis of militarily important viruses and vaccine development
T-cell responses to intracellular bacterial pathogens
Fuctional analysis of the genome sequence of *Deinococcus radiodurans*
Mechanism of neural degeneration following viral infection
Mechanisms in septic shock syndrome
Rickettsial diseases: rapid diagnosis, risk assessment, vaccines, antibiotic prophylaxis, and
     treatment
Protection against malaria by attacking infected hepatocytes
Transmission of *Bartonella bacilliformis* by bites of phlebotemine sand flies
Antibiotic treatment of Gulf War veterans' illnesses
Flagellar regulation and *Salmonella* virulence
Molecular genetic analysis of chlamydia pathogenicity
Sequencing of patient HIV-envelope genes
T-lymphocyte signaling and function
The role of NK cells in stimulating humoral immunity
Expression of DSHV/HHV8 mRNA and viral antigens
Adjuventing response to protein-polysaccharide vaccines
Development of a new small animal model for typhoid fever

In recent years, USU has become increasingly aware of the Department of Defense's need for additional professionals trained in all aspects of infectious diseases. After discussions with the military services' Surgeons General, the Dean of the School of Medicine organized a committee to address the possibility of developing an interdisciplinary program in "new, emerging, reemerging or prevalent infectious diseases." The University Board of Regents reviewed and approved the proposal for this new Graduate Program in Emerging Infectious Diseases for implementation in the academic year 1999–2000.

The new EID program is tailored for students who plan to pursue a Ph.D. degree in one of the academic tracks within the broad field of Emerging Infectious Diseases. The interdisciplinary faculty consists primarily of full-time members of the Departments of Microbiology and Immunology, Pathology, and Preventive Medicine and Biometrics, Pediatrics, and Medicine. Designed for students interested in the pathogenesis, host response, and epidemiology of infectious diseases, the program combines formal coursework with research training. A unique aspect of the Graduate Program is that it also provides opportunities for physicians to complete the research portions of their Fellowships in Infectious Diseases.

The EID Graduate Program's required curriculum includes core courses, electives, training rotations, attendance at Journal Clubs, and a Seminar Series. For the first year of training, students are required to complete a series of mandatory courses (Table 8.2). After completing the core coursework, students select one of three tracks—Microbiology and Immunology, Pathology, or Preventive Medicine and Biometrics—upon which to focus the remainder of their coursework and thesis project. Advancement to Ph.D. candidacy occurs after students have satisfactorily completed their formal coursework, laboratory rotations, and a combined written and oral Qualifying Examination.

TABLE 8.2. Core courses for first-year Emerging Infectious Diseases (EID) graduate students at USU.

Fall quarter	Medical Microbiology and Infectious Diseases
	Fundamentals of Infectious Disease Pathology and Laboratory Diagnosis
	Techniques in Cellular and Molecular Biology
	EID Journal Club
	EID Seminar
Winter quarter	Fundamentals of Infectious Disease Pathology and Laboratory Diagnosis
	Models of Emerging Infectious Diseases I
	Cell Biology I
	Genetics
	Lab Rotation
Spring quarter	Models of Emerging Infectious Diseases II
	Cell Biology II
	Genetics
	Lab Rotation

Completion of an original research dissertation is an integral part of the Program and the final step. As part of their dissertation research, students present an annual departmental seminar based on their original projects. The written dissertation is prepared under the guidance of a major faculty advisor, and the dissertation defense is delivered in the form of a public seminar followed by a private oral examination.

With the addition of the interdisciplinary Emerging Infectious Diseases program, the School of Medicine has increased its capacity and commitment to instruct students in the biology of infectious diseases, especially in the areas of interest to military medicine. Interested students can now be specifically prepared to serve in military and government laboratories, conducting research or providing services that will protect military personnel as they travel the world to ensure the security of the United States. Graduating students will be more broadly based and will have a competitive edge in dealing with the increasingly complex world of science. These traits will be particularly important, given the overlapping nature of most basic sciences today, and the knowledge of resources that derives from an integrated and interdisciplinary approach to infectious diseases will be unparalleled. Thus, this program can serve as a model for the private sector medical schools and graduate programs that want to broaden the educational experience and training of their students.

Conclusion

In this chapter, the authors have given a detailed description of what a dynamic medical school is undertaking as we enter the twenty-first century. The Uniformed Services University of the Health Sciences is leading the way as a standards bearer for the public and private sector medical and nursing schools in the United States. As the preceding examples have illustrated, the innovative, technology-intensive initiatives in the School of Medicine and Graduate School of Nursing are exemplary. The new medical simulation center and the patient simulator laboratories are state of the art and, in some cases, one of a kind. The new department of biomedical informatics, with its broad outreach initiatives toward a virtual faculty and access to some of the best resources in the world, is bound to be superlative. The learning resource center, accessible 24 hours a day, has more online books and journals than most health sciences libraries worldwide. The innovative and successful applications in telehealth and distance learning are being replicated throughout the other health sciences centers in the nation as well as abroad. Finally, the new interdisciplinary graduate programs, such as the latest in emerging infectious diseases, represent the most innovative and forward-thinking initiatives in education. They are well supported by the enabling technologies that provide access to knowledge when, where, and how it is needed—at the bedside and the research bench, in the field of military action, and in the classroom.

The innovative programs initiated at the Uniformed Services University will forever change the way medical and nursing students are trained and the way they practice. In this new millennium, USU will do more than play a major role in training healthcare professionals for the DoD and United States Public Health Service. The school's programs and vision will serve as a formidable example, one that should be emulated by all other medical education centers around the world.

Acknowledgments. The authors gratefully acknowledge the assistance of Faye Abdellah, Emmanuel Cassimatis, Richard Conran, Peter Esker, Val Hemming, Richard Kyle, Charles Macri, Eleanor Metcalf, Leon Moore, Gil Muniz, Aron Primack, and William Sefton.

Readings

Fenton, C. 1998. Patient Simulator. *USU Quarterly* Summer:5–7.
Issenberg, S.B., McGaghie, W.C., Hart, I.R., Mayer, J.W., Felner, J.M., Petrusa, E.R., Waugh, R.A., Brown, D.D., Stafford, R.R., Gessner, R.H., Gordon, D.L., Ewy, G.A. 1999. Simulation Technology for the Health Care Professional Skills Training and Assessment. *JAMA* 282:861–866.
Uniformed Services University of the Health Sciences. 1997. *USUHS Celebrates 25 Years of National Public Service.* Bethesda, MD: USUHS Reference/Historical Document.
Uniformed Services University of the Health Sciences. 1998–2000. *F. Edward Hebert School of Medicine Bulletin.* Bethesda, MD: USUHS.
Uniformed Services University of the Health Sciences. 1998. *Good Medicine In Bad Places.* Bethesda, MD: USUHS Reference/Historical Document.
Uniformed Services University of the Health Sciences. *Graduate Education in the Basic Medical Sciences,* Vol. 14. Bethesda, MD: USUHS.
Vidmar, D.A. 1999. The History of Teledermatology in the Department of Defense. *Dermatol Clin* 17(1):113–124.

9
Optimizing the Military Healthcare System

CAPT William M. Heroman, Col. Michael D. Parkinson,
Kathryn A. Burke, COL Thomas Broyles, COL Frank Berlingis,
RADM(s) Donald C. Arthur, COL Raymond Burden,
COL Daniel Blum, CDR Wyatt Smith, COL James D. Fraser,
CAPT Charles Davis, and COL Sandra Wilcox

With a downsized military and an aging beneficiary population, the Military Health System (MHS) is reinventing itself in an effort to optimize its resources and provide quality care. Their task is daunting: incorporate and value the cultures of the three military services healthcare systems, standardize and implement best clinical and business processes, and optimize the use of contract services to support military medical treatment facilities (MTFs).

The MHS runs the largest integrated healthcare delivery system in the world, with 8 million beneficiaries, 100 hospitals, 500 clinics, and an operating budget of $16 billion. In addition to addressing the usual market forces and management challenges, MHS must fulfill its principal missions to support and deploy a medical force for wartime, contingencies, training, and humanitarian assistance. Clearly, it faces far greater challenges and competition for resources than other healthcare systems.

The transition in 1995 from CHAMPUS to TRICARE was intended to implement a comprehensive system composed of military MTFs and civilian healthcare partners to improve the quality, cost, and accessibility of services for MHS beneficiaries. The most difficult task in transitioning to the Department of Defense (DoD) was putting forth a unified Triservice effort on behalf of the MHS, something that had never been done under the previous CHAMPUS benefit.

The MHS Optimization Plan

In November 1998, the Surgeons General, Deputy Surgeons General, and Health Affairs/TRICARE Management Activity executive staff chartered a Triservice team of six senior officers to conduct research, oversee working groups, integrate initiatives, and recommend strategies and operational plans. As the Reengineering Coordination Team (RCT), they were assigned the task of developing a MHS Optimization Plan.

The plan was to build on the inherent strengths of a prevention-oriented military culture that has historically emphasized fitness and medical readiness. The vision, stated briefly, is clear:

"The Military Health System is responsive and accountable to the Department of Defense (DoD), line leadership, and beneficiaries to ensure force health protection and optimize the health of MHS beneficiaries by providing best value health services using best clinical and business practices."

The vision, when realized, will make MHS the national benchmark for health service delivery systems and the option of choice for its beneficiaries. It will shift the focus from providing interventional services to preventing injuries and illness and improving the health of the entire population while reducing the demand for costly tertiary treatment services.

This vision promises significant health status improvement and cost avoidance, through the implementation of three underlying tenets:

- Effectively use readiness-required personnel and equipment to support the peacetime health service delivery mission
- Reallocate resources to provide as much health service delivery as possible within the MTF
- Use the evidence-based clinical and population-based practices to ensure highest quality services producing best clinical outcomes

To operationalize these tenets and realize the vision, the RCT defined a process, consisting of eight major components, and chartered eight workgroups. Each workgroup developed a plan of action and established milestones specific to the component being addressed. Although several of the workgroups already existed, they all benefited from the newly integrated focus and the Triservice commitment, including active senior leadership involvement. Timelines varied. Some of them were nearly complete, while others still had several months to finish.

Throughout the process, the RCT will provide weekly interim reports to the Deputy of Tricare Management Activity (TMA). The objective is to define and program for the most effective organization, facility by facility, until the MHS is populated with the best solution in both business and clinical practices.

The components of the MHS Optimization Plan, as listed below and illustrated in Figure 9.1, are as follows:

- Triservice Readiness Model
- Readiness Costing Model
- Triservice Enrollment Model
- Triservice Workload Model
- Triservice Resourcing Model

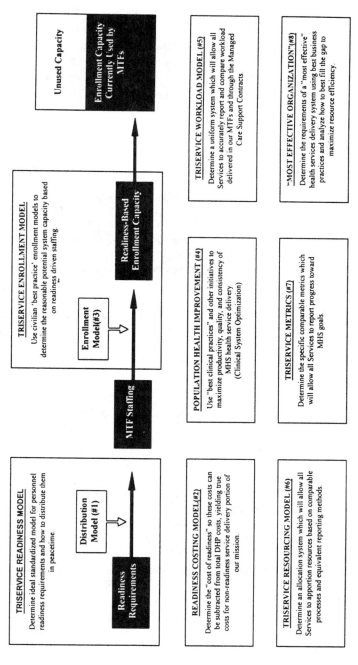

FIGURE 9.1. Components of the MHS Optimization Plan. While several of the MHS initiatives can produce significant cost avoidance in the short term, MHS reengineering and resource realignment can only be accomplished in the POM (DoD's six year financial plan) cycle. Therefore, major components of this plan will be incorporated in the FY2002–FY2007 POM submission.

- Triservice Metrics
- Fulfillment of Requirements for "Most Effective" Organization
- Population Health Improvement

The eight components are discussed fully in the following sections. Population Health is treated last, as it warrants a more detailed discussion. The summaries for each component reflect progress to date toward affordability and accountability for the MHS.

Triservice Readiness Model

Goal: Determine ideal standardized model for personnel readiness requirements and how to distribute them in peacetime.

The wartime requirement for active duty military medical personnel is a straightforward sum of personnel assigned to operational platforms or units during combat, according to individual Service doctrine concerning use of active duty versus Reserve component members. In analyses like the Section 733 Study and the Section 733 Study Update, determining the minimum active duty medical personnel requirement involves specifying both the wartime and the supplemental requirements, the latter often referred to as the Sustainment and Training (S&T) base. The requirement does not include overseas or remote personnel, a rotation base, or training pipeline; it is merely a snapshot of peak operational medical end strength requirements at various points along the war plans timeline.

In assessing total requirements, active duty medical personnel may be organized into six categories:

- Those required as primary and augmenting medical staff of operational units
- Those committed to providing services for the beneficiary population overseas (OCONUS)
- Those committed to providing services for the beneficiary population in medically isolated areas of the continental United States (CONUS)
- Those needed to meet mobilization requirements beyond categories already mentioned, including casualty replacements, research and development personnel, and residual personnel needed to offset the active duty medical force temporarily unavailable for deployment
- Those required beyond mobilization to serve as a peacetime "rotation base" for like personnel assigned to OCONUS, CONUS, or operational billets
- A sufficient number of medical personnel in education and training pipelines to maintain a fully trained medical force that meets the foregoing requirements

Determining active duty medical personnel requirements is based solely on operational requirements and those circumstances in which competent civilian health services are unavailable to care for active duty military members and their families. There is no consideration of care requirements for other beneficiaries or cases in which active duty providers may be more cost-effective.

The MHS maintains more medical end strength in the active component than wartime missions require for several reasons. One of the most important is the need to staff medical facilities that serve military populations posted in locations with very limited or no access to civilian healthcare facilities. Examples include operating locations overseas and some extremely remote sites in the continental United States. This "peacetime operational requirement," added to the wartime estimate, yields a sum that generates two additional sustainment requirements. The first is a population with which operationally based medical personnel will normally rotate (known as the "rotation base"). The second is a training pipeline to feed the sum of all these requirements (wartime, peacetime operational, and rotation base).

Military manpower allocation decisions must account for both of these requirements by building a core readiness capacity that supports the operational mission according to each Service's doctrine, and then optimizing health delivery by distributing additional civilian and military manpower in support of this readiness core. Health services required in the local catchment area beyond the capacity of the military medical treatment facility are then purchased in the private sector.

Organizing an efficient, cost-effective health services system around a readiness core is financially beneficial. Manpower and infrastructure needed for the readiness mission are fully financed as a direct cost of maintaining a ready medical force, and the associated costs are readily identified as a "fixed cost" of readiness. Therefore, the medical services provided by this fixed cost readiness core is a direct benefit of readiness training and is financed as a cost of readiness. Services provided in a military medical treatment facility (MTF) beyond what is required for readiness training may then be compared to services purchased at full cost in the private sector.

Based on the Service staffing levels determined by the DoD Sizing Model, each Service will craft its staffing distribution model. These plans will be different to fit the needs of each Service's operational missions, treatment facility sizes and locations, and demographic demands.

Readiness Costing Model

Goal: Determine the "cost of readiness" so these costs can be subtracted from the total Defense Health Program (DHP) costs, yielding the true costs for the nonreadiness service delivery portion of our mission.

The MHS faces the unique challenge of operating and funding a high-quality and cost-effective peacetime health services system and simultaneously managing the only HMO that can deploy, go to war, and support the increasing demands of "operations other than war." The cost of accomplishing medical readiness is often either buried or absorbed in our MTF operations and distorts civilian sector comparisons. More importantly, with medical readiness and Force Health Protection our primary missions for the MHS, resourcing peacetime health services cannot erode essential and military unique medical mission requirements. In a cost competitive environment, the MHS must be able to identify both its peacetime and readiness costs.

Critical to demonstrating MHS cost-effectiveness is an ability to clearly and accurately articulate the cost of maintaining Service readiness. The MHS total costs are slightly higher than some competing programs like the Federal Employees' Health Benefits Plan (FEHBP). However, we must consider the cost of factors unique to the military, factors that competitors never encounter. These include deployments, personnel readiness, readiness training, and such "costs of readiness" as additional immunizations and eye exams, clinical training for medical personnel, and enlisted medical specialist training. Increasing emphasis on Total Force readiness means that medical and dental support for Reserve Components will become a larger proportion of our health services expenditures. With increasing deployments, the cost associated with shifting health service delivery to managed care support contractors must also be identified when we deploy active duty staff.

When these costs of readiness are subtracted from the MHS total health service delivery costs, the remaining "true costs" can be compared with those of civilian benchmarks. Figure 9.2 illustrates a favorable comparison of actual per-member-per-month costs for the DHP, FEHBP, and a typical U.S. HMO. Accurate readiness costing will allow us to make direct

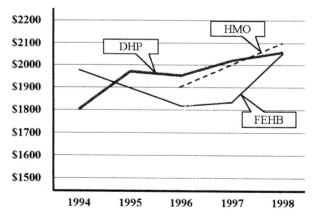

FIGURE 9.2. Comparison of per user costs. (From Center for Naval Analysis Study, 1998.)

comparisons of the isolated health service delivery costs, unencumbered by readiness mission elements.

Military personnel costs and infrastructure/direct health services expenditures are captured in our Medical Expense and Performance Reporting System (MEPRS) with varying degrees of accuracy. Even more difficult is capturing necessary (but high) inefficiency costs associated with time away from the clinic for "military unique" obligations like physical fitness training. Support to other forward deployed locations from a CONUS base, as well as the effects of having a military medical presence regardless of the level of utilization, must also be accounted for and explained.

Triservice Enrollment Model

Goal: Use civilian "best practice" enrollment models to determine the reasonable potential system capacity based on readiness driven staffing.

Reengineering must involve appropriate resourcing of DoD facilities. A major part of that resourcing is personnel, specifically providers. Because of Permanent Change of Station (PCS) and end strength constraints, personnel allocations have long-term implications and must be viewed from a systemwide perspective. Poor allocation of providers among facilities will result in underserved areas with reduced access, low satisfaction, and high bills for purchased services. Areas rich in providers may be inefficient and have high internal costs.

Before TRICARE, efforts to allocate personnel were hampered by the inability to define the precise population for which a facility was responsible. All services were provided on a "space available" basis, and so long as patients filled the appointment logs, facilities could "earn" their providers. TRICARE Prime, with its emphasis on managed care and actual enrollment of beneficiaries, enables precise allocation of providers. A key distinction of TRICARE Prime is the introduction of Primary Care Managers (PCMs), the focal point of an enrollee's interaction with the health system. The PCM treats patients for routine illnesses and injuries, serves as the referral point for specialty services, and is responsible for preventive services and the health promotion of the enrollee.

One challenge in determining the capacity of the MHS is measuring the appropriate ratio of PCMs to enrolled populations. Some studies have estimated panel sizes of 1,300, while others have exceeded 2,000. Our goal is to provide a tool with which MTFs can model beneficiary enrollment under differing scenarios, compare that capacity with current enrollment figures and user estimates, and examine the geographic and specialty distribution of providers. It will begin with PCMs.

Family Practice, General Medicine, General Pediatrics, General Internal Medicine physicians, and Physician Assistants and Family Practice Nurse

Practitioners will be considered PCMs in a practice panel model. Using authorization numbers for these specialties by facility and applying panel sizes of 1,300 to 1,900, the enrollment capacity of each facility can be accurately estimated. This enrollment capacity will then be compared to the number of enrollees currently served by the facility, with an allowance for bases with student/trainee populations that are not "enrolled" because they are on temporary duty. The remaining (unused) capacity will be compared to estimates of potential enrollees. It will consider both Medicare-eligible beneficiaries who do not have an opportunity to enroll (except at subvention sites) and users opting to remain with TRICARE Standard.

Another version of this model will examine the effects of using risk adjustment (equivalent lives based on age and gender adjustments) modified for population disease severity. Epidemiological data for a catchment area population can be applied to normative workload projections to yield demand estimates. The estimates will predict the epidemiology of disease that a given population will produce, and this will form the basis of the make/buy decisions for obtaining necessary services.

This modeling tool can also be used to examine:

- The equitable distribution PCM allocations across the MHS
- The enrollment capacity (supply) and enrollment potential (demand) at specific locations
- The effects of the distribution of PCMs on other variables such as access and referral patterns

Another tool will be developed for examining specialty mixes. Starting with enrolled populations by location, specialty ratios taken from civilian benchmarks will be applied to populations to determine the number of specialists the population could support. If demand for a specialty cannot be justified, then no specialist would be assigned to that facility. Applied over all facilities, this model will be used to examine the distribution of specialties across facilities and among specialties. This model could also support cross-service provider and staff utilization strategies. Further analysis would start with differing scenarios of user populations to account for continued "space available" services.

Once the primary care, specialty care, and operational support models are developed, they will be used for programming decisions in the FY 2002–2007 Program Objective Memorandum (POM) to distribute personnel to enrolled populations. The following model was crafted from all the aforementioned considerations.

MHS Primary Care Enrollment Capacity Model

The MHS primary care enrollment model will allow facilities to perform four tasks:

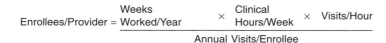

FIGURE 9.3. Enrollee/provider ratio.

- Predict the portion of the catchment area population that can be enrolled
- Identify factors that could be improved to increase enrollment capacity
- Receive financial resources that match capacity and predicted workload
- Monitor performance and improve determinants of enrollment capacity

The number of beneficiaries who can be enrolled to a single primary care provider can be estimated using the determinants in the following formula. Altering these variables will produce significant increases in the enrollee/provider ratio in Figure 9.3.

Numerous factors will determine enrollment capacity and must be addressed to optimize clinic productivity, decrease inappropriate or excessive utilization, and produce better patient outcomes:

- Direct clinical support staff
- Number and availability of exam rooms per provider
- Clinical and business support tools
- Information management and demand management tools
- Demographic factors
- Reserve integration
- Community support
- Operational unit organic medical support

Each facility commander/commanding officer must examine all these factors to determine their impact on enrollment capacity. Enrollment rates above 1,300 beneficiaries per primary care provider may readily be accomplished if factors that reduce productivity are identified and minimized and existing staff is realigned and supplemented to optimize provider/support staff ratios. Expectations are as follows:

- 1,500 beneficiaries enrolled per primary care provider
- 3.5 support staff per primary care provider
- 2 examination rooms per primary care provider
- 25 patients seen per day per primary care provider

Triservice Workload Model

Goal: Determine a uniform system that will allow all services to accurately report and compare workload delivered in our MTFs and through the Managed Care Support Contracts.

The MHS Optimization program depends on our ability to compare costs throughout all DoD facilities. Measuring performance and cost-effectiveness within the MHS, comparing alternatives, and making informed management decisions is predicated on standardized, timely, consistent, and accurate information. As the MHS moves toward standard resourcing and measurement models that enable us to benchmark and resource our healthcare system, we must put increased effort into data quality management and oversight.

Triservice Resourcing Model

Goal: Determine an allocation system which will allow all services to apportion resources based on comparable processes and equivalent reporting methods.

To be a fully integrated health services delivery system, the MHS must appropriately resource the military services and their MTFs in a stable environment that ensures appropriate incentives to optimize MTF capability. Resourcing is the driving force that supports MTF infrastructure, military personnel assignment and performance appraisals, use of civilians and contract support, and day-to-day operations and maintenance expenditures for consumable supplies like pharmaceuticals. The optimized MTF is resourced to be cost-effective and to take advantage of all the factors of production. In the global sense, appropriately capitating MTFs for improving population health maintenance is the resourcing imperative. How each of the services and TMA conduct their business activities, with their different command structures and financial reporting systems, provides the major challenge to equitably distributing resources and monitoring performance.

The Resource Management (RM) Breakthrough Group, chaired by the Deputy Assistant Secretary of Defense (DASD) for Health Budgets and Financial Policy and constituted in April 1997, focuses on defining the evolving Service expectations, establishing a structure and process for decision making, and providing a uniform system to support a structured decision process. The workgroup's primary focus has been establishing and documenting a uniform DoD/Component-level decision to increase effectiveness of the resource decisions. The task as stated is to develop an integrated POM/Budget and allocation model (PPBES) based on a capitation method. Recent efforts to integrate the processes emphasize the need for an incentive-based allocation model; thus far, the main focus has been on developing a full asset visibility model.

The Resource Management Steering Group, the current structure for addressing Service and TMA resource issues and proposed policy and program initiatives, will review progress on meeting the MHS Reengineering objectives. The timeline for systematic changes reflected in the

Program/Budget cycle is the FY2002–FY2007 POM. Some resourcing, allocation, and measurement tools can be employed in concert with other components of facility optimization once the "Most Effective Organization" facility model is determined. Capitation and other Service-specific policies could incentivize MTFs to share or swap production factors to optimize MTF capacity and increase MTF enrollment.

Triservice Metrics

Goal: Determine the specific comparable metrics that will allow all services to report progress toward MHS goals.

The Triservice Metrics Workgroup works under the auspices of the RCT to develop measures that quantitatively assess the performance of reengineering efforts using indicators selected from five areas for targeted change established by the RCT:

- Customer Responsiveness
- Force Health Protection
- Population Health Improvement
- Best Clinical Practices
- Best Business Practices

The workgroup will analyze available products and develop a standardized set of core metrics that can be used to assess MTF optimization. Their efforts will incorporate the principles of utilization/quality management into the MHS. Data will be drawn from existing systems, and a proliferation of performance information will be gathered through web technology.

The goal of Triservice common core metrics is to allow patients, providers, and payers to monitor and benchmark MHS performance in force health protection and population health improvement. Currently, civilian integrated delivery systems monitor the health of enrolled population through HEDIS measures. Force health protection requires readiness measures unique to military populations.

Fulfillment of Requirements for "Most Effective" Organization

Goal: Determine the requirements of a "most effective" health services delivery system using best business practices and analyze how to best fill the gap to maximize resource efficiency.

The MHS must have an energized strategic planning process that articulates a vision, builds plans and programs directly tied to the vision, allocates resources linked with desired outcomes, and measures progress toward achieving its goals and objectives. Organizational structures and processes must be continually reviewed and improved to ensure rapid progress is made toward achieving the vision. MHS enterprise-level decisions must be defined and facilitated in areas that cut across organizational lines to maximize efficiencies. As a "learning organization," the MHS must embrace change and continually incorporate best practices. The "most effective organization" will fulfill all these requirements and facilitate smooth business relationships among MTF commanders, Lead Agents, and Managed Care Support Contractors.

To expand on this brief description, the MHS must have the following capabilities:

- Clear definition of responsibilities for all organizational components and clear performance milestones to incentivize health services delivery platform commanders
- Focus on customer needs and expectations about access to health services and information about health services
- Use of applicable accrediting agencies from the civilian sector as well as best clinical and business practices
- Streamlined oversight and management of information systems
- Organizational structures, responsibilities, and processes that ensure enterprise-wide decision making and minimal cycle times for implementation of plans, policies, and tools
- Standardized performance measures with timely feedback to all levels of the enterprise for rapid quality improvement
- A computerized patient record to gather and track individual and population-based clinical data and convert it to information that will enable business decisions

Computerized patient records are a particularly important component of the "most effective" organization. In August of 1996, DoD published the "Military Health Services System (MHSS) Information Management/Information Technology (IM/IT) Program Plan." In this plan, signed by the Assistant Secretary of Defense (Health Affairs) (ASD [HA]) and the Surgeons General of the Army, Navy, and Air Force, the MHS addressed the need for a CPR as follows:

While TRICARE is a medical force multiplier, it will also demand greater attention from IM/IT for data standardization and interoperability to ensure that the distributed computer-based patient records (CPRs) are easily accessed and totally compatible around the world. Special contractual and security arrangements will be necessary to ensure that TRICARE support contractor systems can support the distributed CPR capability with standardized data, allow authorized users to have ready access to MHSS hosted portions of individual CPRs, and support fast response to MHSS originated CPR and care assessment queries.

The goals of CPR access are improving the quality of care, moving from illness intervention to proactive wellness care, improving efficiency, and reducing cost to the MHS. The CPR will provide the DoD with a health-care record that links to external knowledge sources and provides clinical decision support and rationale for care rendered.

The Composite Health Care System (CHCS) II is one tool that can provide the right information at the right time through a CPR. CHCS II will be a confidential, complete, and longitudinal documentation of care provided across the operational continuum. Applied throughout an individual's military service from induction to loss, CHCS II will be a comprehensive record of care provided, immunizations received, and exposures to hazards. It will provide the following capabilities:

- Beneficiary health history
- Clinical documentation
- Order entry
- Encounter coding
- Alerts and reminders
- Reporting
- Role-based security
- Enterprise Health Record
- Master Patient Index
- Consult tracking
- Beneficiary self-assessment data entry
- Scheduling
- Dental charting and documentation

CHCS II is intended to be an enterprise system for health management that integrates beneficiary data from different times, providers, and sites of care and displays a comprehensive view of an individual beneficiary's health at the point of care. The system will automate Clinical Practice Guidelines (CPGs), enable documentation, measure clinical outcomes, and support FHP/PHI requirements. Providers will be able to access timely feedback on clinical outcomes, costs of care, and other pivotal metrics related to the processes of healthcare delivery for individuals and populations (e.g., the *Tri-service Common Core Metrics* and civilian best practice measures in the Health Plan Employer Data and Information Set [HEDIS]).

The mature CHCS II will contribute to the enterprise-wide success of FHP/PHI in many ways. For example:

- Health information directly impacting individual soldier readiness, and by extension unit readiness, will be completely available, with appropriate scanning, reporting, and alerting tools.
- Standardized and accurate enrollment information will be available to responsible health service providers who will then be able to manage the health of their enrolled beneficiaries.
- Availability of clinical information needed by providers for decision making will be limited only by operational communications restrictions.

This practice will help ensure that individual clinical decisions lead to the most effective and efficient care possible.

- Standardized self-reported beneficiary health assessment reports will be automated, rapidly transmitted to the computerized patient record, and available to providers. Providers will receive timely individual and aggregate reports.
- Where appropriate, collection and reporting of standardized performance measures will be based on and comparable to civilian performance benchmarks. Access to care standards, provider services monitoring, beneficiary satisfaction, clinical outcomes, cost efficiency, and readiness-related standardized metrics will be automated, available, and visible across the enterprise.
- Marketing and education programs, self-care programs (healthcare information lines, web-based approaches and books, educational interventions), and disease and demand management practices and tools (clinical practice guidelines, clinical pathways, referral guidelines, etc.) will be available or referenced in a standardized fashion.

We anticipate continuous improvement and refinement of our policies, practices, and processes. Incorporation of evolving technology will be required for the MHS to become a "most effective" organization. After we identify needs, we must perform make/buy decisions (business case analyses) and find ways to assemble the necessary staff. In some cases, service-specific readiness staffing requirements will need to be supplemented with additional resources.

Population Health Improvement

Goal: Use the "best clinical practices" and other initiatives to maximize productivity, quality, and consistency of MHS health service delivery (Clinical System Optimization).

Two cardinal missions of the Military Health System are to ensure the wellness and readiness of the fighting force and to optimize the health of MHS beneficiaries, including active duty members, retirees, and their family members. The MHS can fulfill these goals through population health, in which all enrolled beneficiaries are considered, not only those who seek access to health care. Refocusing the MHS on population health increases the quality of care through standardized management of beneficiaries, increases the clinical effectiveness of interventions, drives down unwarranted treatment variations, and controls costs. This healthcare paradigm, far more desirable than the traditional model of individualized acute care intervention, clarifies the expectations and delineates the responsibilities of patients, providers, commanders, payers, and managed care contract partners.

Population Health Improvement (PHI) balances awareness, education, prevention, and intervention to improve the health of a specified population. These activities underscore the physical, emotional, spiritual, intellectual, social, and environmental behavior changes needed to optimize health and enhance fitness. They support an individual's ability to practice self-care and modify disease and injury risk, while still supporting the provision of appropriate clinical interventions.

Population Health Improvement requires the following:

- A focus on product lines organized around a disease process or clinical condition, from prevention through management of care.
- Demand management strategies and practices, which further reduce the incidence and prevalence of premorbid conditions and diseases and optimize the appropriate use of health services. Healthcare delivery must be prioritized to meet the needs of the population, and clinical and community leaders must be able to modify resources and processes.
- Useful information for the providers to make appropriate decisions. Analyzed data must be provided to decision makers at all levels to enhance the quality, support change, and audit the effectiveness of human and financial resources.
- Education and assimilation of these principles throughout the MHS. The strength of the MHS is its control over the military clinicians' educational process from undergraduate to professional, and from basic military education through technical training.

The MHS's PHI model unites individual and community-based interventions with the public health and medical approaches through primary, secondary, and tertiary prevention to reduce morbidity and premature mortality. This PHI plan creates a learning organization with a support center that merges concepts of best practices with lessons learned, disseminates them across the system, and uses feedback not punitively, but as a tool to improve the quality of patient care. As PHI matures, most of our traditional Utilization Review and Utilization Management tools will be incorporated into the PHI process and diminish in importance as separate entities.

Figure 9.4 demonstrates the relationship of the various process elements associated with PHI. There are two factors to the equation: the demand on the system and the capacity of the system to complete the mission. Basic laws of economics predict that a gap will exist between these factors; doctrine or management paradigms exist to minimize this gap. The subsections following the figure explain the process elements in greater detail.

PHI 1: Enrollment Processing

The process begins with the first element, enrollment processing, which accurately identifies and defines the people who use the system.

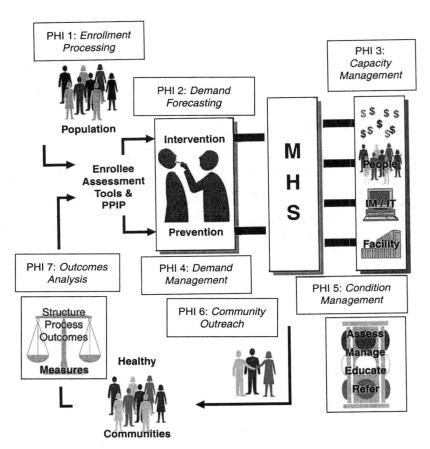

FIGURE 9.4. Force health protection/population health improvement (PHI) critical processes.

Standardization of this process is required to assure continuity of care and to minimize inefficiencies across the vast geographic and Service regions.

Managing the health care of beneficiaries requires timely enrollment in the health plan and the assignment of a Primary Care Manager (PCM). The enrollment process begins when an eligible beneficiary chooses to receive health care under the auspices of TRICARE Prime. The process has two steps, administrative enrollment and Health Enrollment Assessment Review (HEAR) survey completion. Administrative enrollment requires the beneficiary to complete a standardized TRICARE Enrollment Application, which includes specific identification of a PCM and key demographic information. The HEAR Survey or like stratification surveying tool will aid in the assignment of a PCM and must be completed within 60 days of arriving on the station. This step will help the PCM manage care for their enrolled populations by providing information related to health risks and needs and projecting the demand for services.

PHI 2: Demand Forecasting

This element requires the stratification of the enrolled population to forecast the demands for acute and chronic intervention and long-term health promotion and prevention needs. Simply put, a demand forecast is an estimate of the volume of care required by a given population, based on best clinical and business practices. The data that contribute to demand forecasting are the prevalence of disease within a given population, the clinical practices used to treat a given disease, and the system or operationally defined required care. It is critical that the data that supply demand forecasts be accurate to ensure that facility sizing and staffing decisions are appropriate, resulting in maximum value, optimal quality, and efficient access.

The MHS will develop accurate demand forecasts at both the catchment area and facility level. Once complete population data are obtained from the HEAR survey, the enrollee's medical record, or an automated system like the ambulatory data record, each MTF will conduct demand forecasts along two platforms: healthcare demands of the population and operationally defined and system required demands. Information from individual MTFs will be submitted and coordinated at the Lead Agent Office/relevant Intermediate Service Commands (ISC) to conduct and evaluate regional forecasts. The forecasts will then be sent to the respective ISCs to consider appropriate financial and staffing levels. At the MTF level, techniques described in the section on Demand Management will be integrated into the reengineering process.

PHI 3: Capacity Management

Improving cost and access outcomes depends on active management of patient volume, clinical practice, facility size, and staffing. Capacity management means that finite resources must be allocated to minimize the gap between demand and resources. Capacity management is the number of patients that a facility actually or potentially has the ability to receive and treat.

The challenge the MHS faces is how to dynamically link population demand and delivery system capacity by actively managing the demand for services. The MHS can do this by identifying gaps between forecasted needs and medical service capability, linking strategic goals with daily operations, building decision support tools, and establishing explicit performance targets based on best clinical and business practices.

Active capacity management takes advantage of the organizational structure of the MHS—the MHS owns its staff and facilities. This is a complex problem and will require sophisticated decision support tools from the industrial engineering and operations research professions.

PHI 4: Demand Management

Unmanaged demand creates unnecessary bottlenecks that slow the delivery of health care. Demand management is the tool to maximize the appropriate utilization of finite resources. In the short term, these management strategies can encourage efficient use of health services and decrease unnecessary or marginally effective health care. In the long term, self-care and wellness activities will help eliminate harmful environmental conditions and behaviors, reducing the overall need for health care.

Demand management interventions include the HEAR Survey; patient-based preventive care tools; shared decision-making programs; the Put Prevention Into Practice (PPIP) initiative; Preventive Health Care Application (PHCA); and primary care triage systems and self-care programs (e.g., advice lines, health information lines, web-based approaches, and age-specific self-care books). Demand management reflects the activities of a health system designed to create a healthy environment, decrease morbidity and mortality, and encourage the use of effective decision-support and self-management tools.

PHI 5: Condition Management

Condition (or disease) management (CM) is directed at acute and chronic conditions that place the greatest demand on the system. Until behavior of the population changes to embrace the prevention mantra, the greatest cost will be in this arena. Tools such as clinical practice guidelines (CPGs), clinical pathways, case management, and discharge planning will be essential.

CM coordinates and improves all the services provided to patients with a given set of medical conditions. It supports the utilization management/quality management (UM/QM) process by ensuring that the right care is delivered to the right person at the right time. It targets high-cost, high-volume, complex diseases and conditions using performance metric tools to focus on key processes and outcomes. CM also encourages patient–provider collaboration and the use of information technology and feedback from health risk stratification tools to develop optimal care plans.

A successful CM program employs nationally accepted best practices and evidence-based medical practice, but extends beyond merely implementing clinical practice guidelines (CPGs) or critical pathways. When properly executed, CM is customer focused, proactive, and promotes the efficient delivery of high-quality services. It reduces unwarranted variability in provider practice patterns, improves clinical outcomes, satisfies accreditation requirements, and contributes to the satisfaction of the enrollee, patient, and clinical staff.

MTFs within the MHS will institute a process for the implementation of CM programs. The DoD-VA Clinical Practice Guideline (CPG) Working Group is currently working to adapt and field selected evidence-based guidelines across the MHS.

PHI 6: Community Outreach

As the factor with the greatest impact on community health, public health efforts involve many facets of the community, not just the medical faction (e.g., the recent decrease in suicide rate within the USAF). A healthy community continually improves the physical and social environment of its members. Its members embrace a shared commitment to modify behavioral, social, and environmental risk factors that impinge on one's health. Its leaders unite to solve health issues that require a cooperative effort. To create a healthy community, therefore, we must engage its population in process, planning, and education.

Community involvement concepts extend beyond medical interventions focused on an individual or a population with a particular disease. Outreach includes improving and educating people about local environmental quality and hazards; quality of housing, education, and transportation; spiritual, cultural, and recreational opportunities; social support services; diversity and stability of employment opportunities; and effective local government. A Community/Installation Population Health Council consisting of line, command, healthcare providers, and community/installation agency representatives will help address community-wide (installation) programs targeting the health of the community.

Impacting these elements requires long-term and dedicated planning and cooperation between the local military commanders and civilian community leaders. Such efforts should be modeled after successful cooperative programs developed by local, state, and federal governmental health agencies; schools of public health and other academic institutions; local business coalitions; community action groups; etc. Similarly, already developed community health outcome metrics (e.g., Healthy Communities 2010) will be evaluated for adoption. Policy guidance from the DoD Prevention Council needs to ensure implementation of community health improvement activities across all military installations.

PHI 7: Outcomes Analysis

For any system to excel and remain on course, comprehensive measures of the structure, process, and outcomes that lead to success must be developed. Standardized performance measures will be used for evaluating the performance of the healthcare delivery system, the health of the population, and the quality of the clinical services provided to our beneficiaries. With performance measures in place, facilities will be able to identify and prioritize clinical areas requiring reengineering, conduct critical analysis of the health needs of their enrolled population, provide education to identified populations, and improve clinical outcomes. Performance will be continuously monitored at the provider level, and measures will evaluate both the effectiveness of clinical interventions and the effectiveness of the evidence-based practice.

The five key performance measurement areas are customer responsiveness and accountability, force health protection, population health improvement, best clinical practices, and best business practices. To eliminate duplicative efforts, the services will attempt to integrate preventive services and condition management measures with indicators already required and collected for quality assurance programs like the Joint Commission on Accreditation of Healthcare Organizations (JCAHO) or the DoD National Quality Management Program. The use of National Committee on Quality Assurance (NCQA) Health Plan Employer Data and Information Set (HEDIS) performance indicators will allow standardized comparison across the MHS system. Special interest and/or Service specific metrics may be added to this common core.

Service Medical Departments and TRICARE Management will be held accountable to support this population health initiative. In doing so, these departments will fulfill the mission and vision of the MHS. They will help identify and close gaps between current clinical practices and optimal practices.

Next Steps for Population Health

To ensure success of the PHI plan, the creation of a Military Health System Support Center (MHSSC) is crucial. The MHSSC will identify, adapt, implement, and sustain best clinical and business practices to help guide the reengineering of military medicine and optimize the health of the population. It will operationalize the MHS optimization plan and PHI plan and integrate separate activities in the MHS to assess population health data, health surveillance, and program management.

The MHSSC will be divided into four major activities: a Resource Center, Program Support, Patient and Staff Education, and Performance Enhancement Support. The Resource Center will provide centralized help desk support, centralized health services analysis support, management decision support for policy decisions, and IM/IT coordination for implementation strategy. Program Support will include the HEAR program, PPIP PHCA, and condition management. Patient and Staff Education will include central and on-site training using web-based technology. This activity will also facilitate clinical reengineering and integration with IM/IT products deployment and training.

The first step in creating the MHSSC is assembling the Population Health Implementation Team (PHIT). The PHIT will help implement the MHS Optimization and Population Health Improvement (PHI) Plans throughout the MHS. Concurrent with the development of the implementation strategy for the Optimization and PHI Plans, the support needs will be assessed and an analysis of current Service and DoD assets and activities will be performed. The Military Health System Optimization Team, in conjunction with the Population Health Improvement Workgroup and with the help of the PHIT, hope to have the MHSSC fully functional by January 2001.

The MHSSC will greatly benefit the MHS and support the concept of population health. It will allow the MHS to provide a single face to the customer for supporting and executing the programs, tools, and surveillance systems to measure and improve the health of TRICARE Prime population. It will increase efficiencies and decrease variation through collaboration among Service efforts at all levels of program management, education and training, health services assessment, and research. It will also allow the services to affiliate and integrate activities and agencies like the Triservice Medical Systems Support Center (TMSCC), the U.S. Army Center for Health Promotion and Preventive Medicine (CHPPM), the USAF Population Health Support Office (PHSO), and the U.S. Navy Environmental Health Center (NEHC). Most importantly, the MHSSC will help the services develop a common focus on outcome measures for the MHS.

Conclusion

In November 1999, the GAO reviewed the optmization plan and expressed full support of this initiative. Among their key recommendations were the following:

- The MHS should emphasize MTF beneficiary enrollment as a key element of the triservice strategy and make every effort to enroll as many current MTF users as possible.
- The MHS should work with the line commanders and such key stakeholders as cognizant congressional committees and key members, advocacy groups, and others to obtain support for the strategy.
- The MHS should periodically report progress toward developing and implementing the strategy to cognizant House and Senate committees.

In accordance with its mission, the MHS is obligated to ensure force health protection and optimize the health of MHS beneficiaries by producing the best value health services using the best clinical and business practices. As the population health mindset takes hold, we will move from focusing primarily on interventional services to preventing illnesses and injuries throughout the entire life cycle. The MHS must respond to readiness missions, meet Service readiness requirements, and support Service personnel readiness requirements. The system must achieve maximum efficiency and cost-effectiveness. Staffing must adhere to readiness missions, and prevention programs must be robust. We must also remember that the other MHS reengineering initiatives are critical: policies on pharmacy redesign, role and number of lead agents, redesigned managed care support contracts, and the need for an integrated clinical information.

We can make several generalizations about the MHS system's near future:

- Customer service will be paramount: the MHS system will respond to beneficiaries' needs, enrollment will be easy, and benefits will be uniform and transportable. Beneficiaries will be full partners in all their health decisions.
- An effective Utilization Management program will be implemented, and best clinical practice guidelines will be universally adopted to reduce variance and improve quality.
- Clinicians will use easily accessible evidence-based clinical decision-making tools and receive timely professional improvement training.
- Costs of goods and services will be readily ascertained, and costs of the readiness mission will be separable.
- Data analysis and tracking functions will robust and responsive. The patient record will be computerized, and the combination of data tracking programs and the computerized patient record will give providers timely feedback on costs and clinical outcomes.

- Prevention and screening programs will be fully deployed and measurable. Well-established performance metrics will provide incentives and feedback.

The MHS Optimization Team firmly believes that in the decades to come, systemwide implementation of the optimization plan will make this future vision a reality. Full implementation of the plans described in this chapter will manage costs, improve staffing and other resource allocations, and profoundly improve MHS service delivery methods.

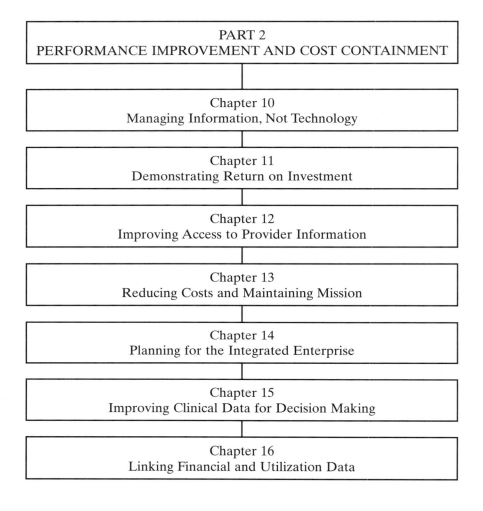

PART 2
PERFORMANCE IMPROVEMENT AND COST CONTAINMENT

Chapter 10
Managing Information, Not Technology

Chapter 11
Demonstrating Return on Investment

Chapter 12
Improving Access to Provider Information

Chapter 13
Reducing Costs and Maintaining Mission

Chapter 14
Planning for the Integrated Enterprise

Chapter 15
Improving Clinical Data for Decision Making

Chapter 16
Linking Financial and Utilization Data

Part 2
Applying New Models for Improvements and Cost Containment

10
Building the Knowledge-Enabled Organization: Beyond IT Infrastructures to IM Infostructures*

Maj. Detlev Smaltz, Maj. Roger Price, Col. Paul Williamson, and Peter Ramsaroop

Webster's definition of the word "challenges" suggests that they require "full use of one's abilities or resources." Such an expenditure of time, money, personnel, and energy is a daily fact of life in the multifunctional and multiservice integrated operation of public sector health care. Much like private sector health care, the Military Health System (MHS), the Department of Defense's healthcare system, is faced with the challenge of delivering timely, quality healthcare services at a reasonable cost in a dynamically complex environment. Success in such an environment requires matching levels of complex human and technological infrastructures. Regardless of how the MHS's healthcare delivery operation is defined (i.e., group practice, group practice without walls, physician/hospital management organization, or staff model HMO), the need for timely, reliable information remains a common denominator in the calculation of success. Controlling cost while enhancing the timeliness and quality of care delivered from cradle to grave is supremely important and must be objectively, not anecdotally, demonstrated.

Intuitively, healthcare professionals in the public sector feel confident that their acute care and health promotion strategies are making a difference in population health. However, from a business analysis perspective (i.e., using accurate, reliable data sources), we are challenged to show definitive improvements in outcomes, efficacy, or cost containment. Has the public sector's shift to insurance carriers, as opposed to direct provision of medical care, improved clinical outcomes? Has it reduced the cost of healthcare delivery? Has it improved the health of the public sector beneficiary population? In our highly regulated, fiscally austere operating environment, clinical and financial outcomes must be justified with some degree of rigor to all the enterprise's stakeholders (e.g., beneficiaries, corporate

---

* The views expressed in this chapter are those of the authors and do not reflect the official policy of the United States Air Force, Department of Defense, or the U.S. Government.

headquarters, Joint Commission on Accreditation of Healthcare Organizations [JCAHO], Health Care Financing Administration [HCFA]).

To do this, executive management teams at all levels of the enterprise need highly accurate and timely information within the context of their clinical and business operations. In short, they must be "knowledge enabled." Ironically, although our enterprise is loaded with talented individuals and modern information technology (IT) tools that produce an abundance of *data*, we have historically lacked timely, reliable *information* to guide the decision-making process. Simply put, we are data rich but information poor. The public sector healthcare system now faces the challenge of building on its IT infrastructure with a vigorous focus on establishing an information management (IM) *info*structure—that is, an information-based infrastructure that enables quality decision making throughout the enterprise. In fact, a knowledge-enabled organization cannot exist without both a solid IT infrastructure and a solid IM infostructure.

IM Infostructure Versus IT Infrastructure

Many executives use the terms computer systems, management information systems (MIS), information management (IM), and information technology (IT) interchangeably. Most recently, the acronym IM/IT has come into favor to represent all things concerned with information management and information technology. However, IM and IT are distinctly different functions with distinctly different organizational implications. In simple terms, IT is focused on hardware, software, and functionality, whereas IM is focused on people, process, and capability. Both are crucial components of a knowledge-enabled organization and permit quality decision making throughout the enterprise (Figure 10.1).

To expand on the simple definition, IT forms the basic computer technology foundation that automates many routine processes in the healthcare enterprise. IT includes but is not limited to telecommunications networks and servers; mainframe and mini- and microcomputers and the software that runs them; and a technical staff able to program and troubleshoot these technologies. In addition, it forms the foundation without which true IM capabilities cannot be sustained. Therefore, IT is a necessary—but not sufficient—tool for building a knowledge-enabled organization.

IM, on the other hand, refers to the value-adding functions that leverage the enterprise's investment in IT. Specifically, IM comprises the people and processes that optimize the data input, administration, integrity, quality, integration, and informatics analysis processes, thereby providing a true information capability to support enterprise managers and decision makers. It aligns full-time resources focused on optimizing information-based processes (such as medical records, data quality, data analysis, and clinical informatics) horizontally across the organization, marking a shift

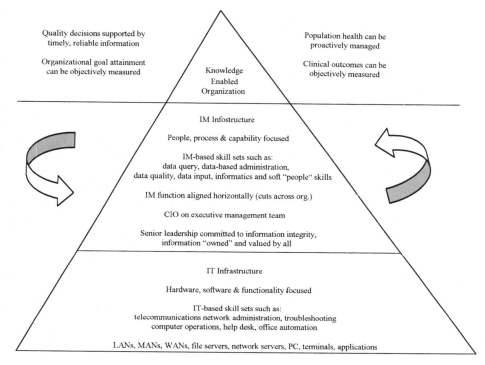

FIGURE 10.1. The foundations for a knowledge-enabled organization.

from traditional, stovepiped vertical structuring arrangements. In addition, organizations have established an executive-level information officer position to help them develop an IM infostructure. This officer would participate fully on the enterprise's senior executive team.

Challenges of Building a Knowledge-Enabled Military Health System

Many information-intensive industries clearly demonstrate, via their organizational and process structuring arrangements, an understanding of the difference between IT and IM. However, public sector health care still seems largely unaware of the distinction. For many in public sector health care, IM and IT *is* "the systems department." IM is not, in most cases, a comprehensive, enterprise-wide, executive management responsibility. Although there is a great deal of talk about the importance of IM in public sector health care, the lack of structures, processes, and incentives to support true IM indicates that more action needs to be taken. Despite inroads made to public sector health care during the late 1980s and early 1990s by the quality movement, with its process measurement–information focus, the "reinvention of government" is ongoing. Entrenched ways of doing business die hard. Institutions die hard. Bureaucracies die hard.

One criticism of the MHS is that it is still highly compartmentalized and that its agencies do not work together well enough to effectively use the IT infrastructure in place. At the risk of oversimplifying, we note that the Information Systems Office of the organizations that make up the MHS has focused on offering technical solutions and keeping networks operating efficiently—in short, it has been primarily IT focused. Furthermore, at the hospital and clinic level (where the actual healthcare "rubber meets the road"), chief information officers (CIOs) historically have not been empowered or resourced to integrate and optimize the processes that provide and distribute information. Within the MHS, this has precipitated a prevailing view of Information Management/Systems as a provider of faster/better hardware, infrastructure, and capacity to communicate. This view has been accepted and promulgated throughout the MHS for years. While the MHS continues to excel at building and renewing its IT infrastructure, decision makers throughout the enterprise remain skeptical about the value gained from IT investments.

To be fully understood, this statement requires further clarification. Few within the MHS would dispute the value gained from IT investments to support acute care decision making. The MHS's integrated hospital information system provides excellent patient appointing, admissions, discharges, transfers, ancillary test ordering, and results reporting in support of physician decisions relating to acute care. However, realization of MHS investments in IT fall short when attempting to truly assess population health, to manage disease processes within that population, to analyze variation in practice patterns, to determine the efficacy of long-term health promotion programs, or to gauge the benefit of outsourcing to other healthcare providers.

Interestingly, the IT functionality (for the most part) currently exists to make such analyses. However, responsibility for ensuring that the IT assets are used effectively and efficiently has primarily fallen on users who, in general, know little about the systems or their capabilities. This limitation makes it impossible to fully realize the IT benefits. Because users must become more proficient, a major challenge now facing the MHS is to build on its excellent IT infrastructure by augmenting the people-based processes of an IM infostructure.

Some organizations within the MHS are beginning to transform themselves by building IM infostructures. The rest of this chapter further explores the process of building an IM infostructure, expanding on the incentives, structuring arrangements, and the importance of senior leadership commitment and developing a data quality culture. In each section, we weave in the relevant experiences of one organization within the MHS, Keesler Medical Center.

Building an IM Infostructure

Organizational Incentives

Clearly, there are motivating forces for decision making revolving around direct patient care—that is, a physician simply would not make a clinical intervention without highly reliable test results. Despite its importance, however, there are currently few incentives or penalties for decision making at the business process level. Although enrollment-based resourcing mechanisms, if properly implemented, could bring a significant "carrot on the stick" incentive structure to decision processes in the public sector, the current operating environment of the MHS provides little incentive to hospital and clinic CEOs to manage care effectively. From a process perspective, if patients are moved out of the CEO's hospital into a network partner's facility, there is no real incentive for the CEO to actively oversee that patient's care or make an attempt to retrieve that patient at the earliest clinically feasible time.

Within the MHS, individual CEOs and executive teams like those at Keesler Medical Center are implanting, through their focus on managing the continuum of care, an incentive basis that drives information-based analyses. However, these types of incentive structures are only effective for so long as executive management is focused on them. Incentives implemented by executive mandate do not build the long-term motivating foundations for building a true IM infostructure.

To achieve the goals of optimizing cost, access, and the quality dynamic and shifting to a population health model, the MHS must implement fair and appropriate incentives. If excellent business decisions are not appropriately and consistently rewarded and poor business decisions do not negatively and consistently impact an organization's bottom line (at least from a budgetary standpoint), the impetus for transformation disappears. Only if business decision outcomes matter in a palpable manner will organizations be driven to build their IM infostructures and transform themselves into knowledge-enabled organizations where quality decision making reigns.

Senior Leadership Commitment

Building an IM infostructure requires a significant reengineering of the culture, processes, and organizational structures within an organization. For an organization to truly advance from an IT functionality to an IM capability within an organization, several changes are important.

First, senior leadership must commit to an organizational structure that both integrates the information processes within their organization and ensures that IM is not marginalized. Horizontally incorporating the key information management functions within a healthcare organization and ensuring that IM has a seat at the executive level accomplishes important tasks. It empowers the CIO and officially makes him/her responsible for integrating and optimizing the information-based processes within the organization. This integration also ensures that both clinical decision processes and business decision processes are supported at an organizational level, and it builds the foundation of an IM infostructure.

Second, senior leadership must commit to managing by fact rather than factoid. Information-based decision making must be embedded into the culture of the organization, and senior management must insist that all proposal reviews and business process analyses are absolutely supported by accurate information. In cases where reliable information cannot be obtained quickly, management must be committed to following up with relevant information process owners for resolution. In short, they must insist on fact-based decision making on the part of all their subordinates.

Organizational Structuring Arrangements

Much has been written regarding strategic structuring arrangements, which can be summed up briefly in the phrase "form follows function." What this means is that the organizational structure must be set up in a way that facilitates organizational goals and strategies, and the hyperturbulence of the healthcare industry demands that the structure be flexible and adaptive.

The approach taken by Keesler Medical Center attempts to align all the IT- and IM-related functions in the medical center under the organization's CIO (Figure 10.2). Traditional IT functions (computer operations, computer security, network administration, and systems administration) are joined with such IM functions as clinical informatics, data quality and analysis, and medical records.

By integrating both the IT and IM functions under a single department and making the CIO accountable for building the IM infostructure, Keesler Medical Center has horizontally structured itself with respect to the information flow processes. This is a crucial step toward becoming a truly knowledge-enabled organization.

Another important structuring arrangement concerns CIO membership on the organization's executive management team. We believe that a knowledge-enabled organization cannot exist without a CIO who is very much in tune with the rest of the organization. Recent research indicates that although a high-placed reporting relationship does help ensure that the CIO is in alignment with executive management and organizational strategies, it is even more important to ensure that the CIO is a full-fledged

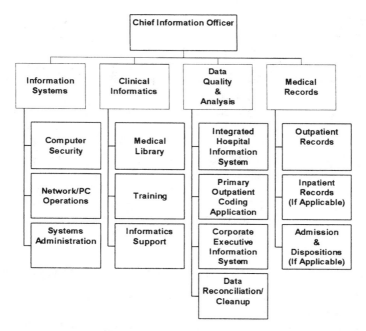

FIGURE 10.2. Proposed Keesler Medical Center IM/IT organization chart.

member of the organization's executive management team. Lack of full acceptance by executive management minimizes the CIO's influence and does not position the IM/IT department to address key organizational issues. In a recent study by this chapter's first author of 154 not-for-profit healthcare CIOs, fully 69% of civilian CIOs were members of their organization's top management team, compared with only 31% of MHS CIOs. These differences in the two populations of CIOs were highly significant ($p < 0.001$), suggesting that there are systemic differences between how civilian not-for-profit healthcare organizations view the importance of CIO membership on the executive management team and how MHS organizations view it.

Currently, Keesler Medical Center's CIO reports to the organization's COO (Administrator). This arrangement provides the CIO with first-hand and daily contact with a member of the organization's executive management team. However, Keesler's CIO, like the majority of MHS CIOs, is not a formal member of the organization's executive management team. Although counterintuitive to building an IM infostructure, this is not an uncommon structuring arrangement within the MHS. The problem lies in the rank structure embedded within the MHS.

As noted earlier, IM/IT was highly IT-centric until recently. With such a long-standing IT focus, there was no perceived need for the MHS to bring resources perceived as purely technical into the executive circle. As such, most of the MHS's rank and file CIOs typically are lower-ranking members of the military, while their executive peers hold higher military ranks. Because the executive management team has historically been composed of each organization's highest ranking (in a military sense) members, it is difficult for many higher-ranking executive team members to see the value of having a lower-ranking member on the executive team.

In addition, many of the MHS's CIOs become their own worst enemies by continuing to foster the IT-centric view of their own role. More than a few focus on technical innovations but have not stayed current with business or clinical practices, making them ill equipped to "talk the talk and walk the walk" of executive management. Both Keesler Medical Center and the MHS would likely benefit from bringing CIOs into the executive team and mentoring their development into executive-level information managers.

Importance of Developing a Data Quality Culture

In addition to structuring arrangements, an obsessive commitment to data quality assurance is the second fundamental building block of an IM infostructure. Historically, the accuracy and timeliness of the data provided to Keesler Medical Center's management was questioned for a number of reasons. First, few if any feedback mechanisms were in place relating to questions of data quality. In addition, no measures focusing on data accuracy and timeliness were tracked, and the management consequences of having poor data quality were not emphasized.

Today, Keesler Medical Center, a tertiary teaching hospital with more than 60 specialty clinics and 95 operating beds, employs one full-time staff member and six part-time staff engaged in data quality functions (e.g., data reconciliation, cleanup, validation). Clearly, Keesler understands that building an IM infostructure requires quality data for quality decision making. In addition, Keesler Medical Center employs five additional full-time staff to assist functional users throughout the medical center with data analyses (e.g., pulling data from multiple data sources, integrating the data, and assisting users with data validation and presentation).

The ability of an organization to effectively accomplish analyses cannot be underestimated. In the IT infrastructure-centric model, the focus was on fielding information systems, training users, and then essentially leaving them alone to attempt their data analyses. Without a sound understanding of the dynamics involved in ensuring data validity and the methods of extracting data from disparate systems, users produced suboptimal data analyses that formed the basis of business process decision making. In the IM infostructure-centric model that Keesler Medical Center has adopted, informed decisions are made by numerous full-time staff who fully understand the sources of data, its validity, and how to extract it. This practice has an orders-of-magnitude leveraging effect on the ability of Keesler's knowledge workers to objectively and rigorously assess their processes and strategies.

Besides committing significant resources to the pursuit of data quality, Keesler Medical Center also recognized that data quality could not be centrally controlled. Rather, it had to become the mantra of everyone in the organization to ensure a solid information foundation for decision making. Particularly important were data input sites to Keesler's information systems, where most data quality problems originate. From a human resources perspective, it is important to note that the MHS, like many healthcare organizations, entrusts a most important function (i.e., data entry) to "information warehouses." Although these data will form the basis of enterprise decision making, data entry is placed in the hands of individuals in jobs that are among the lowest paid and are often seen as undesirable. To overcome the natural complacency that these jobs induce, Keesler focused attention on the continuum of data and information flow processes by developing the Quality Decision Making continuum (Figure 10.3). Data entry clerks throughout Keesler were required to adopt a zero-tolerance policy for poor data entry.

The purpose of the Quality Decision Making continuum is to help decision makers throughout the organization understand how to efficiently and effectively obtain accurate data. The CIO has the responsibility to develop this process to ensure quality data input. This process involves providing data feedback and developing and communicating a process to correct deficiencies (championed by its Data Quality and Analysis branch). Correcting deficiencies usually requires training (Clinical Informatics and Medical Records Elements branch) and hardware/software, security, and infrastructure improvements (Information Systems branch).

For instance, for the key information system it operates, Keesler Medical Center's IM/IT department routinely conducts staff assistance visits with its clinics to validate the Quality Decision Making process. An example of such a staff assistance visit checklist can be found in Table 10.1, which concerns Keesler's Ambulatory Data System. This checklist encapsulates the quality decision-making process relating to the Ambulatory Data System, representing all the items that must work correctly to produce accurate and timely information. After personnel have been presented with the process and training has been provided, continuous monitoring of the output is required to ensure that personnel are abiding by guidelines and that new personnel are properly indoctrinated into Keesler's information-based culture. Once this is done, facility leadership is much more assured that accurate data are available for making data-driven decisions. Regulatory agencies like HCFA and JCAHO will be pleased to see a structure and documentation for assuring quality data through the computer systems, making sure the organization's information "looks as good as it really is."

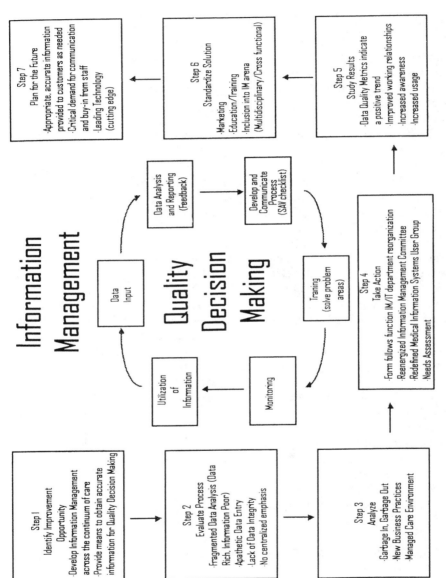

Figure 10.3. Keesler Medical Center's IM quality decision-making continuum.

TABLE 10.1. Staff assistance visit checklist.

Clinic:	Date:

Section 1: Overlays

☐ 1. Clinic is aware of procedures, and has the ability, to modify and commit overlays?

☐ 2. Active appointment types identified in the CHCS clinic profile also assigned to overlay form in ADS?

☐ 3. Efficient use/number of appointment types? (*comparison between "count" CHCS and ADS*)

☐ 4. Overlays include clinic's most frequently used ICD-9 codes, CPT-4 codes, and E&M encounter types? (Promote removal of "unspecified" diagnosis form overlay)

☐ 5. Clinic tracks the use of Lab, Pharmacy, and Radiology orders in the "clinic use only" area?

☐ 6. Appointment types properly identified as "count" or "non-count"?

☐ 7. Clinic has default overlay form established for each MEPRS code utilized?

☐ 8. Number of overlays used by the clinic?

☐ 9. Sample of completed Bubble Sheets reviewed for correctness?

Section 2: Training

☐ 1. "Superuser" received formal training?   "Superuser" rank/

☐ 2. Technicians received formal training?   name/phone_____

☐ 3. Users competent in utilization of the encoder grouper?

Section 3: Security

☐ 1. Password protection promoted?   By what means?_____

☐ 2. Users have correct level of access (HCP for superuser, clerk for standard user)

☐ 3. Is there a "community" password that subverts formal training?

Section 4: Equipment

☐ 1. Scanners routinely calibrated?   Most recent

☐ 2. Clinic provided calibration handout?   calibration?_____

☐ 3. Users know how to power cycle Milan Box (printer driver)?

☐ 4. Printer alignment checked?   Calibration

☐ 5. How many PCs have ADS connectivity?   schedule?_____

Section 5: Standard Operating Procedures

☐ 1. End of day (EOD) processing procedures in place. (EOD processing policy letter provided)

☐ 2. EOD processing importance emphasized, effects of data corruption/absence of data?

☐ 3. Editing procedures consistently practiced and scanning/coding errors corrected per "scanning error sheet"?

☐ 4. Bubble sheets are being physically corrected before being sent to Third Party Collections for billing?

Continued

TABLE 10.1. *Continued*

Clinic:	Date:

☐ 5. ADS sheets completed/scanned edited *daily—in their entirety?*

☐ 6. Walk-ins completed daily in EOD procedures?

☐ 7. CHCS info verified when appointment is made? (phone number, SSN, address, third party insurance info)

☐ 8. Telephone consults entered and monitored in CHCS?

☐ 9. Ambulatory Data System (ADS) bubble sheets generated *and* scanned for telephone consults?

☐ 10. Are backup tapes installed nightly as part of EOD process—if no, procedure explained?

Section 6: Contingency Planning

☐ 1. Equipment failure procedures identified?

☐ 2. "Sample forms" maintained for each clinic overlay to be utilized during system or network downtimes?

Section 7: Feedback

☐ 1. Date scheduled to provide SAV feedback to clinic?   DATE:_____

☐ 2. Clinic provided feedback on information needs?

Keesler Medical Center's CIO found that, although personnel in the outpatient clinics were skeptical at first, they began to appreciate the interest in the information they produced once they realized that the staff-assistance visits intended to ensure that credit is given for all the care provided. In addition, individual clinics began using their own data for studies focused on continuous quality improvements of their services. Ownership has taken place because the clinicians have been involved in making sure their data makes them "look as good as they are." A paradigm shift has occurred in the clinicians' view of their job; now, entering accurate data in the computer system is a natural part of seeing each patient. More importantly, by providing a means for the lowest echelons of the organization to accomplish introspective analyses of their own operations, true organizational transformation and flexibility are made possible.

Informatics in Population Health

Deployment of a population health strategy in the public sector is fundamental to its financial survival. Although the private sector has experienced a slight trend in population health via managed care models, the public sector cannot afford the cost of the current system. In all probability, therefore, healthcare outcomes will suffer. Disease management and demand management play a key role in today's healthcare environment, but while we keep the foundations of utilization management in place, we must explore methods of keeping young people healthy through population health strategies. Without meaningful incentives for healthcare providers, tactical deployment of informatics to profile and measure costly outcomes, and a sound population health strategy, the delivery of health care will become a major financial burden to the citizens of this country.

Informatics is key to a population health strategy. As one can glean from the contents of this chapter, executive leaders must promote the deployment of informatics. Organizations lacking the insight to do so could seal their financial fate, because survival of healthcare organizations in this new century will depend on informatics methodologies implemented today.

Future Considerations

Like its counterparts in the private sector, the MHS is faced with an intensely dynamic and complex operating environment. With a sophisticated enterprise-wide IT infrastructure in place and processes in place for its continued renewal, the MHS must now turn its attention to building a sound IM infostructure if it hopes to transform itself into a knowledge-enabled organization. The brass rings of population health management, disease management, clinical outcomes management, and objectivity cannot be attained without enterprise-wide, executive-level focus on IM processes. We have highlighted here one MHS organization's quest to transform itself into a knowledge-enabled organization, but the majority of the structuring and process arrangements of MHS organizations indicate a continued IT-centric focus. We believe MHS organizations would do well to learn from and adopt Keesler Medical Center's IM-centric focus to aid their own knowledge-enabling transformations.

11
Assessing and Achieving Value in Information Technology

Martin Belscher and William L. Sheats

As the information technology (IT) industry experiences explosive growth, it is offering organizations a steady stream of new systems, tools, and functionalities. The miniaturization of hardware, the increasing capacity of processing and storage capabilities, and the introduction of new technologies have all merged to decrease costs and increase functionality. Internet access and the significant investment in businesses that leverage the Internet have redefined many organizations and compounded the IT industry's growth over the past few decades. IT appears to offer unlimited possibilities, and it represents a powerful opportunity to solve the business problems facing global competitive markets.

The healthcare industry has taken advantage of the new capabilities afforded by the IT industry and has increased its spending on IT solutions. Historically, healthcare providers and insurance companies have been paper-intensive organizations. From insurance claim forms to handwritten orders for securing medical interventions in hospitals, the paper-based nature of the industry is known to create inefficiencies, bottlenecks, and errors. Lack of automation has impacted the ability to capture and analyze data quickly and efficiently.

Healthcare executives, like their counterparts in other industries, recognize the critical importance of information for making decisions. Reduced funding for healthcare services and increasing competition from other players within the industry have created an urgent need for informed decision making. To compete, executives require access to information that can be quickly and appropriately analyzed in a format that facilitates decision making. The healthcare and IT industries have found each other and are pursuing a path of mandated coexistence.

Health care's rush to improve and invest in IT became frenetic in the shadow of Y2K. In early 2000, the IT industry in general and health care in particular suffered from a spending and Y2K hangover. They paused to assess IT investments and focus on ways to achieve IT value, two crucial concepts that this chapter discusses in detail.

The first part of this chapter clarifies current trends in IT spending and sets up the challenge: aligning IT with business objectives and demonstrating value. The second part discusses ways of assessing current IT environments, including the IT organization's processes, performance, installed applications and technologies, governance, and strategy. The third part focuses on ways to achieve IT value and offers a framework organizations can follow.

Current IT Spending and Value

According to a focus group of chief information officers (CIOs) conducted by College of Health Information Management Executives (CHIME) in February 1999, the typical private sector integrated delivery system spends approximately 2.8% of operating funds and 30% of their capital budget on IT. During 1996, the Department of Veterans Affairs spent slightly less than $1 billion on IT with $324 million, the largest category, going to IT equipment (Gartner Group 1997). Worldwide, the research firm Computer Economics projects that total IT expenditures for all industries will exceed $1.1 trillion by the year 2001. Hardware is expected to represent over one-third of the $1.1 trillion expenditure, a reflection of the expected increase in IT investments in Europe and Asia. (Computer Economics 1999).

According to the CIO focus group just mentioned, 84% of IT investments fail to meet their original projections. The group attributed this high failure rate to difficulty in getting senior leadership to ensure that information systems were properly implemented with the necessary process changes. On a larger scale, the Gartner Group indicated in 1996 that the net average return on IT for the period 1985–1995 was 1%, all factors included. Reasons identified for the low return were "project changes, inability to realize intrinsic benefits not immediately capturable, under-specifying the infrastructure, and failing to reinvest in applications" (Gartner Group 1997).

The inability to demonstrate achievable benefits from IT investments occurs early in the life cycle of an IT initiative. Besides the reasons specified in the Gartner Group study, several general factors hinder the realization of IT value. Organizations are preparing themselves for disappointment when the following situations prevail.

- **IT is not integrated with operations.** Traditionally, the perception has been that merely automating current processes or operations is the solution to business problems like high staffing levels and slow processes. IT solutions have been implemented with little input from their daily users and without the integration of IT and operations. This limits IT's potential. When IT does not enable operations or processes, staff tends to use less than its full capability. Rather than reducing workload, the new IT solution creates more work and more problems: it dictates unfamiliar actions for the staff and creates a parallel work stream.

Because the extraordinary flexibility of IT solutions allows users to configure the system to meet their unique requirements, it is relatively easy to configure the system in a way that conflicts with current operations. An example is an outpatient clinic that wants to collect patient copayments at the point of scheduling but configures the registration system to record copayment collection at the point of care. Although the scheduler knows to collect the copayment via a credit card while the patient is booking a clinic appointment, the system does not follow this kind of workflow and will not allow documentation of the patient's payment. This is a relatively benign example, but it reflects the level of flexibility in current IT solutions and the problems that arise when IT is at odds with operations.

- **Staff training is insufficient**. When budgets are tight or deadlines are imminent, organizations tend to sacrifice staff training. On more than one occasion, the rationale for reducing staff training has been attributed to "the ease and power of the new IT solution and the ability of staff to quickly learn new things." Without solid experience to back up this claim, new IT solutions are rolled out and meet immediate resistance from the staff they were intended to help. Lack of effective staff training when operations or processes are changed continues to be a significant barrier to demonstrating how IT enhances the organization's performance.

- **Old processes are still in place.** Purposely eliminating the traditional way of doing work reinforces the need for staff to adjust to the new way of doing it. So long as the familiar way of performing the work exists, staff members who remain frustrated with the new solution can easily become tempted to revert to the comfortable past. Although it is very important to dismantle old processes upon implementation of the new integrated IT solution, doing so mandates that the implementation is complete and that staff members are all properly trained and ready to use it.

- **Value measurement is insufficient.** According to the February 1999 CHIME focus group for CIOs, only 20% of the organizations involved in the group had a program in place to measure the benefits achieved from IT investments. (The section on IT assessment further clarifies the need for measurement and suggests solutions.)

Executives and boards of directors are voicing disappointment in the level of IT value their organizations have received. For example, anecdotal evidence indicates that executives are questioning the Y2K investments they made before the new millennium. With relatively few computer errors surrounding the transition to the year 2000, some are wondering whether Y2K fear was used to allow IT organizations to increase their spending. Although no one knows what would have happened in the absence of these investments, the fact remains that very large expenditures were made to address a relatively simple date deficiency at a time when IT spending is under intense scrutiny for the value it delivers.

Webster's dictionary defines *value* as "a fair return or equivalent in goods, services, or money for something exchanged." Value emphasizes the amount of benefit relative to the investment, not just the amount of the investment. The IT value challenge, therefore, is not focused on how efficiently or effectively the IT department or function operates, but on demonstrating *how* the IT investments have enhanced the operational performance or competitive position of the organization. In other words, what is the organization deriving from the investments in terms of equipment/hardware, applications/software, training, and IT operations? Why should executives continue to invest in IT?

In this new century, both the private and public sectors must demonstrate how IT investments deliver value to organizations. This challenge can be successfully addressed through assessing and measuring value in the current environment and implementing strategies to achieve increased value.

IT Assessment

During the past decade, the federal government has passed legislation and established initiatives that embrace IT assessment and performance measurement. The Government Performance and Results Act of 1993 (GPRA), which holds federal government agencies accountable for achieving program results, is looking to establish program performance goals and measure against them to improve effectiveness. The Information Technology Management Reform Act (also known as the Clinger-Cohen Act) of 1996 aims to establish a culture within federal agencies of managing IT resources as a capital investment. This move would include linking IT planning with budget and performance measurement efforts, managing processes supported by the planned technology, developing and using performance metrics, and ensuring that inefficient and ineffective procedures and work processes are not automated.

Assessing IT-based services is not a new concept; users and executives have been observing and judging IT for decades. What is new is an emerging art and science that provides a more objective and insightful assessment. IT has been a mystery to many who are not directly involved in the field. Users and executives often wonder why IT is so expensive, unreliable, and disappointing in its return, and they want to know why projects take so long and generate so many surprises. Optimistic executives also ask how IT can transform their operations or propel their services and products into the "e-world." Although some IT professionals and leaders have successfully answered these questions, unclear answers have tarnished the image of the tens of thousands of IT professionals who have developed and implemented an incalculable number of high-quality, cost–effective systems.

New assessment methodologies will objectively measure IT from the user and executive point of view. The emerging assessments, a blend of old and new approaches, view IT from the outside as well as the inside and feature assessments of value to the organization, quality, risk, return on investments, and cost-effectiveness.

- **Value to the Organization.** The question of how much value IT is returning to the organization is particularly urgent in health care and related businesses. Investments in IT are perceived to be significant, and efforts to implement IT are seen as lengthy and exhausting. Not surprisingly, executives are asking if all the effort and investment is "worth it." The latter half of this chapter focuses on how to reap the most value from IT implementations.
- **Quality**. A quality-oriented assessment of the information services (IS) organization focuses on the length of cycles (e.g., problem reported to problem resolved), "redos" (e.g., the number of times staff return to desktop workstations before a repair is satisfactory), management and planning disciplines, quality measurement, and continuous quality improvement methods. In a well-led IS organization, every important IS service is measured by a service-level agreement (SLA). The quality-oriented assessment inspects the breadth and depth of the SLA system and asks if the data collected in the SLA system are used continuously to find fertile ground for quality improvement initiatives.
- **Risk.** The "risk" assessor outlines the areas where risk is a consideration and then describes the processes that must be in place in each area to avoid risk. For instance, an IT organization must have an ongoing process to develop an IT strategy aligned with the organization's business strategy. If this is not the case, the assessor would conclude that the organization bears the risk of IT investments diverging from the business strategy. Similarly, risk would exist with these factors:
  - Weak project planning and execution
  - Weak fiscal responsibility
  - Flawed recruitment and retention processes
  - Poor return on investment
  - Weak IS technical infrastructure
  - Ineffective SLA process
  - Unstable IT applications that are prone to errors and outages
- **Return on Investment (ROI) and Other Measures of Value.** All facets of the healthcare community are under extreme economic pressure. Hospitals and integrated delivery networks (IDNs) face the ravages of the Balanced Budget Act. Pharmaceutical companies face not only the pressures of the competitive marketplace but also government initiatives to control Medicaid and Medicare reimbursement. Health plans that have battled

to gain and hold market share on the basis of low premiums are losing operating cash, and Congress is pressuring government health providers to be as cost-effective as those in the private sector. In addition, the cynical world wants to know what it is receiving in return for the perceived Y2K-related "spending spree." Because IT is a major cost and a productivity driver, the healthcare community needs to be reassured of IT value through assessments. The obvious approach tries to pinpoint areas where greater economies are possible, but we must keep the potential impact of this type of assessment in perspective. For IT organizations in the family of providers, plans, and pharmaceuticals, which typically spend 2% to 6% of their total annual operating budget, a 10% savings in IT would yield less than 1% on the bottom line. Obviously, the major returns are in the effective application of IT in the organization.

- **Cost-Effectiveness.** We have all heard the old saying that efficiency is doing the job right and effectiveness is doing the right job. A body of knowledge on IT cost-efficiency has grown as IS has become a profession and a subject of academic discourse, but it is even more valuable to investigate its cost-effectiveness. For example, most computer centers generate truckloads of printed reports. Generating reports in the most economical manner is important, but eliminating reports that are no longer useful is more important. Doing the right job effectively is the goal; doing the wrong job at a low cost is a poor substitute.

    The cost-effective IT service conforms tightly with user needs, responds quickly to changing business requirements, and often requires that installed applications be challenged. For example, although registration systems are often designed to register patients at the front door, many hospitals have revised their services to direct outpatients to ancillary departments for services. However, the tradition of front-door registration and the inflexibility of the installed applications lead hospitals to register patients in both the admissions and the ancillary departments. Driving cost out of the installed technologies would help, but it would be more cost-effective to drive the duplication out of the registration process.

Emerging IT assessments reflect evolution trends in general business ranging from return on investment, cost–benefit analysis, total quality management, strategic alignment, and balanced scorecard. The best contemporary methodologies incorporate the best of each trend. Properly devised and applied, these new approaches will also point to areas where improvement is required.

Who Requires an IT Assessment?

Over time, the success or failure of IT has become more important to the careers of chief executive officers (CEOs). Boards of directors are more cognizant of IT, and they recognize the important role IT can play and the significant cost it has generated. Therefore, boards are more inclined to hold CEOs accountable for IT. Compensation decisions and even terminations are affected by the state of the organization's IT services.

Given this sensitivity, CEOs are often arranging assessments of IS at the time of their arrival in the organization. A metric benchmark of IT is an excellent means of determining the status of IT on the arrival of the new CEO, thus protecting the new CEO from being blamed for the missteps of a predecessor. Similarly, a new chief financial officer (CFO) or chief operations officer (COO) to whom IT workers report often retains a consultant to create a credible benchmark to establish the status of IT, and a new CIO frequently follows the same path for obvious reasons. There are defensive but appropriate rationales for conducting an assessment. Just as good health requires regular and systematic physical examinations, healthy IT must be maintained with comprehensive and regularly scheduled assessments. Every 12 to 24 months is the recommended interval, assuming that any issues that surface are addressed in the intervals between assessments.

Assessments and Outsourcing

In the government sector, Congress and the executive branch have, for more then a decade, embraced the trend toward "privatization." The private sector is held in esteem by many politicians who believe that outsourcing IT functions will prove cost-effective. For components that are not outsourced, there is great pressure to emulate the private sector in terms of cost-effective operations. Contrary to popular opinion, however, many government IT operations are very well led and cost-effective. In those organizations, the leadership occasionally turns to consulting firms to conduct an assessment that will either document excellence or find potential areas for improvement.

The recent and enormous upsurge in interest in outsourcing accounts for some of the contemporary interest in assessments. The motivation varies by player and circumstance.

- **The CEO.** CEOs worry about cost, quality, and agility. They want costs that are predictable and reasonably even from year to year, but they also demand quality IT. Sporadic outages, flawed claims, and unreliable data interfaces make CEOs think about alternatives like outsourcing. Although they may be uncertain about the direction they want the organization to take, they know they will need to move quickly when they do decide. Given the CEO's agenda, a professional objective independent assessment will help determine if IT is able to meet the criteria or if outsourcing should be pursued.
- **The CFO.** Predictably, many CFOs are driven by cost-effectiveness and cost-efficiency. Outsourcing is a means of negotiating and controlling cost

and placing the efficiency burden on the outsourcing provider. To determine if outsourcing is an appropriate prescription, an assessment/diagnostic is a logical next step.

- **The CIO.** In the 1980s, CIOs often tried to "do it all and control it all," and some viewed outsourcing as a sign of weakness and failure. During the past decade, CIOs have become more comfortable with outsourcing as they have found niche providers to provide specialty services (e.g., implementation support, data center management, network management, help desk management). Another reason enlightened CIOs are embracing broader outsourcing is that the number of IT professionals in the marketplace is grossly disproportionate to demand. Because of the ever-changing kaleidoscope of skills required, it is difficult to acquire, recruit, and retain IT professionals.

- **The Outsourcing Provider.** When an organization begins serious discussions with an outsourcing provider, an early task for the outsourcer is to conduct an assessment with intensive evaluation of present and future cost. Driving the cost issues are all the basic criteria: alignment, governance, project planning and execution, and infrastructure management, to name a few.

How to Conduct an IT Assessment

Thus far, this chapter has discussed a number of factors to examine in an assessment: value, facility, risk, return on investment, and cost-effectiveness. It is not necessary to choose among these factors. A well-constructed assessment can address the essence of all of these.

Assessments are based on benchmarks, which are based on either normative databases or best practices. Normative data for the broad-based assessments we are discussing are not generally available. Gartner, GIGA, Computer Economics, and other research organizations have developed performance metrics, most of them based on cost or FTE count. Generally, most of the data are representative of the IT industry. Healthcare-specific metrics and norms are scarce, but where they are available, they should be employed. The alternative assessment methodologies compare the organization's performance to best practices, a valuable approach. As interesting as comparisons with the competition may be, the more important question is how an organization's performance compares with best practices.

The essence of a comprehensive assessment revolves around 10 areas of inquiry, listed in Table 11.1 along with the crucial factors to be considered with each.

First Consulting Group has developed a series of questions based on best practices for each of the categories in Table 11.1. Each question is weighed based on relative importance, and each area is scored based on the

TABLE 11.1. IT assessment areas.

Assessment area	Crucial factors
Strategic planning and continuity	Planning and communication Business knowledge of IS; IS knowledge of business
Governance and policy	Steering committee with IS and senior executives Consensus for priorities and budget Architecture and standards Service request process
Project execution and delivery	Standard project management methodology Interdependence of projects Quantifiable project ROIs
Application management	Development, maintenance, enhancement Database and interface management Security and confidentiality Quality and production change management
Operations and data center management	Upgrade and change management Customer service
Infrastructure (networks, servers, desktops)	Local area and wide area network Remote access Back office Voice communications Internet/intranet Help desk and user training
Fiscal responsibility and management	Budget linkage to corporate operating plan Timely, accurate budget reports Clear accountability for budget Cost related to results
Staff development and leadership	Staffing plan Skill assessment Recruiting Staff development Performance review Staff retention program
Service levels	Establishment of application service levels Service level experience tracked with costs against budget Service level impact on productivity CQI Program Benchmarks for SLA performance Customer satisfaction survey
IT value	Document IT investment request Review and evaluate request Monitor IT investment

degree to which it is accomplished. Data required to answer each question are found in documents, files, and interviews, gathered from IS leadership, and cross-checked with users and executives. A score comparing the organization to best practices is calculated for each area. Although the size and complexity of organizations is great, a sound assessment can be prepared by a seasoned team of three to six consultants over a period of 1 to 2 weeks.

Achieving Value from IT Investments

After the current level of IT value is measured and assessed, the second part of the challenge remains: how do organizations go about maximizing and maintaining that value? The first principle to achieving value from IT investments is that IT enables operations or processes, not vice versa. IT is not the solution in and of itself. Enabling operations and processes with IT increases efficiency and effectiveness, which in turn enhances operational performance and demonstrates value. The value of IT can then be quantitatively determined by measuring the change in performance of the enabled operations and processes.

Achieving value from IT investments requires a disciplined approach to viewing and managing IT as a scarce resource. In the subsections that follow, we offer a framework that has proven to be highly effective in providing the mechanics to derive value from IT in a wide range of organizations. Organizations must remember, however, that the specific approach adopted is less important than establishing IT value achievement as one of the organization's management principles.

Step 1: Defining Tools

A number of straightforward tools can reinforce the management principle and provide structure for the organization's approach to achieving value from IT. Each organization needs to determine which will be used and how they will be applied within the overall framework for achieving IT value. The tools include the following:

- **Business Case.** The business case can be as complex or simple as required to establish the business imperatives for pursuing the IT initiative. Within the business case, there should be a description of how the initiative supports the organization's overall strategy and business objectives and the compelling business reason for engaging in the effort. The business case clearly articulates how the IT investment enables or supports a business need identified by the organization's executive leadership. Business cases should be as quantitative as the requestor can be; that is, if the business case can demonstrate the expected impact on the overall performance of the organization, it becomes a more compelling argument for investing in IT. An integral part of the business case is the discussion of how IT will be integrated with operations and the organization's future visions.

- **Return on Investment (ROI).** ROI is a means to represent the financial value of the investment with a single number. ROI compares the cost to the benefit and results in a ratio of the latter to the former. For example, an ROI of 7 indicates an expected benefit seven times greater then the expected cost. ROI is an important tool to use when attempting to prioritize multiple IT investment requests competing for a limited pool of funds.
- **Payback Period.** Payback period is a calculation that adds the dimension of time to ROI. The calculation of payback period assesses the timeframe in which expected benefit will equal the total expected cost of the IT initiative. For example, a payback period of 6 years indicates that within that period of time, expected benefits will equal the cost of the initiative. Payback period is an effective tool for prioritizing requests and is often used in conjunction with ROI. Both can be calculated relatively easily with estimated values, but there are limitations on their accuracy.
- **Benefits Profile.** The benefits profile identifies the expected type of benefit, performance metric, baseline, and target data points for the metric, expected value, and efforts required to achieve the benefit. This tool quantifies the value of the expected benefit and delineates, at a high level, the operational and technology changes required to achieve the benefit. The benefits profile also establishes expectations regarding the amount of change required. Profiles can be prepared at varying levels of detail and should be tailored for the point at which the IT investment proceeds through the lifecycle.
- **Cost–Benefit Analysis.** The final tool is the traditional cost–benefit analysis (CBA), which can involve a significant amount of effort to develop and use. A useful tool to help track progress and performance, the CBA identifies detailed cost and benefit data for the initiative and may include the calculation of an ROI and a payback period at a higher level of accuracy than either can offer. The CBA level of focus should be restricted to very expensive initiatives or those IT investments that have been approved for funding.

Step 2: Identifying Executive Commitment

Perhaps the most important requirement to achieving value from IT lies with securing sustainable commitment from the organization's executive leadership. Commitment originates with establishing the achievement of IT value as a management principle. Executives who clearly, consistently, and continually articulate the importance of deriving value from IT will demonstrate the importance of this management principle to the organization.

As a part of this commitment, executive leadership holds themselves and their management group accountable for achieving value from IT investments. Ensuring accountability includes aligning individual and group incentives with achieving value and not approving any IT request that has not been through a valuation process. Achieving value from IT is a shared responsibility of the organization's senior information and operations executives.

Sustaining executive commitment and organizational interest requires continual reinforcement of the importance of IT value; this can be accomplished by including IT valuations in the annual budgeting process and communicating successes at achieving IT value to the organization's constituencies.

Step 3: Defining the Plan for Achieving Value

As with any effort, without a plan for achieving objectives, the likelihood of failure is high. A commitment to achieving value from IT alone will not generate the desired outcome. Using the benefits profile described earlier, organizations should develop the plan for how the expected benefits will be achieved. The plan should include responsible parties, definitive action steps, timeframes, and means for measuring progress. Achieving benefits from IT also requires a clear understanding of how operations and IT will be integrated and leverage each other. The plan should have linkages to and be synchronized with the IT initiative's implementation work plan to ensure dependencies are properly recognized and managed.

Identifying linkages between IT and process can generate significant benefits. For example, if the performance objective is to reduce medication costs, IT functionality can combine with the provider's decision-making process at the point of initiating care orders to provide an automated prompt of less expensive alternative medications. Orders placed electronically can easily be prompted to provide alternatives, whereas paper-based manuals can be difficult to use and access. This automated capability can be enhanced by easily making related medication information, such as efficacy experience and potential patient complications, available electronically.

Assumed within this approach is the need to clearly define how a process will function; that is, who will be accomplishing what tasks, where, and in what order, needs to be understood before identifying the enabling IT functionality. The organization's overall strategy and business objectives must drive the design of the process that identifies the enabling IT. Understanding the capabilities of IT when the process design is in its formative stage helps bring out the full potential of the enabling IT.

Step 4: Establishing a Mechanism for Measuring and Monitoring Value

The final component of a framework for achieving value from IT investments is establishing and implementing an ongoing monitoring mechanism that allows for the periodic measurement of performance and reporting of progress. Measuring and monitoring IT value are essential to sustaining it. Recent experience shows that process models, which have been identified for both healthcare provider and payor organizations and used to design more efficient and effective operations, can also serve as the basis for measuring performance. Process performance is typically measured using a combination of metrics: cost, cycle time, customer satisfaction, revenue, and clinical quality.

Using the "Access to Care" process as an example, we can describe typical performance metrics. The Access to Care process represents the activities involved for a patient from the point of contacting the healthcare provider to the point at which care is rendered. This process includes such activities as registration, insurance verification (coverage, eligibility, and preauthorization), financial counseling, clinical preparation and education, and appointment scheduling. Efficiently and effectively completing these activities before the patient arrives for care allows the provider to prepare more completely for rendering service.

Cycle time reduction can be measured by the length of time the patient waits for care on the day of service; length of time the care providers wait for previous medical records or patient test results; and the overall number of patients the clinic can accommodate in a given period of time (capacity). Cycle time reductions that eliminate delays positively impact customer satisfaction. Revenue enhancement can be measured by the number of denied claims for payment due to lack of insurer preauthorization, clinic cash collections around due copayments and collectibles, and days in accounts receivable. Although these performance metrics are not a complete means of measuring the Access to Care process, they do give some indication of the potential for measuring the process.

The potential benefits for clinical care quality and cost are illustrated by the "Document Care" process. As its name indicates, this process involves the activities undertaken to ensure that all care, whether diagnostic or therapeutic, is recorded and available to all care providers. (A significant challenge within care settings is ensuring effective communication among the healthcare team members.) Metrics that track duplicate order requests, adverse medication interactions, and timeliness in results reporting can improve the quality of clinical care and reduce its cost.

Monitoring progress should not be laborious or overly complex. The intent is to have an objective means for defining progress and showing the organization the results of efforts. Adopting a monitoring mechanism provides the organization with easy access to periodic information for purposes of communicating to various constituencies.

Conclusion

Information technology is changing at a phenomenal pace and providing organizations opportunities to accomplish business objectives in ways never imagined in the past. However, while there is clearly a luster to technological innovation, executives will require clear demonstration of value from any investment in IT. Executives, boards of directors, consumers, and taxpayers will continue to demand that IT functions are operating effectively and efficiently. Competition for fewer and fewer healthcare dollars is not expected to subside in the near future, and in both the private and public sectors, healthcare organizations will have limited funds available to support IT. To ensure that all investments are fully aligned with business needs and contribute to the overall mission and vision, organizations must assess the current IT environment and implement a sound framework to achieve, measure, and monitor value.

References

Computer Economics. 1999. Total Worldwide Information Technology Spending to Exceed $1.1 Trillion by 2001. Press Release, 2/10, www.computereconomics.com
Gartner Group. 1997. Information Technology Spending Trends FY 1994–1996. Research review. Stamford, CT: Gartner Group.

12
Improving Provider Performance: An Integrated Approach and Case Study on Privileging and Credentialing

Lt. Col. James Williamson, LT Edwin Rosas, and Lori B. Blades

The Military Health System (MHS) has long endured the cumbersome and time-consuming task of maintaining different processes and systems for the U.S. Army, Navy, and Air Force. Before the start of the project discussed in this chapter, there was no one system that could be accessed to indicate that a provider was credentialed and list his or her exact privileges. This lack of integration caused significant inconveniences for all involved. If an Army physician were to walk across the street to a Naval facility, the staff would have no idea who he or she was, and the subsequent application process for credentialing and privileging would sometimes take weeks.

Through a case study detailing the MHS development of the Centralized Credentials Quality Assurance System (CCQAS), this chapter discusses ways to improve access to provider information to enable efficient credentialing and privileging of providers, regardless of where they are working in the MHS. Before continuing, however, it is important to clarify the principal terms we use.

In the healthcare arena, terms are often used interchangeably even when their meanings differ somewhat. The terms "credentialing" and "privileging" are widely used throughout the industry, but almost never are they clearly defined. Because of this, they are used differently by different authorities, the MHS included. Very simply, the word credentialing is defined as the process of verifying that an individual has the appropriate education, training, and experience to meet the defined standards for medical staff membership. Privileging is a separate process used to determine what specific patient care services a provider can practice at a given facility.

Private Sector Model

In the private sector, it is not unusual to have a totally integrated system that resembles Figure 12.1. This model, which the MHS is very close to achieving, allows for total integration of all functions.

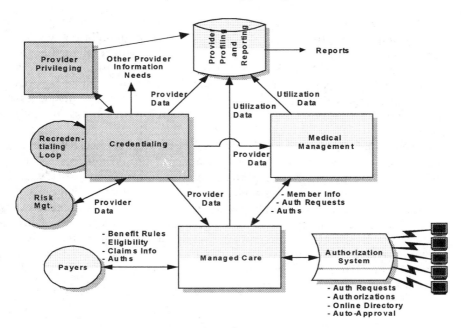

FIGURE 12.1. Integrated system model.

The key concept of this type of model is to appropriately manage care and provider data. It provides the ability to preserve the confidentiality of risk management, a very important issue. It allows for customization of the processes or data at service levels. It also helps support standardization of data for consistency and reporting. The business processes can be supported at the local service operations level. The model also allows for correspondence management and the centralization of data storage for ease of data management.

The MHS currently has the credentialing and risk management modules in place and is working on the privileging portion. They will then decide whether to integrate these modules and potentially some of their other functions. Once the entire system has been completed, it will be the most comprehensive credentialing and privileging system in the federal government.

Background on MHS

The Military Health System (MHS) supports the Department of Defense (DoD) and the nation's security by providing medical and dental care during peacetime and wartime operations. It is one of the nation's largest healthcare systems, offering benefits to approximately 8.3 million people at an annual cost of $16 billion. TRICARE, the DoD regionalized managed care program, is the overarching umbrella under which all healthcare services are provided. TRICARE brings together the healthcare resources of the Army, Navy, and Air Force and supplements them with networks of civilian healthcare professionals and facilities to provide better access and quality care while maintaining the capability to support military operations.

The MHS mission is to provide top-quality medical services, whenever and wherever needed, to active duty members of the Armed Forces and their families, retired military and their families and survivors worldwide. These services are provided through a system of 94 military hospitals and medical centers and 53 freestanding ambulatory clinics worldwide, employing 144,000 full-time military and civilian personnel and more than 90,000 medical personnel in the National Guard and Selected Reserves. The civilian managed care subcontractor provides a network of additional support to the MHS TRICARE system with 113,000 healthcare providers, 1,980 hospitals, and 22,000 pharmacies.

Impetus for Automation of Credentials

Each service has an office that is charged with the mission of validating and maintaining the credentials of their military or civilian healthcare providers as required by DoD directives and the Joint Commission on Accreditation of Healthcare Organizations (JCAHO). They are further charged to ensure that providers act within established standards of conduct within the scope of their training and current competency. Quality management personnel also periodically assess provider performance for the purpose of continuing staff appointments and privilege awards. Efficient management of provider information is essential to the rapid deployment of privileged healthcare providers during peace and war times.

Following the Persian Gulf War, the DoD Inspector General (IG) initiated a review of DoD Medical Mobilization Planning and Execution. The purpose was to evaluate the DoD's ability to provide adequate medical support for military mobilization contingencies. A comprehensive inspection of the mobilization process for health care was performed. One of the major findings was that availability of medical personnel during contingencies was hampered by shortfalls in the credentialing process. Specifically, provider credentials files were found to be outdated or incomplete, mainly in the Reserve and Guard components, and there was no automation of credentials to support the process. These inadequacies delayed healthcare providers from engaging in their duties and required additional staffing to support the process of bringing credentials files up to date. As a result of these findings, the DoD IG recommended improving the accuracy of credentials files, establishing a centralized DoD automated credentialing system that would be interoperable across all Active and Reserve components, and incorporating privileges into the system. Implementing these recommendations would enhance efficiency and expedite movement of medical personnel between Service hospitals or in times of deployment into theaters of operation. The recommendations were the primary catalyst that led to development of the Centralized Credentials Quality Assurance System (CCQAS).

Approach

Following the DoD IG report, a Tri-Service credentials working group was established to formulate a strategy for implementing the DoD IG recommendations. The first order of business was to facilitate the sharing of credentials information between military medical facilities. A standardized letter was established as a stopgap measure to accomplish this task and was labeled the Inter-facility Credentials Transfer Brief (ICTB). Before implementation of the ICTB, each facility had been required to "prime source verify" providers' credentials as they moved from base to base within their service or among other services. The ICTB eliminated the need to prime source verify credentials at every location.

The services were using service-specific information systems that captured information to support the credentialing process, but each system had significant shortfalls. The next task for the working group was developing a standardized automated credentialing system encompassing the functionality of three legacy systems: the Army's Medical Quality Assurance System (MQAS), the Navy's Centralized Credentials Database (CCDB), and the Defense Practitioner Data Bank (DPDB), maintained at the Armed Forces Institute of Pathology/Department of Legal Medicine. The workgroup examined the existing functionality and defined additional requirements that would capture unique needs among the services. The June 1995 Office of the Assistant Secretary of Defense/Health Affairs memorandum, "Policy Guidelines for Medical Staff Appointment and Privileges in DoD," implemented a uniform policy for appointing and privileging across the services, eliminating barriers to interservice provider sharing. The concept of CCQAS as a tool to facilitate standardization developed from these efforts.

CCQAS Task Statement

The development of a standard DoD information system is a monumental task from beginning to end. The approach was in accordance with the standard procedures established by the Military Health Service System (MHSS).

A task statement for the CCQAS Executive Agency was issued by the Office of Assistant Secretary of Defense for Health Affairs, and the Principal Deputy Assistant Secretary of Defense (Health Affairs) approved the Executive Agent process and the designation of Navy as the agent for the CCQAS Program. The Navy was then responsible for managing the overall execution of the CCQAS Program in support of the MHSS mission. The CCQAS mission statement at the time was this:

In order for the military services to meet their mission, they are required to maintain specific credentials and privileging information on all licensed health care providers and medical practitioners. CCQAS will provide a standardized, centrally managed automated microcomputer-based system for decentralized Tri-Service use. This information tool will empower TRICARE agencies to maximally utilize provider resources. The system will operate in a Client/Server, Corporate Information Management-compliant, network environment. The services are committed to:

- Readiness of healthcare provider during peacetime and wartime
- Provision of top-quality, cost-effective health care
- Innovation and application of new and emerging technology
- Readiness of health care provider during peacetime and wartime

CCQAS Objectives

The initial CCQAS objectives were as follows:

- To provide interoperable databases of verifiable credentials for all DoD Health Care Providers (HCP) in a timely manner (as defined in DoD Directive 6,025.1 l including active duty, National Guard, Reserve Component, Civilian, and contract employees)
- To improve the posture of the services in response to medical readiness requirements
- To expedite transfer of privileged providers for temporary or permanent change of assignment
- To provide a means to collect and manage risk assessment of torts/claims and adverse privilege actions data
- To provide a means to document current competence and compliance with accepted standards of practice and support overall healthcare analysis as valid and reliable measures become available
- To meet federal, state, and other agency provider reporting requirements
- To reduce the time required to query the National Practitioner Database before appointing and privileging HCPs
- To optimize accuracy and efficiency of Credentials Review and Clinical Privileging activities

Development of CCQAS

Initially, $2 million was allocated for the development of CCQAS. The workgroup realized that the best way to answer the DoD IG report was to develop something quickly. The Navy's CCDB was selected as the "Best of Breed" for modification to full CCQAS functionality. The Naval Medical Information Management Center, Norfolk Detachment, developed the initial CCQAS 1.0–1.5. This application automated the provider credentials side of Quality Management (QM). The functional capabilities, including the collection, tracking, and reporting (ad hoc and standard reports) of healthcare providers' credentials, limited medical readiness training information by the appropriate authority at the Military Treatment Facility (MTF).

This xBase application, written in Clipper 5.2, was essentially a standalone database that could be networked within the facility with multiple users accessing the same database. The initial development began in 1995, was completed in 1 month, and was deployed via disk to the services. The initial usage required all active duty sites to input all privileged providers within 1 year of the deployment and all Reserve Component providers within 2 years. CCQAS 1.5 was officially sent to more than 700 sites worldwide, more than any other application in the MHS.

The development and deployment of CCQAS 1.5 was considered phase I of the implementation. Phase II was to develop a true client–server application with a centralized database of all privileged providers' credentials using replication. The central database would eliminate the need for sites to send their data to the service headquarters on a quarterly basis to be inputted into the service databases. This concept also addressed the issue of data integrity.

Before development of the application began, an initial study was conducted to answer the age-old question of commercial off-the-shelf (COTS) versus government off-the-shelf (GOTS) products. The analysis would determine which route would truly satisfy the functional needs in the most cost-effective manner. GOTS became the initial solution due to cost and timelines and the scaled-down requirements. The analysis concluded that the limited systems on the market would not support the need. The astronomical initial investment, costs for customization, lack of code ownership, and a significant funding tail made the decision clear. In 1996, CCQAS 2.0 was sanctioned to be a GOTS product using COTS whenever possible.

CCQAS 2.0 application programs were designed to run at as many as three levels, constituting a three-tier architecture:

- Level One is the basic level of input; it is at the MTF where data will be recorded and managed on a PC. The credentials custodian at the MTF will enter data for civilian providers at the time of employment.

- Level Two involves the Service HQ. A consolidated database for all components of the service will reside on an appropriately sized computer. Basic data on a provider will be validated by personnel records at this level. The initial input of data for a military provider will be done at the Service HQ level when the provider is screened for accession.
- Level Three is a larger capacity system for consolidation of all services' data. Application programs for DoD-level reporting and cross-service searches would be available.

CCQAS Functionality

CCQAS data will be gathered at both the Service HQ and the MTF level. When a provider leaves the facility for reassignment or separation, a "summary" record for that provider will continue to exist. When a provider reports to a facility, the provider records will automatically be sent to the new MTF database. All updates to a provider's record will be applied to the Service HQ database.

Because each military service performs some parts of its mission using different methods, CCQAS seeks to automate functions that can be identified as procedurally uniform. The governing body for determining CCQAS functionality will be a tri-service committee of credentials' managers. As policy changes and uniform requirements are identified, some additional functions may be added to CCQAS. Functions that remain service specific will not be incorporated into CCQAS.

Additional functionality planned for CCQAS 2.0 includes the following:

- A consolidated database of all DoD healthcare providers, allowing the generation of aggregate reports for DoD review
- The ability to electronically transfer data for the Inter-facility Credentials Transfer Briefs (ICTB). The ICTB has been approved by JCAHO and is the preferred method of credentials transfer between DoD MTFs for temporary assignments
- Operational control over National Practitioner Data Bank queries. The date of last query will be stored so that repetitive and unnecessary queries are not made
- The ability of MTFs to review all validated credentials of assigned providers

Issues and Challenges

Moving from a concept to a tangible product is always a challenging task, and development of CCQAS was no exception. The issues facing the CCQAS Configuration Control Board (CCB)/Functional Workgroup were many, which created a domino effect in the entire program. Among these were programmatic—specifically, funding and technological/contractor—issues, plus functional issues pertaining to service-specific requirements.

For a program to be implemented successfully, sufficient resources must be allocated. This is a standing issue within the Military Health System (MHS). To cope with this continuous challenge, the members of the CCB and Functional Workgroup became extremely active participants in the CCQAS Program.

Funding was an ongoing issue because of the uncertainty invariably associated with government funding from year to year. Budgets are planned well into the future, but shortfalls commonly affect the entire MHS. IM/IT is just one of many departments in the system and must also share the burden by making adjustments. Although the MHS spends approximately $650 million a year on automated information systems, it is not that much considering its size, and any shortfalls are usually felt across all systems. The other piece of the equation is competition for funding among all the systems currently in development or already deployed (maintenance money required).

Automated information systems must be racked and stacked annually to give funding priority to systems that provide the most benefit to the overall enterprise. CCQAS was considered important enough to continue funding each year, but resources received were not always at levels requested. This lack was because more complete funding was allotted for the development, upgrade, or maintenance of flagship systems on which the enterprise was more dependent.

When the funding levels received are not equivalent to the levels requested, a two-part problem unfolds. First, cost becomes the major constraint when considering development proposals, design, testing, and implementation. Every stage of the software development life cycle requires resources to maintain a proper balance of cost, schedule, and performance. These challenges are true of any development effort. If funding levels are decreased, the project manager has limited choices—reducing functionality and shortening testing phases are just two of these options. CCQAS continues to struggle with this constraint.

The second issue when development funding is reduced is maintaining the legacy system. Annual maintenance costs for the legacy system continue to rise, because the replacement version is not available and the life of the legacy system is extended. Therefore, functional users continue to be haunted by the limitations of the existing system while overall business practices and technology improve.

Technology challenges were numerous in this project, particularly because of inadequate funding and the magnitude of the development. Initially, CCQAS was intended for approximately 454 sites worldwide, a number that grew to more than 700 sites. When development began in 1996, the infrastructure for each site varied from remote Reserve/Guard installations with a 2,600-baud modem to large networked medical centers. It is difficult to develop a system for bare minimum requirements when technology improves exponentially, and the system design needed to somehow address this issue. Based on the functional requirements, a web-based architecture seemed to be appropriate; however, web technology in 1996 was not as mature as it is today, and the infrastructure could not support it. The final decision was to design a client–server application.

Technology is changing so fast that by the time an application is developed and ready to deploy, it may be passe, inappropriate, or an inferior solution. The client–server format for CCQAS was generally able to meet the functionality requirements of the services and the MHS, but it carried high cost disadvantages for deployment, maintenance, and application updates. As deployment approached for the second version of CCQAS, the technology issue came into play, forcing a decision. The client–server issues, the fact that technology for web-based applications was proving dependable and cost-effective, and the action of other major organizations moving related applications to web-based architecture were catalysts for the CCQAS CCB to reevaluate the information technology.

Unique requirements by each of the services were discussed regularly, because the nomenclature and data requirements required to perform credentialing, risk management, and privileging were different for each of the three military departments. Generally speaking, however, the services had much more in common than not. Rather than fail to support the needs of sister services, the three departments usually reached consensus via compromise or by capturing unique requirements.

Contractor performance was a major problem, and it had to be constantly monitored. Although the performance of a contractor may start off well, the agreed-upon performance requirements may not always be fulfilled. Contractor performance may wane, resulting in significantly delayed or unacceptable deliverables. CCQAS is currently on its third contractor because of such problems.

System Design

The first version of CCQAS was deployed in the summer of 1996 to more than 700 Active Duty, Reserve, and Guard sites worldwide. CCQAS 1.5, essentially a stand-alone application capable of being used on a LAN, was developed using a nonrelational database and was Windows compatible. The functional capabilities of the system included the collection, tracking, and reporting (ad hoc and standard reports) of the healthcare provider's credentials and limited medical readiness information by the appropriate authority at the military Medical Treatment Facility (MTF). Data collected at the MTF level were forwarded via modem or floppy disk to their service (Army, Navy, Air Force Surgeons General level) for aggregation each quarter. Information collected on individual healthcare providers included demographics, specialty/subspecialty details, professional and additional training, affiliations, licensure/certifications, and malpractice insurance.

Loading of credentials and medical readiness information into CCQAS for all privileged active duty and civilian personnel healthcare providers was completed by January 31, 1997. Nonprivileged licensed/certified providers will be loaded into the second version of CCQAS after its deployment. CCQAS was approved by the Joint Commission on Accreditation of Healthcare Organizations (JCAHO) as a technical solution for electronic transfer of prime source verified credentials data and other related material.

Development of CCQAS 2.0 began in June 1996. Requirements for CCQAS version 2.0 added malpractice and adverse privileging action modules to the program. Additional functionality included storing historical data on all MTFs where a provider has worked, capturing continuing medical education, and formatting queries/reports to the National Practitioner Data Bank to eliminate double keying. Again, one of the greatest challenges was accommodating the disparate infrastructure of all 700 sites.

The Department of Legal Medicine (DLM) at the Armed Forces Institute of Pathology will be tapping into the CCQAS 2.0 central database to develop rates and trending analysis on the risk management data for DoD. The central database will serve as a replacement for the old malpractice/adverse privileging actions database software, called CLIN2/TORT2, which DLM used for the DoD Defense Practitioner Data Bank.

The goal of CCQAS 2.0 was to create a client–server database that allowed each site's credentialing information to be fed into a single consolidated database. The CCQAS 1.5 databases at each site would also be converted into the CCQAS 2.0 databases, eliminating double entry of data and retaining historical data. To accomplish this goal, a number of decisions had to be made.

The first limitation was hardware. One of the primary assumptions when the CCQAS project began was that the services would be responsible for ensuring that the required hardware was available at each site. However, the project was not given funding to provide the hardware necessary to support the application. Minimum hardware requirements were defined, and CCQAS was required to be operational on Windows 3.11/95/NT on the client side and Windows NT Server on the server side. After hardware, the next decision involved choosing the relational database management systems (RDBMS). Oracle, Informix, and Sybase SQL Anywhere were examined, with cost a looming factor. Another important capability of the RDMBS was to provide a mechanism to replicate CCQAS data from the local MTF to the service level and then to the consolidated databases. The Sybase product was chosen on the basis of these requirements.

Again, the design and architecture were based on the infrastructure limitations imposed on the project. E-mail based replication seemed to be the most reasonable, cost-effective, and efficient solution. The Sybase software also supported this capability. Building a replication system on top of a message system meant that CCQAS could use a single, dedicated e-mail account to transfer updates to the consolidated database and accommodate the three-tier architecture. Each message would be encrypted and customizable to a maximum of 50 K, and the site could also schedule replication to occur mostly at night or on demand. Another benefit of e-mail based replication was that sites not connected via LAN could use a dial-up connection to an Internet Service Provider to replicate changes made to the local CCQAS. This provision avoided the need for a constant remote or direct-dial connection into the consolidated server.

Outcomes

Eventually, the final architecture of the project became two tiered to simplify replication issues. Development was completed in May 1999, and beta testing began in late May–June 1999. CCQAS 2.0 was tested at approximately 15 sites of various sizes and locations. The beta test did exactly what it was intended to do: uncover difficulties with the installation procedures and with actual deployment support.

Estimated deployment of the client–server application was 6 months to 2 years, depending on the military service. The deployment was intended to take full advantage of service CCB members by forming a CCQAS "Tiger Team" to handle the deployment and postdeployment support with limited assistance from the contractor. The CCQAS installation software and documentation would be sent to each site via certified mail, and the deployment would be scheduled as sites were available to begin data conversion. This step eliminated the need for a contracted deployment team.

The CCB realized that deploying a client–server application as complex as CCQAS was extremely difficult. Complicating matters was the question of funding—although limited funding required innovative solutions, this task was too great for the services alone to support. This realization, coupled with the lack of support available at each site, created problems.

The best solution to mitigate these risks to the program was to redevelop CCQAS as a web-based application; this would reduce the time and cost for initial deployment and subsequent releases of the application. Configuration management and version control would be easier to manage, and maintaining the application would become a central management issue. CCQAS has always been a top candidate for a web application.

Development of a web-based application is currently being pursued under the caveat that it can meet certain performance requirements, although it is understood that the expectations cannot be the same as the client–server architecture. The performance of the web-based application relies on the Internet connection and central database architecture. The client–server version has been put on hold and is available if potential issues exist with the web-based application. CCQAS will be the first Tri-Service application to be converted to a web environment. At the time of this writing, the timeframe for release was targeted for full deployment immediately following the Y2K moratorium.

Lessons Learned

With this project, the main lesson learned revolves around developing functional requirements for an application. We believe this is the most critical step in the entire process. If done thoroughly, it is easier for a project manager to balance cost, schedule, and performance by reducing the number of changes required during the development phase of the project life cycle. Requirements creep is one of the most prominent risks to the success of a development project. Unfortunately, gathering all the requirements and articulating them in a formal document is easier said than done: After the development process is under way and functional representatives see the application taking shape, the initial requirements may be exposed as inadequate. Additional requirements or changes may start creeping into the development equation, delaying delivery time and increasing costs.

Encouraging the developers to interact closely with the functional team will allow for an easier translation of functional requirements to system requirements. Not all functionality may be anticipated until the program becomes tangible, but a balance must be reached in which only adjustments critical to the program's functionality will be made. Other noncritical system changes should be put on hold until the next software release, even though changing the program in an attempt to make it "perfect" is a difficult temptation to resist. Software development is a dynamic task, and so long as everyone understands that the program will *never* be perfect, most can accept postponing nonessential changes to maintain the development schedule.

Another lesson learned is that compromise is the key to successfully navigating the development process; without it, making progress becomes impossible. Many people involved in the process are from the functional side of the house and bring specific requirements to the table. These requirements may not always act in agreement with others, a discrepancy that can lead to conflict. The best solution is a thorough discussion of the issues involving all interested parties. This basis will foster a better understanding of the requirements and will usually lead to consensus. If the functional representatives are not able to compromise, program development becomes extremely difficult.

Future Directions

The next step for CCQAS will be adding and integrating privileges into the program. Currently, each service and corresponding Reserve Corps has individual privilege lists for each provider specialty, which are uncoded. The plan is to put common language privilege lists for each provider specialty into CCQAS and map them to ICD9CM and CPT4 codes. The purpose of this is to place all the services on the same list of privileges to facilitate the amount of resource sharing that occurs between them and will increase in the future. The coding will facilitate provider profiling and dovetail with the use of such codes in other MHS systems. However, before this goal can be achieved, the privilege lists of each provider specialty in each of the services and Reserves must be matched up with each other to develop the common language privilege lists. First Consulting Group has been hired to perform this task and is working in concert with the software developer, Sybase.

Also on the drawing board are plans to address medical incident reporting integrated within the risk management module of CCQAS and interfaces to support provider profiling and medical readiness and reduce double keying of such data as provider demographics.

CCQAS will continue to participate in the Federal Credentials Program, which aims to expedite the credentialing process across all federal agencies involved in resource sharing through electronic transfer of credentials. The underlying goal, which is one of the original intents of CCQAS for the military, is to eliminate the redundant and costly process of primary source verification every time a healthcare provider moves from location to location within the federal system. The MHS currently has many instances involving the Department of Veterans Affairs (DVA) in which healthcare providers are shared within the same facility (e.g., joint ventures) or work at other facilities. In an effort to promote this initiative, an electronic sharing mechanism has been developed in the second version of CCQAS for use between the MHS and the DVA.

Although CCQAS implementation proved to be a difficult project at times, lessons learned from its early phases were invaluable. We believe converting CCQAS to a web environment will solve the problems we pinpointed. Through its rebirth as a web-based application and continual revisions and additions, CCQAS will fulfill its overarching objective: to maintain specific credentials and privileging information on all licensed healthcare providers and medical practitioners in support of the military services and their mission.

13
Cost Containment: A New Approach and a VA Case Study

CYNDI KINDRED, DON PRATT, AND KIMBERLY MILLER

The healthcare industry has recently experienced an onslaught of pressures to reduce costs, a demand fueled by a host of factors shaping and changing the current healthcare market. These familiar factors include, but are not limited to, the following:

- Increased managed care discounting
- Tightened government reimbursements as a result of the Balanced Budget Act of 1997
- Losses on bad physician and HMO investments
- The 1983 inpatient hospital prospective payment system and the corresponding change from reasonable cost reimbursement for inpatient hospital care
- Audits that introduced a wave of scrutiny into billing and coding practices in the Medicare system

Over the past few years, these factors have caused such serious financial problems that some public hospitals have been forced to close or be sold to investor-owned corporations as private nonprofit entities. According to the American Hospital Association, the number of publicly owned hospitals has decreased significantly in the last decade, from 1,509 in 1987 down 17% to 1,260 in 1997. A similar trend of hospital mergers and closings has emerged in the private sector, as healthcare providers struggle to stay afloat in the changing healthcare market.

In response to all these financial pressures, public and private healthcare institutions are struggling to find ways to reduce their operating and fixed costs. Predictably, public healthcare organizations are using some traditional methods of cost containment taken from the private sector. However, many traditional methods of cost containment that work well in the private sector may not be appropriate for use in the public sector, or they may result in reduced operational efficiency, reduced patient and employee satisfaction, and archaic information systems and equipment. As costs are cut through reductions in personnel, IT investments, and other methods, the overall strategic goals of the organization may not be considered.

One of the biggest concerns when cutting costs in the healthcare industry is the potential impact that reduced costs will have on patient access to care and the delivery and quality of care. Recent findings indicate that managed care and other cost containment methods impact access to healthcare providers and affect public opinion of the quality of care in the U.S. (Donelan et al. 1999). Specifically, more than half the respondents in a recent survey cited insufficient funds or insurance to pay for necessary care. The United States incurs the most expense per capita in health care ($4,090 per capita in 1997), and the majority of Americans do not have the financial means to supply their own private health insurance. Although quality and access to care are high under traditional (fee-for-service) coverage, those in managed care plans reported much lower satisfaction and ability to see specialists.

Clearly, a combination of adequate insurance and public-assisted health care is necessary to meet the needs of the American public. The public sector must develop a new model for reducing costs without compromising quality or access to care. At the Veterans Health Administration (VHA) in particular, this task will be challenging; as we will further explain in this chapter, issues surrounding patient care are extremely complex because of the cross-delivery of care and services between VA and non-VA providers. Although initiatives have been instituted to address some of these concerns through the use of information technology and other process improvements, cost management with no degradation of quality requires a new business model.

Traditional Cost Containment Model in the Private Sector

During the past 35 years, healthcare organizations within the private sector have participated in a phenomenon commonly referred to as the "corporatization of medicine." Spurred by the government's establishment as a major purchaser of health care for the elderly and medically indigent U.S. populations (through Medicare and Medicaid), hospitals began to apply the traditional cost reduction techniques that had been used successfully in manufacturing industries for years. They have also developed sophisticated corporate finance and industrial engineering departments. These departments, staffed by individuals skilled in the highly specialized areas of Medicare reimbursement, budgeting, legal and regulatory compliance, and motion and time study, have focused on incorporating the discipline and structure previously found in manufacturing and industrial settings into the management of healthcare providers.

The traditional cost reduction techniques of healthcare providers have mimicked those of manufacturers and industrialists throughout

American business history. Traditional cost containment methods include these:

- Reducing variable costs by massing purchasing power
- Reducing fixed costs
- Increasing volumes while holding fixed costs constant or relatively constant

Reducing Variable Costs

The first category of cost reduction techniques involves reductions in an organization's variable costs. Variable costs in healthcare organizations typically include items that are "consumed" during the course of treating a patient. Examples include medical and surgical supplies, pharmaceuticals, and the like. Initial attempts at cost reduction generally focus on massing the purchasing power of institutions through centralization of the materials management, or purchasing, function. The positive impact of centralization is often magnified through the organization's participation in group purchasing initiatives sponsored by various membership organizations (e.g., Voluntary Hospitals of America, American Hospital Association) that are able to negotiate steeper discounts from vendors.

Reducing Fixed Costs

The second type of cost reduction technique involves a focused effort on reducing or eliminating fixed costs. To understand the approach most often used by healthcare providers when attempting to reduce fixed costs, we must examine the typical cost structure of a healthcare organization. Within the cost structure of healthcare providers, with hospitals being used as a proxy for all providers, the single largest element of fixed overhead is composed of salaries, wages, and related costs (including employee benefits), which equal approximately 81% of total costs. Administrative costs total approximately 11%, whereas maintenance and occupancy, pharmacy and central supply, and housekeeping and dietary costs equal approximately 2% each (HCFA Medicare Cost Report Public Use Files 1996). For nonhospital providers, the percentage of costs related to personnel tends to be higher because smaller institutions and noninstitutional providers usually are not burdened with the same physical plant and infrastructure requirements as hospitals.

Given the cost structure just described, most organizations will initially target personnel and administrative costs when attempting to achieve significant cost reductions. Of these two focus areas, personnel cost reductions (by way of reducing staffing levels) are easier to implement, given that cost reductions in administrative functions typically involve an initial investment in technology or equipment to streamline operations before any meaningful cost reductions can be demonstrated.

Increasing Volumes While Holding Fixed Costs Constant

The third cost reduction category involves an organization's ability to increase its volume of patients while holding its fixed costs stable. Organizations that are able to accomplish this will experience a reduction in *cost per unit* rather than a reduction in *total cost*. Effective strategies for increasing volumes in healthcare organizations typically center on attracting new patients or establishing new service offerings. For these strategies to be successful without incurring additional costs, the organization must have excess capacity or underutilized resources.

Lessons Learned

Because reduction of fixed costs tends to be the most targeted area for cost containment in the private sector, it has been heavily used in the public sector as well. When GA-based Sumter Regional Hospital was in dire financial straits, they hired CEO Jerry Adams, who immediately ordered cost-cutting measures through labor force reductions and renegotiating vendor contracts (Taylor 1999). Sumter was successful in turning its financial situation around as a result of changes, but not at a small price. For 5 years, the 221-bed hospital delivered services with only 50% of its normal medical staff, and has required neighboring hospitals like Phoebe Putney to share oncology and cardiology services.

As evidenced by the closing of many publicly owned hospitals in the United States, when costs need to be cut, staff are reduced and services are discontinued or consolidated among multiple sites. As hospital beds are underutilized and appropriations are cut from the federal and state budgets, public organizations will move in a similar direction. There has never been a financial incentive to reduce costs in the federal sector, and the tendency has always been to cut staff when cost-saving measures were employed, either until the next fiscal year or until the budget has been reallocated. This method can no longer be the standard operating procedure if the VA's budget hold until 2005 is any indication of the major changes that await.

Although methods that simply reduce labor costs may result in "quick-hit" savings and an immediate change in the bottom line, they do not have long-term positive results unless processes are changed as well. Cost reduction measures should be significantly aligned with the goals of the healthcare organization to be truly effective. As the labor force is reduced, there is often noticeable operational inefficiency, low morale, and reduced employee satisfaction, as well as an overburdened workforce. In response, the healthcare provider is often forced to rehire staff as a result of high turnover and employee absenteeism. Long-term solutions, therefore, need to encompass more than just short-term savings in fixed operating costs. Especially in the case of federal public providers such as the VA and Department of Defense (DoD), those short-term savings will not penetrate the organization or make lasting changes to business processes.

Long-term changes require process redesign in the organization, which will help it run more efficiently, automate certain functions through technology so that personnel may focus on care delivery, and use the resources of the organization in the most efficient way possible. All these changes should eventually increase the quality of care provided and bring about long-term savings through reduced employee turnover and integration of core business functions.

As the private sector has seen over time with its many hospital mergers, acquisitions, and mass consolidations into large integrated delivery networks (IDNs) single providers can no longer afford to run their businesses as they once did. Through these difficult lessons, the public sector has an opportunity to learn from the mistakes of others and affect change for the future of public healthcare delivery in the United States.

Differences in Public Sector Health Systems: A Case for Change

Public healthcare organizations should approach cost containment through careful planning and long-term solutions rather than the "quick-hit" solutions that may simply require recovery periods and more changes. Before we can present the new model, the differences between the public and private sectors need to be addressed. These differences are crucial to our understanding of how change drivers are affected by these two systems and how process improvement needs to align with the differing strategic goals of each. Through the following distinctions between the public and private sectors, we present a new approach for traditional cost containment procedures for use in the public sector:

- Funding in the public sector is not revenue driven as it is in the private sector. Financial budgets are allocated through congressional or state budgets and may change given the political and financial situation of the constituents. One of the reasons cost containment was never a major incentive for federal healthcare providers is that if they reduced their expenses in one year, their budget would decrease rather than increase the following year. This disincentive has permeated organizations.
- Populations of patients served by the DoD, VA, and other public entities may have different needs than does the general population. They may

also have more complicated financial and geographic situations, which makes the delivery and recording of their patient files more challenging than it is within the private sector.

- Rates of reimbursement are even more heavily affected by the Balanced Budget Act, because as much as 40% or 50% of a public hospital's revenues may come from Medicare reimbursements. Because public providers rely on Medicare reimbursements more heavily than do private providers, this has had tremendous impact on providers. Medicare billing has come under intense scrutiny in billing and coding practices.
- Government healthcare providers like the VHA have not always had the authority or ability to bill Medicare. The VHA was granted the authority to submit bills for certain Medicare-eligible veterans in 1998, but the cost recovery system is still deciding on how to truly become a revenue-driven part of the organization.

Given these distinctions between the private and public healthcare sectors, we can understand why some traditional approaches to cost containment may need to be modified for the public sector. We have the opportunity to anticipate what some potential consequences of cost containment may be and to try to achieve the best, most long term results for the organization. The conceptual model presented in the next few sections introduces that new approach to traditional cost containment.

Public Sector Cost Containment: A New Approach

The new model for cost containment stresses the importance of identifying process change before cost reduction and aligning any cost reduction procedure with the strategic objectives of the organization. The model focuses the areas of cost reduction "discovery" (i.e., determination of the areas where cost containment should take place) to the core processes and subprocesses of the organization. Furthermore, the model emphasizes the importance of defining a plan for performance measurement to ensure that levels of improvement identified at the onset of cost containment are sustained throughout their implementation.

The new model for cost containment is presented as a target whereby the internal influences on the healthcare organization are contained within the target, and the external factors impacting the organization are located outside the target. The arrow signifies that performance measurement activities are completed throughout the life cycle of any cost containment procedure. The new model is presented in Figure 13.1.

This model demonstrates the importance of understanding the external and internal influences impacting public healthcare organizations before making decisions about cost containment. Rather than mapping out a step-by-step process, this model is intended to serve as a guide that identifies the most crucial factors to be understood. The external and internal influences

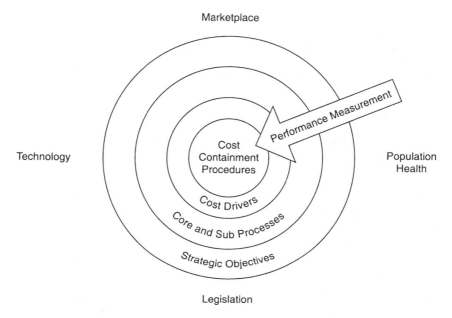

FIGURE 13.1. New model for cost containment.

are defined in the sections that follow, and a discussion of the practical application of this "target" approach is presented through the lessons learned at the VHA.

External Factors

Before determining cost containment procedures, the organization must have a clear understanding of its external influences. These influences impact all aspects of the organization, from the delivery of care to financial management to administrative processes. Changes in these external influences can have a dramatic impact on the organization's method of cost containment.

As depicted in the model, the external factors typically influencing the public sector are the following:

- **Marketplace**: the current state of the healthcare industry in the organization's geographic area, including the private sector "competitors" and providers of care
- **Technology**: the current tools available to enable processes to be streamlined and integrated across care settings and geographic regions
- **Population Health**: the health of the population in the organization's geographic region; especially influential in the public sector, where some providers may see populations with high proportions of the elderly,

chronically ill, and those with severe mental illness and veteran-related disabilities

- **Legislation**: current public policy and legislation changes (such as the Balanced Budget Act of 1997 and Medicare/Medicaid legislation) that have a direct impact on reimbursement rates and funding

Internal Factors

Several fundamental processes within organizations must be understood before deciding on a cost containment method. These areas are explained in more detail in the sections that follow:

- Strategic Objectives
- Core and Subprocesses
- Cost Drivers
- Cost Containment Procedures

Strategic Objectives

Too often, organizations undertake cost reduction measures independent of their strategic objectives. For example, an organization may reduce customer support personnel to minimize administrative costs while identifying an increase in customer satisfaction as a key strategic objective. Failure to align cost containment procedures with strategic objectives may result in an inability to fulfill the overall vision of the organization.

In addition, strategic objectives often pinpoint the areas in which cost containment should occur. For example, an objective like increasing access to care may result in a technology investment that educates customers more efficiently about where to go for certain procedures. This approach can reduce costs associated with inappropriate care while aligning cost management efforts with a strategic objective.

Core and Subprocesses

Likewise, the core and subprocesses that drive the day-to-day operations of the organization must be clearly defined and understood. The practical application of the strategic objectives within these processes must be articulated and communicated throughout the organization. The core and subprocesses represent the areas within the organization where cost containment will occur. This approach includes evaluating performance metrics to determine areas where improvements can be made and identifying cost drivers that can be improved upon through technology (see cost drivers). In addition, relating the core and subprocesses to the strategic objectives can uncover areas that do not align with the organization's vision. Once the core and subprocesses are understood, the cost drivers within them are analyzed.

Cost Drivers

Cost drivers represent those factors that cause the organization to incur costs. Cost drivers include staffing, management, materials, etc. For each cost driver there may be an opportunity for cost savings. An analysis of the cost drivers may result in the redesign of inefficient processes, the introduction of technology, and the elimination of processes that do not add value. These activities result from an examination of the inefficiencies related to the core and subprocesses. If inefficiencies are identified, the process is further investigated to determine the specific cost containment procedure required. Throughout the analysis of the cost drivers, proper alignment with the strategic objectives must occur.

Cost Containment Procedures

The cost containment procedures are a direct by-product of the cost drivers. They may include the specific steps in a process redesign or the functional changes that result from a technology implementation. To achieve the long-term benefits of cost containment procedures (whether they are improvements in technology or in staff training), there may be an initial investment of time and capital. The key is to determine whether the organization has the ability to make that investment to achieve long-term results. Once again, the alignment of the cost containment procedure with the strategic objectives will aid in the realization of the organization's vision.

Performance Measurement

It is important to measure the performance of the organization both before and after any cost containment efforts or improvements in technology so that progress can be monitored and goals can be realized in an objective way. This plan helps to not only educate the organization about the impacts of a cost containment procedure, but also to measure the extent to which performance has been improved.

VA Case Study: Cost Containment Through Centralization of Services

Business Problem

The Veterans Health Administration Rocky Mountain Network was established in March 1996 as one of the 22 Veterans Integrated Services Networks (VISN). The role of the VISN is to deliver, coordinate, and manage the care of veterans who live within the defined geographic area. The Rocky Mountain Network, VISN 19, spans more than 450,000 square miles across several states and is one of the largest networks in terms of geography. It services veterans in the entire states of Montana, Utah, Wyoming, nearly all of Colorado, and portions of Idaho, Kansas, Nebraska, Nevada, and North Dakota.

Healthcare delivery in VISN 19 is influenced by many factors, including the large geographic area, a wide range in population density, and the socioeconomic status of the population. Significant portions of the population have an income below poverty level, and much of the service area is designated as "Health Manpower Shortage Areas," especially for primary care and mental health services professionals. To provide a full spectrum of services to veterans in remote areas, the VHA uses the services of private sector providers. This type of care is commonly referred to as non-VA provided care, or fee-basis care.

Delivering, coordinating, and managing health care is uniquely challenging in an environment that is geographically dispersed and has wide variation in healthcare delivery capability. To be successful, the VISN must have information that identifies the healthcare needs of its population and indicates how these needs can be met. Having this information available allows the network to proactively plan for services that must be provided outside the VHA system and manage the cost of those services.

The major business problem facing VISN 19 was that information regarding services received outside the VHA system did not become available until after the service had been delivered. The timing for receipt of this information prohibited the network from controlling both the cost and quality of care received by veterans outside the VHA system. VISN 19 was unable to do the following:

- Control variable costs by negotiating fees with a private sector provider before care was delivered
- Control variable costs by preventing the delivery of unnecessary or duplicative services
- Control fixed costs by eliminating duplicate processes

The goal of the cost containment effort for VISN 19 was to reduce overall operating costs. This change would allow the network to provide an increased number of services to veterans while remaining within budget.

Historical Approach to Managing Non-VA Provided Care

Before establishing the VISNs, the VHA functioned as a decentralized organization with operations focused at the Medical Center level. This type of organizational structure led to duplication of effort and services within the VHA enterprise. The management of non-VA provided care is an example of the duplicate efforts and inefficiencies commonly observed in a decentralized system.

Historically, veterans who required services outside VHA facilities would identify a non-VA provider and obtain the services. Once the service was delivered, the provider would submit a claim for the service to the local medical center. The claim was processed by Medical Administrative Services (MAS) personnel based at each medical center. The steps to process a claim included determination of medical necessity, identification of the reimbursement rate for the service, and approval of payment. Customized software designed to capture service-specific information and the amount of payment was available at each medical center.

At regular intervals, the information was batch processed from the medical center to a central facility. The central facility was accountable for these steps:

- Maintaining the VHA workload database
- Editing the claim information for accuracy
- Approving payment for the service
- Providing reports to the medical centers indicating the amount of payment that was approved

Each medical center used this information to update their budget for non-VA provided care. Despite the presence of standardized software, each medical center had developed its own process for managing and monitoring non-VA provided care. Variations in the criteria for determining medical necessity, the process for approving claims, and the skill set of personnel reviewing the claims existed across the medical centers.

The Solution

VISN 19 developed a plan to more effectively manage the non-VA provided care that was based on existing private sector health plan models. Specific components they focused on included provider network management, preauthorization of services, and case management. To realize the plan, VISN 19 was required to design new processes, acquire new skill sets, and select enabling technology.

The Process

The network established a central Network Authorization Office (NAO) to support and administer the new process. When a veteran contacted the NAO, they had immediate access to a nurse who could provide education, medical advice, and preauthorization for a service outside the VHA system. When providing a preauthorization, the NAO nurse determined the medical necessity of the service using established criteria. Services determined to be medically necessary were preauthorized, and authorization information was retained and used for claim adjudication and as a reference database for services required outside the VHA system. By providing the authorization before the service was delivered, the NAO was able to contact non-VA providers and negotiate a discounted rate for the service.

Frequently, veterans called the NAO simply to have access to medical information and advice. Personnel working within the NAO became very familiar with the health issues of specific veterans and used a case management approach when dealing with these individuals. A segment of the veteran population previously unidentified within VISN 19 was composed of veterans with spinal cord injuries who were clustered in a defined geographic section of the network. Having information funneled through a central source allowed the NAO to recognize the existence of this group and arrange for services specific to their needs.

The People

The new process required skill sets and work experience that simply did not exist within the VHA. The preauthorization process and case management approach required skill sets frequently found in a managed care environment. To quickly fill the gap, nurses with managed care experience were brought into the NAO. Existing staff members were provided with a significant amount of training related to the principles of managed care, the new procedures, and the new equipment.

The Technology

The existing software for non-VA provided care did not meet the requirements or workflow of the new process. A vendor application that was DOS-based and designed to support case management and authorization tracking was selected. In addition to the software, the NAO was equipped with standard desktops and phone lines with 800 (toll-free) capability.

The process changes that were designed and implemented by VISN 19 and the benefit that can be realized from the change are outlined in Table 13.1. The VISN 19 plan was presented to VHA leadership and approved for pilot implementation. It was agreed that the pilot would be evaluated at 6- and 12-month increments. Based upon the results of the evaluation, the pilot would be considered for roll-out to the other VISNs within the VHA enterprise.

Implementation Barriers

Implementation of the new process for non-VA provided care faced multiple barriers throughout the course of the pilot.

- The DOS-based application that was selected to support preauthorization and case management required the development of multiple inter-

TABLE 13.1. Process changes and benefits for VISN 19.

Cost containment approach	VISN 19 process changes	Expected benefit
Control variable costs	• Establish contracts with non-VA providers for discounted rates • Determine medical necessity before service delivery • Triage services to VA provider if appropriate • Coordinate care through case management to reduce duplicate services	• Decrease non-VA provider reimbursement • Reduce inappropriate services • Reduce cost of care • Reduce duplicate services
Control fixed costs	• Eliminate duplicate claims processing capability at Medical Centers • Outsource services when applicable (triage and medical advice)	• Reduce salary expense • Reduce facilities and equipment expense

faces to the existing VHA information systems. Each time a change was made to one of the existing VHA information systems, a new interface had to be developed. One of the major interfaces was to the VHA billing system that feeds the national workload database. This database is used to establish VISN funding for the following fiscal year. The disconnect between the national workload database and the new VISN 19 application led to a temporary underreporting of VISN 19 workload.

• The need to obtain authorization for a service before receiving the service was perceived by veterans as the creation of an administrative roadblock. It was met with resistance by Veteran Service Organizations and almost led to discontinuation of the pilot. Implementation of the new process was slowed to allow for increased communication and education of veterans regarding the need for and purpose of the new process.

• The new process was initially established for a small portion of private sector care, but it was rapidly expanded to include all private sector care. The volume of requests coming through the NAO was far greater than the NAO's capacity to administer the requests. As a result, segments of the veteran population were turned back over to the VHA Medical Centers.

• There was resistance to change from the local medical centers that did not want to give up ownership of the process. To reduce this resistance, each facility was allowed to maintain a portion of the process. This allowance had a direct impact on the ability of VISN 19 to standardize the process across the network. The result was that duplication of services remained and fixed costs could not be reduced as originally projected.

The pilot was evaluated at the 6- and 12-month postimplementation landmarks. The results of the pilot demonstrated an increase in the continuity of care to veterans and an increase in veteran satisfaction, the latter of which was directly related to the veterans' ability to speak to a clinician and obtain advice for medical inquiries.

Improvements in the quality of non-VA provided care data were not as significant as anticipated. The ability to improve data quality was negatively impacted by the lack of process standardization across the network. Cost containment efforts were very difficult to measure, because the network lacked baseline information and specific performance metrics and targets were not established before implementation.

Lessons Learned

The major lesson learned through this experience was that a change of this magnitude requires significant planning and communication before implementation. In hindsight, some of the issues encountered by VISN 19 could have been more effectively managed through the establishment of a communication plan and change management strategy, system integration planning, and a performance measurement plan. Based on this experience, we strongly recommend that any organization seeking to transform operating practices focus on these areas:

- Identifying the key stakeholders that will be impacted by the change and developing targeted communication strategies
- Creating incentives for making the change and communicating those incentives to the constituencies impacted by the change
- Identifying expectations for the new process and establishing a plan to measure the benefits that are achieved
- Striving to achieve standardization

Vision for the Future: Bridging the Gap

Managers in the public sector today are facing many unprecendented circumstances that will cause them to view their management problems from a completely different perspective. New changes, particularly in the federal sector, have increased the necessity to adopt new ways of thinking and managing to effectively run healthcare organizations. If this new model for cost containment is to be used, then it will cause managers to evaluate problems in ways that they have not previously used. Eventually, as the gap between business practices diminishes, healthcare organizations will behave in increasingly similar ways across public and private lines.

The gap between public and private organizations is a result of traditional practices like cost containment, which cannot be directly applied in the public sector. In the past few years, cost containment has increased existing employee workloads, diminished available training and education resources, and increased the incentive to inflate financial data integral to determining funding levels. Managers have been faced with even more complex situations as Congress has straightlined Departmental budgets through Fiscal Year 2002. There has always been concern with the Congressional appropriation process, which provides departments like the Veterans Health Administration with their operating budget for any given year. When personnel costs consume most of the budget, fixed appropriation greatly reduces a manager's ability to make strategic decisions.

On the other hand, knowing what funds will be distributed in the future can improve planning. The fixed budget concept has caused all public sector managers to become more accountable. Even the lowest level manager must adhere to management guidelines imposed on the operation, and diagnostics measures should be developed that provide comparison with progress in the private sector. Benchmarking studies that can accurately compare public to private sector performance metrics need to be improved and published on a regular basis. Likewise, routine performance indicators should be compared with targeted goals to ensure that these goals are being achieved.

Cost containment methods are a major factor driving changes within the public sector, but they should be combined with an effort to reengineer business processes and generate nonappropriated money as a way to supplement the budget and introduce greater flexibility within the federal system. Without significant improvements to business operations and greater efficiencies within the existing system, any cost containment methods we use will only exaggerate the problems. As public and private systems share such resources as money, personnel, consumers, data, and technology, a combined effort to reduce costs while maintaining quality will be the key to a more effective and efficient healthcare system for the United States public.

References

Balanced Budget Act of 1997. United Stated Congress, Washington, DC.

Donelan, K., Blendon, R.J., Schoen, C., Davis, K., Binns, K. 1999. The Cost of Health System Change: Public Discontent in the Five Nations. *Health Affairs* May/June. Results of Commonwealth Fund's 1998 International Health Policy Survey, conducted by Harvard School of Public Health and Louis Harris & Associates.

Health Care Financing Administration (HCFA). 1996. Hospital Wage Indices. From *http://www.hcfa.gov/stats/pufiles*. Washington, DC.

Health Care Financing Administration (HCFA). 1999. Hospital, Employment, and Price Indicators for the Healthcare Industry: Second and Third Quarters 1998. From *www.hcfa.gov/stats/indicatr/analysis.htm.* Washington, DC.

Taylor, M. 1999. Conversion Eases Financial Woes: Public Facility is in the Black after Converting to Private Operation, Escaping Bureaucracy. *Modern Healthcare* 29(29):36.

14
Process-Oriented Strategic Information Management Planning

Col. Sue Chiang, Col. Bruce Oksol, Col. Patricia Lewis,
Maj. J. Zarate, Barbara Hoehn, Beth Ireton,
and Alex Mustafaraj

As the healthcare provider market migrates from freestanding care centers to integrated delivery networks (IDNs), the strategic, operational, and economic focus of these organizations is radically changing. Organizations are transitioning away from segmented care provision and toward managing care and wellness services across the continuum. Primary care groups are replacing hospitals as the centers of the delivery systems, organizations are becoming flatter and more successful, and IDNs are becoming knowledge-based organizations. In the midst of this change, the importance of the information management infrastructure—that is, the operational strategies, resources, technology, and integration mechanisms needed to support business strategy—cannot be overstated. The ability to rapidly gather, communicate, analyze, and act on enterprise-wide information will be a crucial factor in the successful development and ongoing management of integrated delivery networks.

Industry trends show that the primary influences in the development and successful deployment of an integrated delivery system are these:

- The level of clinical integration among the individual entities of the system
- The managed care penetration in the geographic marketplace of the IDN
- The degree of physician-system integration
- The culture of the system

These influences are depicted in Figure 14.1.

Clinical Integration

Clinical integration is the extent to which patient care services are coordinated across the IDN for the purpose of maximizing the value of services delivered to patients and members. It can be argued that clinical integration is the key to providing seamless care across the continuum and the basis of all integrated delivery systems efforts. As organizational and tech-

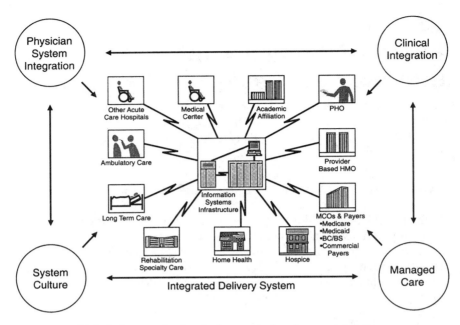

FIGURE 14.1. Influences in the deployment of an integrated delivery system.

nological linkages expand into ambulatory and alternate care delivery sites, as well as the homes, schools, and employment centers of the community, the degree of coordinated clinical efforts broadens into the total integration of wellness and illness services.

As clinical protocols and critical path initiatives develop, IDNs will need to identify the clinical and demographic data elements needed to coordinate care within the enterprise and facilitate patient care follow-through between patient visits. They will need to specify the clinical information components of an ambulatory health record and how they can be best captured, processed, and analyzed. They will need to define how the acute care record and ambulatory record will evolve into the computer-based medical record. They also must support case management and initiate organizational process changes to support uniform patient management into and within the health system.

To do this, IDNs will have to identify the best strategic and tactical approaches for expanding hospital-based technology while identifying common system functionality across all providers. They must address the unique information and technology needs of the individual provider organizations, and they must identify technology mechanisms for bringing hospital-based information to physicians at all sites of care delivery. This advance will improve the decision-making process and facilitate the communication of patient data captured in the physician's office, among the other care delivery settings.

Key information management initiatives to facilitate and support clinical integration include consolidating patient history into a single medical record and developing an enterprise-wide patient identifier, unified registration, interentity critical paths, and clinical protocols.

Managed Care

As managed care continues to penetrate the healthcare marketplace, efforts in cost management are intensifying. Information analysis and sharing will be key to IDNs in effectively negotiating and managing a capitated environment. Organizations will need to define the information management tools needed to communicate effectively within the system and with employers and payors. They will also need to identify what information is needed to "get the business" and "keep the business" and how technology can support these two distinct initiatives.

Physician–System Integration

As the relationship between physicians and the system evolves into risk-sharing partnerships, the ability to track and share clinical, administrative, and financial information among the partners becomes fundamentally important. All providers assuming risk must efficiently and effectively manage their resource utilization and understand their individual and collective roles in providing high-quality care to patient populations. To be successful, IDNs will need to define what clinical, business, credentialing, and utilization information is needed to manage the physician–system relationship and evaluate both parties' performances.

System Culture

The ability of the system to view itself as a single network with a common vision gives IDNs an advantage as they start identifying the enterprise-wide information technology support needed, both now and in the future. Initial efforts in systemwide collaboration include developing a unified vision and mission, exploring opportunities for cost-effectiveness, establishing affiliations, addressing community mental health issues, and jointly enhancing information services.

Given the importance of information management to IDNs, the need for insightful long-range information management planning has never been greater. Mounting demands on current information systems, coupled with dramatic technology developments, have increased the information technology options available to healthcare providers. This technology is rapidly evolving to a stage where healthcare professionals can, for the first time, see clear benefits from their investments. These gains do not come without inherent complexities and cost, and charting the correct course demands a level of executive participation not traditionally associated with information technology planning efforts.

In response to the strategic and tactical efforts under way, IDNs seek to develop an organization-wide strategic information management plan to guide decisions for the next several years. The major focus of this planning effort should be to establish guidelines and an overall framework for developing an integrated portfolio of information systems to support the IDN's changing business environment. The information management (IM) plan should effectively synchronize the changes in processes and information technology investments with the organization's strategic business direction and strategies.

Examples from the private healthcare sector indicate that IM planning, not information technology (IT) planning, has better positioned IDNs to successfully implement enabling technologies and achieve long-term performance improvements. There are several reasons:

- Information management planning is driven from the business strategies of the organization.
- It engages the senior leadership of the organization and is oriented to the key business and clinical processes associated with these business strategies.
- It is focused on a shorter planning timeframe so that it can be adjusted rapidly to the dynamics of the business environment.
- The output of the planning process is the identification of information management solution sets that incorporate process design, organizational change, and information systems.

Perhaps the most significant part of information management planning is that it sidesteps the traditional focus on acquiring information systems and focuses on improving the performance of key processes needed to achieve the business objectives. Information systems acquisition becomes an essential component, rather than the goal itself. This approach leads to more innovative uses of multifunctional technologies (e-mail, Internet, faxing, *and paper*) as interim and possibly permanent solutions to information management needs.

IM Planning Approach

Figure 14.2 presents an example of a sound IM planning approach, described in the subsections that follow.

Overall Approach
Strategic Information Management Planning

Develop alignment, consensus, and buy-in

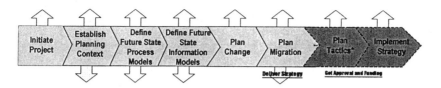

Identify and launch "NOW" projects

FIGURE 14.2. IM planning approach.

Step I. Project Initiation

During step I, the project goals, organization, participants, and schedule are finalized; expected outcomes are established; and the communication plan for status reporting and interim recommendations is defined.

Step II. Establishing the Planning Context

Three factors have a major influence on the information management strategies and tactics of an organization: the demands of the market, the business strategies of the organization, and the current status of information support. During step II, the core planning team works with the senior leadership to develop a shared understanding of these elements and set the context for developing the IDN's information management strategy.

Step III. Define/Tailor Future State Business Process Model

During step III, the executives responsible for the operations of the organization further refine the processes determined to be essential in achieving the stated business objectives. These processes typically are identified as Access To Care, Provision of Health Services, Population Health Management, and Business Management. The future state of each core process required to achieve stated business objectives is defined, and a high-level self-assessment of current performance levels is performed or confirmed. For each major process, IDNs establish key performance measures that will enable the organizations to monitor progress against the plan.

Step IV. Defining the Information Management Models

During step IV, the future information management needs and attributes for each process are defined in concrete, actionable terms. As an outcome, the overall requirements to support the business process models are translated into application, infrastructure, and organizational/governance models needed to provide the information support.

Step V. Change Planning

Throughout the planning process, a substantial number of gaps that must be filled to achieve the desired level of information support are identified. Given limited time and resources, these gaps must be set in priority order. To begin this process, gaps will be arranged into logical groupings, or "change initiatives." Typically, change initiatives will involve both information process (business) changes and changes in information systems support.

To set priorities, each change initiative implication should be reviewed for cost and resource implications, prerequisites, risks, and business value (benefits stated in terms of anticipated improvement in performance criteria). Change initiatives should then be rated against the evaluation criteria that were previously established and set in priority order. In a stable world, priority initiatives could be translated directly into a migration plan. However, because requirements will continue to evolve in the rapidly changing healthcare environment, each initiative should also be examined to determine the technical risk and existing barriers to implementing the changes.

Step VI. Migration Planning

During step VI, the strategic planning effort is completed by sequencing the high-priority change initiatives, identifying the implementation timeframe and associated resource implications, and developing a communications plan to facilitate plan roll-out. Major components of the IM strategy should include plans for technology, process change, organization, and macrolevel resource requirements.

Because the strategy is developed by the executive leadership team, marketing the plan for understanding and commitment is an essential part of the rollout. The linkage from strategy to performance metrics to information changes is designed into the planning process, so all the initiatives will be directly tied to the achievement of a business goal. This approach should make education and approval of the plan easier, because once there is buy-in for the overall business strategies, there is philosophical buy-in for the information management initiatives. However, it will also be important to identify the implications of the plan's changes, challenges, and benefits for each major consistency.

Step VII. Tactical Planning

There has been ongoing debate about the relationship between strategic and tactical planning. Some argue that tactics have no place in a strategy, while others strongly believe that there is a need to bring the strategy down to implementable terms. The approach of First Consulting Group (FCG) involves a compromise. As part of the strategic planning process, tactical plans for two types of projects are developed: "quick hits" and durable, urgent projects (to be implemented as soon as resources are approved and available). Quick hits are changes that are consistent with the overall migration plan and will be implemented rapidly, within current budgets. These projects can begin to be implemented while the strategy is being approved and funded.

The other tactical planning efforts will address urgent priorities that are early in the migration plan, have been shown to be durable (not affected by predictable changes in business strategy or environment), and will provide immediate value to the organization. By developing detailed tactical plans for these projects while overall approval is being secured, implementation of these urgent projects will have minimum delays. This action helps to sustain momentum and makes it clear that the goal of the planning process was not to create a plan but to create change. The project plans developed during this phase will also serve as models for the continued tactical planning of future projects.

Use of Information Management Planning at the Department of Defense

The Department of Defense (DoD) delivers health care and services to the Army, Navy, and Air Force through its Military Health System (MHS). The Military Health System is composed of 12 regions worldwide and supports both internal and outsourced health services. It includes:

- 8.4 million beneficiaries
- 108 hospitals and medical centers
- 113,000 network providers
- 1,980 network hospitals
- 22,000 network pharmacies
- 480 ambulatory clinics
- 144,000 personnel

Order of magnitude is 10 times that of most private sector IDNs, but organizational, operational, and informational issues are the same when trying to bring multiple organizations together under one umbrella—in this case, the MHS—to achieve a single set of objectives. Integration issues are greatly compounded because, in addition to the sheer size of this organization, the participants who will achieve these objectives include members of the three military branches of service, the political appointees, and the government civil servants.

The Military Health System has been tasked with addressing the following goals:

- Cutting unnecessary costs
- Migrating to a wellness focus of health services for both service personnel and their beneficiaries; ensuring the fighting workforce is "ready"
- Becoming the most effective organization through the application of best clinical and business practices demonstrated either in the private or public sector

The MHS recognized that technology-driven solutions were marginally, if at all, successful in achieving these objectives, and that a more business/operational process-based approach driven by the user community was needed. An Information Management (IM)/Information Technology (IT) organization was created to migrate planning from an IT to an IM focus.

The new director of the IM organization was looking for a pragmatic, process-based framework to help move the organization from technology to process-based planning. The director embraced First Consulting Group's (FCG's) core process framework and began taking steps to develop a process-based planning approach (see the process model framework in Figure 14.3).

Approach

A workgroup was created with representatives across all military services and functional areas throughout the DoD. Five work sessions were conducted over a 2-week period, and each work session was approximately 4 hours long. The workgroup session objectives are outlined in Figure 14.4, which further describes the IT-enabled process-based planning approach used.

Although the output of the information management planning process in the private sector consists of solution sets incorporating processes, organizational changes, and technologies, the public sector must also include policy decisions to the solution set. Policy drives processes, so policies must be understood and the solution sets must acknowledge the effort required to change existing policy. The organization must understand how the effectiveness of the solution set will be impacted if the policy is not changed. Figure 14.5 encapsulates the key elements that must be balanced throughout the information management planning process.

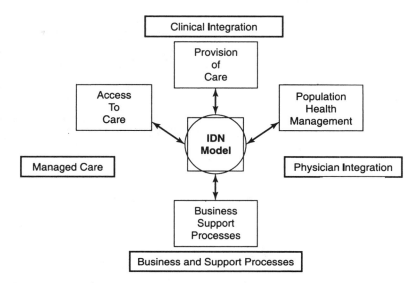

FIGURE 14.3. Core process model framework.

The workgroup's objective was to complete the first three steps of the overall Information Management Planning Approach. Over the course of several weeks, the workgroup developed a common understanding of the MHS's goals and objectives. The group then established the linkage between the organizational goals and the subprocesses that will enable the organization to achieve these goals.

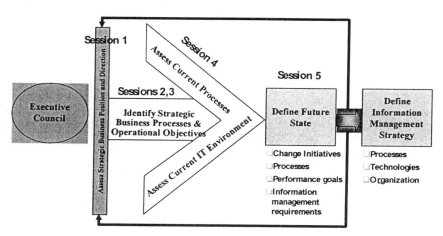

FIGURE 14.4. Process-based information planning approach..

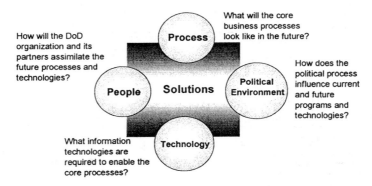

FIGURE 14.5. Elements of the information management planning process.

The core process model framework contained approximately 40 sub-processes, which were assessed based on three factors (Figure 14.6). This exercise would result in a recognition that processes are fragmented, re-dundant, and not optimized across the organization. Rarely did a rating of "good" or "adequate" appear on the worksheet; the usual assessment was "requires remediation." After the assessment, the subprocesses were categorized as "baseline" or "strategic" in nature. A baseline process was a core competency, or something that must be done regardless of strategy. A strategic process would move the organization toward a competitive advantage.

For each process, workgroup members were asked to determine the desired level of standardization. The workgroup overwhelmingly agreed that the majority of processes must be standardized across the MHS organization, or at least standardized within each service. Future state scenarios were discussed for each of the four core processes, which allowed the workgroup members to identify process initiatives to be addressed for

IDN Processes	Representative Sub-processes	MHS Process Prioritization			Sample Performance Measures
		Priority for MHS	Current Assessment	Desired Degree of Standardization	
Engage and Retain Patients/Members					
• Manage Enrollment/ Eligibility	• Verify eligibility • Maintain group policies • Maintain benefits • Maintain enrollment	❏ Strategic ❏ Baseline ❏ Not Applicable to MHS	❏ Good ❏ Adequate ❏ Requires Re-mediation	❏ High ❏ Medium ❏ Low	• Percent of members with current enrollment data • Percent of groups with current benefit history loaded

FIGURE 14.6. Assessment of current MHS processes.

the next 12 months while the information management planning activities continued.

Case Study: Langley Air Force Base–1st Medical Group Access to Care/Population Health Management

Background

The 1st Medical Group is located in Hampton, Virginia, and is part of the Department of Defense (DoD) Region 2. The Tidewater region is unique in that both the Army (McDonald Army Community Hospital) and the Navy (Navy Medical Center, Portsmouth [NMCP]) are within 20 miles to the east and west of Langley AFB. The 1st Medical Group's primary product lines include primary care, obstetrics, and dental care. 1st Medical also provides the only military emergency service and obstetrical service on the Tidewater Peninsula. Because the Peninsula is geographically separated by water from Norfolk, sharing of these services with NMCP is sometimes difficult.

1st Medical Group, along with other Air Force medical treatment facilities (MTFs) has been challenged with aggressively moving from an intervention-based inpatient strategy to a preventive, regional, population health strategy. First Consulting Group (FCG) was engaged to assist 1st Medical Group in devising local MTF strategies to support these Air Force and regional (DoD) goals:

- **Need to increase enrollment.** In an effort to decrease cost, the Air Force is planning to entice users of the direct care system into becoming enrolled TRICARE beneficiaries.
- **Need to increase capacity in the existing MTF system.** Demand for services will rise as the population of enrolled beneficiaries grows. Patient to *primary care manager* (*PCM*) ratios must be at 1,500:1. To meet these ratios, productivity of the PCMs must increase.
- **Need to increase the ease of access to services for enrolled population.** If resources within the MTF are strained, access standards will be missed (e.g., patients calling for appointments may have to wait well beyond standard wait time).
- **Need to decrease the demand for services through management of health and populations.** It will become imperative to move from a reactive, intervention-based system to a more proactive prevention and wellness-based system.

More specifically, the task for 1st Medical Group was not only to achieve the targets outlined as part of the DoD business drivers, but also to align and achieve unity of effort in meeting the organization's more immediate local business objectives:

- To expand enrollment
- To enhance customer service
- To improve productivity
- To manage population wellness/demand for services

FCG brought private sector analysis expertise and knowledge of DoD planning to help devise a coherent, aligned execution strategy that would support local, Air Force (AF), and Regional DoD objectives. The consultant team addressed this challenge by completing the following tasks:

- Validating immediate objectives and business drivers associated with access to care and population health management at 1st Medical Group
- Assessing 1st Medical Group's readiness for change
- Identifying changes in organizational behavior required to position the organization for success
- Assessing the information management environment at 1st Medical Group
- Identifying initiatives linked to access to care and population health and recommend prioritization of projects
- Developing a business case for access to care and population health management

Approach and Scope

At the Department of Defense, the Information Management organization was looking for a process-based framework for information management planning; this would aid in moving the organization from a technology-based planning process to a planning process based on clinical and business vision and associated IM requirements. As a result of a focused effort to develop a process-based approach to IM planning, the DoD embraced several core processes upon which to build the IM plan:

- Access to care
- Provision of care
- Population health management
- Management of the business

FCG provided knowledge of private sector best practices relative to these core processes, while helping the DoD define its vision, goals, and information management requirements. At 1st Medical, FCG used a process-based framework to create a case for action for access to care and for population health management. Figure 14.7 illustrates the process improvement model that was used at 1st Medical Group. Within this process improvement framework, the scope of this engagement included primarily steps I and II. Specific tasks associated with these steps were as follows:

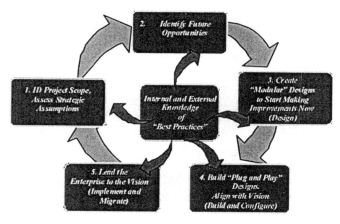

FIGURE 14.7. Process improvement model.

- **Task 1: Review Current Environment.** FCG conducted both executive interviews and interviews with key 1st Medical Group staff. Existing operations were evaluated, and a readiness assessment survey was distributed to selected personnel.
- **Task 2: Analyze Current Environment Findings.** FCG assessed the current environment against IT and process requirements, analyzed the results of the readiness assessment survey, and outlined preliminary recommendations for improvement. These recommendations were presented at an interim briefing meeting to the 1st Medical Group executive team.
- **Task 3: Outline Future State Options.** During this task, FCG worked with 1st Medical Group to begin to outline operational redesign options and to make recommendations for future access to care and population health models based on industry best practices. Projects currently planned and in progress were assessed for their linkages to access to care and to population health management.
- **Task 4: Develop Case for Action.** FCG helped outline recommended options/approaches for how 1st Medical Group could achieve its business targets through care access and population health. Critical success factors and benefits of the various options/approaches were outlined, and a final document was presented to the project sponsor(s) in a final briefing session.

Recommendations

Based on the project approach just outlined, FCG, with the assistance of the 1st Medical Group sponsors and project resources, made recommendations in five key areas: strategy, culture, organization, process/activities, and information management. The following sections cover three critical elements FCG suggested implementing.

Integrated Access to Care

1st Medical Group had many of the core processes necessary to meet their business/clinical targets either in progress or planned at the time this engagement took place. However, these processes were not always integrated or supportive of a common vision. They also did not support another crucial 1st Medical Group goal: focusing on "leading-edge" components relative to access to care in some areas and basic components of access in others. FCG recommended that 1st Medical Group embrace a model that blended basic and intermediate components (e.g., access to appointments, telephone response, triage, creating the ideal patient encounter). Based on the assessment of current and planned practices and processes at 1st Medical Group, this model was more likely to meet the goals of improved access to care, clinical staff productivity, and customer satisfaction.

Another suggestion involved hiring a clinic business manager who would own and be responsible for implementing the 1st Medical Group value-added model in at least one test site or clinic. It would also be necessary to reevaluate the scheduling and triage processes and standards between 1st Medical Group and TRICARE. In the current environment, TRICARE was scheduling some appointments and some of the larger 1st Medical Group practices were scheduling others. Nurse triage was becoming the "complaint center" for patients who could not obtain an appointment, a situation that created a serious backlog and an extra step in the scheduling process. Several other recommendations that reflected best practices in the private sector are currently being evaluated by 1st Medical Group for their applicability in a military environment.

Integrated Population Health Model

At 1st Medical Group, design and preliminary implementation of a population health management flight was well in progress. Based on the approach outlined above, FCG recommended that the programs and processes identified in this flight be integrated with access to care programs and processes. Specific suggestions included conducting focused utilization studies to identify which population health programs should be implemented first, and identifying how limited 1st Medical Group resources could be leveraged to support those programs.

FCG also suggested identifying linkages between access processes and population health processes by analyzing patient flow between population health condition clinics of interest and access to care. For example, if a patient were seen at a population health condition clinic for hypertension, how would that patient's PCM be notified, and vice versa? What should a triage nurse do if a patient calls with a problem is being seen in a population health condition clinic, or is enrolled in a disease management program? How would the triage nurse know what programs and clinics patients are enrolled in? Without looking closely at linkages and shared processes, patient satisfaction, compliance, and the success of these programs could be compromised.

Integrated Population Health Program

Built into these recommendation was the suggestion that 1st Medical Group gain a more in-depth understanding of the enrolled population; this would involve gathering information about their diseases, their demographics, and their cost by collecting and analyzing data by disease state at a regional level.

Critical Success Factors

For 1st Medical Group to successfully change current practices and redesign current processes, a number of critical success factors needed to be addressed. The following section summarizes two of the most critical factors and describes how they were approached.

Commitment of Leadership and Stakeholders

Clearly, 1st Medical Group had to identify and secure a commitment from all major groups of stakeholders. The initial challenge for the consulting team was to gain organizational buy-in and the acceptance of a long-standing executive team. The duty of the executive team and other stakeholders was to reconcile ongoing planning efforts with the consultant's recommendations.

To increase trust and achieve a common understanding of the project objectives, 1st Medical Group leadership, executive staff, and key stakeholders held several offsite meetings at key points during the engagement. At each of these, with the consultant team present, leadership expressed its vision and reaffirmed end-state objectives.

Shortly after the initial recommendations were briefed to the executive staff, several issues became obvious. Not everything could be done at once, and the executive staff needed a process to prioritize efforts. Furthermore, much time was being spent discussing changes to operational issues without the benefit of planning. Executive staff needed a midmanagement Change Management Team sponsored by senior executive staff to harness innovative ideas, prioritize solutions, and channel efforts toward the agreed-upon goals.

Borrowing the notion of "goal champion" from the Air Force Medical Service Mission Support Plan helped facilitate unity of effort. Goal champions act as definitive sponsors for recommendations and help align and integrate strategic planning objectives with locally researched solutions. To ensure success and maximum efficiency, these goal champions (together with the change management team) should be ready to partner with the consultant team and should be committed to developing solutions as recommendations are formulated. The consultant team should be free to use the change management team as a resource to learn the local organizational culture and leverage that knowledge toward long-term success. This should be viewed as a win–win partnership.

Information Management Support

A technical infrastructure, including an information management support structure, was needed to support new strategies and to support collecting data when and where needed. This need has proven to be one of the more challenging aspects of implementing Population Health and Access to Care programs. Flux in the status of regional/local databases and lack of accurate coding of procedures, visits, and records makes the data questionable, in the best of cases. Although valuable data exists, access to these depends on the availability of specialized programmers who can execute the necessary data retrievals. The project team found no consensus among queried resources on what databases would produce a reliable data set for Population Health.

In the case of Access to Care, the data were also available but of dubious value. Multiple appointment processes and widespread use of nonstandardized appointment types made it difficult to gauge routine access and next-day appointment availability. On the positive side, the executive staff realized the importance of data and began building this resource under an Information Management Flight. It has fully supported the addition of coding resources, of clinic template management to increase productivity, and the use of standardized appointment types.

Lessons Learned

1st Medical Group embraced the majority of the recommendations that were presented. Several of the recommendations were not accepted, however, due to timing, staffing, and cultural constraints. On careful reflection and evaluation, 1st Medical Group learned several key lessons:

- **Set and manage expectations.** Setting and continually managing customers' expectations is a key to making progress in any effort. Policy, cultural, and service barriers need to be identified, articulated, and addressed when setting expectations.
- **Develop and execute a communication plan.** Effective, comprehensive, and timely communication is a key success factor when working in the public sector. Formal meetings are insufficient for relaying ideas and recommendations. There are layers of preparatory meetings, prebriefings, and informal briefs that must be executed before a formal meeting;

these may occur within services, across services, or within a MHS organization itself. Interim updates with the consultant team should discuss progress, sensitive issues, and preferred/private industry best practices. "What-if" scenarios should be clearly outlined, discussed, and challenged. Ideas must be formulated quickly and "road-tested" long before the final outcome is determined.

- **Clarify roles.** A preparatory offsite meeting with the consultant team, Change Management Team, and appointed goal champions and other stakeholders should be conducted. During this meeting, clear delineation of the change management process, each player's role, and the project's mission should be clearly reviewed. How the project supports the organization's goals and objectives should be outlined as well.
- **Build a flexible plan that can be segmented in increments.** The MHS is in perpetual transition. There is built-in turnover, from the political appointees (every 4 years) to the military personnel (from 18 months to 3 years). These personnel want to make their mark during their tenure, and recommendations must fit those windows of time. It is a challenge to develop a strategy that can be implemented in incremental chunks and can achieve enough credibility and momentum to transcend personnel turnover.
- **Maintain strong sponsorship.** Plans need sponsorship to be successful. Sponsors may be executives who participated in the development of the plan and can continue to "sell" the vision of the organization. They reconfirm the organization's direction and communicate how each increment of the plan helps the organization reach its ultimate goal. The sponsors see the plan through to completion.
- **Understand and incorporate cultural and political challenges.** Information management planning involves organizational, policy, people, and technology changes. The MHS is composed of two of the oldest institutions in this country: the military and the government. Planners must appreciate the traditions of these institutions and their reaction and readiness to change. Change initiatives that challenge long-standing cultural beliefs will be much more difficult to achieve and may require many incremental steps to be successful. Policy also does not move quickly. Planning constraints must be identified early in the process, and reasonable timeframes for resolving them must be determined.
- **Discuss requirements in terms of business needs and expected value.** The MHS speaks in terms of application acronyms when asked to discuss their needs. The process framework has provided the user community with a mechanism to discuss their business needs with each other. The framework also requires the users to consider what the expected value should be as a result of improving/implementing this process. The talk is now shifting from application solutions to operational objectives and expected outcomes.

- **Work to break down silo thinking.** The MHS has been silo driven. Each branch of service is a silo, the functional areas are silos, and the care delivery sites are silos. Information management planning attempts to break down these silos and move to cross-continuum requirements for information. An organization comfortable with silo thinking will attempt to take the core process model framework and create new silos: Access to Care, Provision of Care, Population Health, and Business Management. Efforts must be made to understand the linkages/integration points for the processes that move organizations from data collectors to knowledge generators.

Conclusion

1st Medical Group gleaned valuable insight and confirmed necessary changes in its strategy. Although it was important to revise the way they conducted operations, they realized that implementing recommendations is still a local, tactical endeavor and is what makes this strategy executable. Implementing changes to processes and practices that affect access to care and population health management requires progressive leadership, including a change management team and goal champions who are responsible for ensuring that approved recommendations are implemented.

The experience of 1st Medical Group can serve as a model for other organizations as they launch their own efforts in strategic information management planning. In this new century, these efforts will be integral to their success. As integrated delivery networks are transformed into knowledge-based organizations, those that fail to keep up will falter in the absence of a sound strategy to gather and analyze timely, accurate enterprise-wide information.

15
Data Quality Case Study

WENDY CARTER AND CYNTHIA FODOR

The poor quality of organizational data is a growing concern, one that is affecting all industries. In health care, this issue is particularly salient. Data are no longer used for only internal purposes; healthcare organizations now depend on externally generated data for clinical decision making, quality assurance, cost and utilization analysis, and benchmarking.

How serious and widespread is the problem of poor or incomplete healthcare data? Merida L. Johns and data quality expert Thomas C. Redman cite studies in which 20% to 80% of patient charts in healthcare institutions were missing crucial data like complete physician notes. Johns cites a 1988 study by Hsia et al. documenting error rates of more than 20% in the diagnosis and coding of patient medical records (Redman 1996, p. xix; Johns 1997, p. 194). Such poor data quality can cost an organization time, money, and the trust of clients or patients. For example, Redman notes that typical error rates are 1% to 5%, which translates to 10% of the revenue for a medium to large organization (Redman 1996, pp. 7–14), or 40% to 60% of service organization expenses (Redman 1996, p. 82). Larry English cites Joseph Juran's work, indicating that poor quality costs an organization 20% to 40% of sales because of customer complaints, rework, and throwaway work (English 1999, pp. 11–12).

By contrast, high-quality data can reduce organizational costs and help make positive contributions to the bottom line. It can eliminate redundant files, databases, and processes; reduce the need for corrections and rework; and provide customers, clinicians, and senior leadership with accurate, timely, and meaningful information (English 1999, pp. 3, 458; Redman 1996, pp. 6–9).

Although healthcare organizations clearly must focus more attention on the quality of the information they use to make clinical and strategic decisions, data quality programs still are not as prevalent in health care as they are in other industries. In many cases, data quality has been so departmentalized that the errors and inconveniences have simply been tolerated. However, now that information is considered an enterprise resource that enables rapid, significant, and strategic decisions, data quality is being recognized as a key to success. The increasing number of data warehousing projects in healthcare organizations is also contributing to this heightened awareness of data quality. According to Merida Johns and Ken Orr, data warehousing projects are the primary reason managers have started to focus attention on data quality (Johns 1997, p. 194; Orr 1998, p. 69). Many recent data warehousing projects have failed, not because of the quality of the coding or table structures, but because of the poor quality and reliability of data sources.

In 1998, the Veterans Health Administration (VHA) identified a need to examine the quality of the data used for decision making and initiated a data quality project in response. The following case study discusses the key issues that generated interest in the project; the Data Quality Summit that marked its launch; roles, responsibilities, and action items of the project's working groups; and plans for the future. Applicable and relevant, this case study should be reviewed by any healthcare professional who recognizes our increasing need for improved data quality.

Background*

The Department of Veterans Affairs (VA) was established March 15, 1989, with Cabinet rank succeeding the Veterans Administration and assuming responsibility for providing federal benefits to veterans and their dependents. Headed by the Secretary of Veterans Affairs, the VA is the second largest of the 14 Cabinet departments and operates nationwide programs of health care, assistance services, and cemeteries: the Veterans Health Administration (VHA), the Veterans Benefits Administration (VBA), and the National Cemetery System (NCS).

Led by the Under Secretary for Health, the VHA is the VA's healthcare system and the largest integrated delivery system in the United States. It includes 172 medical centers, approximately 551 ambulatory care and community-based outpatient clinics, 131 nursing homes, 40 domiciliaries, and 73 comprehensive home care programs. VA healthcare facilities provide a broad spectrum of medical, surgical, and rehabilitative care.

In fiscal year 1999, the VA expects to treat approximately 750,000 patients in its hospitals, 106,000 in nursing homes, and 25,000 in domiciliaries. The VA's outpatient clinics expect to register approximately 35.8 million visits in fiscal year 1999. Nearly 3.6 million individuals will receive care in all VA healthcare facilities in 1999.

The VA also conducts an array of research activities concentrating on some of the most challenging issues facing medical science today: aging,

---

* *Source*: Department of Veterans Affairs website, www.va.gov.

women veterans' health concerns, AIDS, and posttraumatic stress disorder and other mental health issues. A world leader in these research areas, the VA has improved medical care not only for veterans but also for the population in general.

To help maintain its standards of excellence, the VHA has implemented some of the most sophisticated information systems in the country. There are more than 140 VHA enterprise-wide databases and many more local databases. The national health information system used by the VHA is known as VistA.

Over the past 3 years, the VA has restructured its medical system into 22 integrated networks of care, called Veterans Integrated Service Networks (VISNs). Each VISN has medical centers; outpatient, community, and outreach clinics; nursing homes; and domiciliaries. Through the VISN structure, the VA can pool and align resources to meet local needs in the most cost-effective manner and provide greater access to care.

The VHA Data Quality Program: Key Issues

A number of issues led to the development of the VHA's Data Quality program. Data quality is mentioned as a key element in the VHA's strategic plan, the *Journey for Change*, which states that "accurate, consistent, and meaningful data from the VHA's national databases is critical to decision-making, performance measurement, and outcomes assessment." Also, data validity issues at the VHA had been recently identified and documented by both internal and external reviewers. Validity issues included:

- Lack of standard definitions
- Decentralized approaches to data collection and implementation of automated systems
- Local modification
- Lack of knowledge and understanding
- Difficulty coordinating more than 140 VHA databases

Data quality problems associated with medical records coding and documentation particularly affect the VHA. Incomplete, inaccurate coding and inadequate documentation of diagnosis and procedures limit the VHA's ability to benchmark patient care with the private sector. Incomplete coding and lack of documentation affects the calculation of workload and therefore impacts the amount of funding each of the 22 integrated networks of care, VISNs, and facilities receive to provide patient care.

All these issues prompted the VHA's senior leadership to take action. Together with the Chief Information Officer (CIO), the Under Secretary for Health initiated the VHA's data quality project, the Data Quality Journey.

Initiating the Idea: The Data Quality Summit*

The journey formally began when the Under Secretary for Health charged the CIO with the task of organizing a Data Quality Summit. Participants in this Summit would work to identify issues that impact the VHA's ability to produce comprehensive, accurate data and then recommend action plans that would best address the issues. The Data Quality Summit was designed and planned by a steering committee led by the Co-Director of Health Information Resources Services, with key input from the Deputy Under Secretary for Health.

The Summit was held in December 1998 in Washington, D.C. Approximately 150 people attended the Summit, including clinical and administrative stakeholders from Headquarters and the VA field facilities, other federal agencies, and veterans' service organizations. Participants prepared for the Summit by writing a two-page paper on a crucial data quality issue. All papers were then posted on the VHA's Data Quality Summit website so all participants could read and review the issues before attending the meeting. Major issues identified in the papers as problematic included timeliness, completeness, accuracy, and documentation of data.

Summit Workgroups

At the Summit, 12 workgroups were formed to facilitate discussion about the design of a data quality action plan. The groups, designed to mirror different stages of data management, were organized by local, VISN, and national perspectives. Each group attended two Summit sessions, organized around three major tasks:

- Assessing the gap between current data quality practices and the desired data quality practice
- Developing action items to close the gap between current and desired data quality practice
- Identifying and prioritizing the most critical areas to address

Expert Presenters

The perspectives and experiences of industry experts in data quality/ information management set the tone and focus of the Summit. In a presentation on "Understanding the Information Requirements of Healthcare Processes," Barbara Hoehn of First Consulting Group provided an intro-

---

* *Source*: Data Quality Summit Summary Report, January 19, 1999.

duction to current and emerging market trends driving healthcare provider strategies and tactics and discussed the evolution toward Information Management. The process approach set forth in this presentation would ensure top-down and bottom-up alignment by addressing the needs of the patient, the information needed to support patient services, and the model that best supports clinician decision making.

In "Crafting a Data Quality Program: Keys to Getting Started," Thomas Redman of Navesink Consulting Group gave practical advice that would help project members adopt the right approach as they began moving theory into practice. According to Redman, a database can be compared to a lake. Once they become polluted, there are two ways to clean them: use filters or eliminate the pollutant. Because huge quantities of data are produced every day, it is difficult to clean databases with filters, and process improvement is more efficient and cheaper. By focusing on identifying the source of the problem (the pollutant) and eliminating it, organizations can prevent future data quality problems.

In keeping with this advice, the VHA was instructed to study their critical business processes and identify variations in the processes that cause data quality problems. Redman recommended studying the processes with a clipboard instead of a computer, noting that "if you can't make the business process work in that manner, then you can't make it work when computerized."

After all the groups reported on the gaps, ideas, vision, and proposed action areas, the findings were summarized. Redman recommended five action plans to close the gaps between current and desired data quality practices. The resulting project would do the following:

- Create a Data Quality Council and a Standards Process Group that report to the council
- Define process standards
- Define and implement "local accountabilities for data"
- Develop a data quality patient data access analysis and action plan
- Develop a data quality education, training, and communication program

These five action plans formed the basic structure of the VHA's Data Quality program.

Assigning Roles: The Data Quality Council and Workgroups

The structure of project membership was the next major decision to make. The VHA decided that the program would consist of a Data Quality Council (in accord with the Redman recommendations), plus an advisory group and five operational workgroups.

Data Quality Council

The Data Quality Council would act as the advisory group for the program. The roles and responsibilities for the Council were developed at the Summit. Specifically, the Council would provide leadership for the data quality program, interact with other leadership bodies in the organization to prioritize data quality projects, implement change to improve information and process management, set targets for improvement, and establish accountability. The Summit participants recommended that a subteam report to the Council and that a high-level leader like the Deputy Under Secretary for Health chair the Council.

Data Quality Journey Workgroups

Five workgroups were formed, one for each of Dr. Redman's five action plans:

- The Data Quality Council/Leadership Workgroup
- The Standards Process Workgroup
- The Local Accountabilities Workgroup
- The Employee Education, Training and Communications Workgroup
- The Patient Access Workgroup

At the Summit, two chairpersons were appointed to lead each workgroup. The chairpersons, all clinical, administrative, and information systems professionals from headquarters and the field, volunteered to take on this responsibility.

Laying the Foundation: Workgroup Goals and Participation

Membership

Participants from the Summit volunteered to join one or more workgroups. The process was self-selecting—members chose to participate in the group in which they were most interested. The size of the workgroups ranged from 15 to 38 people. The members, who represented Headquarters, VISNs, and the local levels, included:

- CIOs
- Clinical and program managers
- Representatives from the finance office
- Systems and computer specialists
- Planners
- Decision support staff
- Pharmacists

- Education officers
- Medical center directors
- Physicians
- Research and development staff
- Chiefs of staff
- Clinical program managers
- Data architects

Active participation on the teams varied. Because the chairpersons and many of the members were required to travel extensively for their jobs, all members could not attend all the meetings. Many members wanted to participate in an advisory rather than a participatory role.

Vision, Mission, and Goals

During the first phase of the project, the chairpersons came together for one face-to-face meeting. At that meeting, they developed the vision, mission, and goals of the Data Quality Journey (Table 15.1). The workgroup's objectives and action items supported the goals of the project.

Meetings and Communications

Each workgroup decided to hold a standard monthly conference call, the preferred mode of group communication for members located all over the country (most day-to-day workgroup communications would occur over e-mail). Meeting via telephone would minimize the costs and timing issues associated with hosting meetings for such a large number of participants. To direct conversation to the most important issues, one of the chairpersons would facilitate each meeting.

TABLE 15.1. Vision, mission, and goals of the data quality journey.

VISION
Reliable data for healthcare professionals.

MISSION
Make data quality an integral part of all care delivery and business processes.

GOALS
1. Integrate education into every process to improve data quality.
2. Promote employee awareness about data quality—its relevance and impact on their daily work.
3. Promote the belief that accountability for data quality begins with each and every employee.
4. Improve patient access to their data so they can partner in their care.
5. Promote a common understanding of data characteristics.
6. Standardize the approach to data collection and use.

As a tool to encourage further communication between workgroup members and other VHA employees interested in data quality, a Data Quality Journey website was created on the VHA's intranet. Meeting minutes, work plans, issues logs, contact lists, and other documents were posted to the site. This easily accessed, up-to-date information proved to be a critical success factor. Everyone knew where to get current information, and everyone had ready access to their work and the work of other teams. The availability of this information built open communication and trust.

Taking Action: Workgroup Roles and Responsibilities

The first charge for all workgroups was to define the priority action items on which their team would work. The action items from the Summit were analyzed and assigned to one of the five workgroups. Each team ranked the items and chose three or four to work on. The action items had to be aimed at meeting a critical business need, and the groups had to be able to accomplish each within a 6-month time frame. The groups began working on the action items in March 1999 and expected to complete the work by September 1999. Tables 15.2 and 15.3 display the major goals and high-priority action items, and the following section clarifies the roles and responsibilities of each workgroup.

Data Quality Council/Leadership Workgroup

The Data Quality Council/Leadership group assumed the role of the subteam to form and operationalize the Council. This workgroup would:

- Establish a management board that defines data standards.
- Charter a high-level action group that will act as a review board for data quality issues. The group would oversee the work done by the Data Consortium, the Standards Process workgroup, and other VHA groups developing processes/procedures/policies to improve data quality.
- Establish a National Data Validation Task Force to deal with local, VISN, and national levels.
- Create a Data Registration Authority.

Standards Process Workgroup

The Standards Process group, according to the recommendations of Summit participants, would implement standard processes for these items:

- New data elements and data elements no longer accessed for use
- An education, training, and communication program

- Identification of appropriate data sources for information required by decision makers
- Simplification of access to information required by decision makers
- Certification and validation of data

The Standards Process workgroup assumed these responsibilities and worked with other data quality workgroups to ensure that the local levels would receive communication and education on standards processes. This group may stay together after the first phase of the project is completed and report to the Council, or it may become a subteam of another project group, such as the Data Consortium. The Data Consortium is composed of representatives from the Planning, Policy, Information Systems, and Finance departments. They are addressing the establishment of a single point of access, standard data definitions, and an authoritative source for duplicative data.

High-priority action items included the following:

- Compile and synopsize all data standards efforts under way in the VHA. Information (including goals, group leaders and contact information, products, etc.) should be posted on the Data Quality web page. In performing this survey of efforts, the workgroup would establish itself as a data clearinghouse, ensuring that independent efforts would be cohesive. The goal was to minimize redundant data elements and initiatives.
- Develop a VHA-wide business practice requiring ad hoc and canned reports to include specific details about the data contained within them (e.g., originator/contact, source of data, assumptions used, algorithms/ formulas applied, timeframes, run date).
- Provide VHA field elements with national guidance on compliance with national healthcare industry standards for patient care data. This priority reflected the national compliance initiative, with particular focus on the use of ICD-9-CM, CPT-4, and HCFA Person Class designation, in documenting into databases the patient care delivered.

Employee Education, Training, and Communication Workgroup

This workgroup was made responsible for suggesting and implementing methods for educating, training, and communicating data quality initiatives to VHA employees at all levels of the organization. They would coordinate efforts with the Standards Process and Local Accountabilities groups to ensure that the appropriate methods are used to educate and communicate information about data quality initiatives. This group would report to the Council after the first phase of the project was completed.

High-priority action items included:

TABLE 15.2. Data quality journey workgroups: goals.

	Council/leadership	Employee education, training, and communication	Local accountabilities	Patient access	Standards process
Goals	• Articulate the organization's priorities and link appropriate business processes to be reviewed for data quality improvement • Support changes required to promote data quality • Lead efforts for developing a data quality standardization process throughout the organization • Ensure the quality of the underlying data that is used	• Partner with other workgroups and organizations to take advantage of education communication strategies • Communicate the importance of data accuracy from creation and collection to interpretation • Educate employees about the importance of data quality and their ongoing role in it • Establish communication process that includes	• Assign accountability for data from highest level down • Assign accountability at the process level and ownership at the clinical level • Establish a certification process standardizing and validation data • Ensure consistent, reliable healthcare documentation • Establish roles and responsibilities for clinical and administrative	• Use an automated multidisciplinary history and physical • Develop patient focus group to help develop a standardized patient health summary • Provide patients and their families with secure access to their health data by multiple methods • Provide patients and their families with secured information regarding medication, appointments, and preventive care	• Develop/recommend a standardized process for certifying data and identifying a veteran • Develop performance measures on data quality, similar to patient safety • Create a standard policy that states data used for decision making purposes must be certified • Review coding practices • Recommend a standard definition of encounter times • Define data needs using industry standards • Recommend/redefine

TABLE 15.2. *Continued*

Council/leadership	Employee education, training, and communication	Local accountabilities	Patient access	Standards process
for performance measurement • Establish appropriate subgroups, defining specific policies/procedures and an implementable plan • Define accountability for data quality at the VAMCs, VISNs and Corporate levels	standards for the data user community • Recommend a competency certification process for employees • Provide tools for transforming raw data into usable information • Create skilled subject matter experts • Identify and provide for educational needs specific to clinicians and providers	issues at each level • Establish clinical ownership for data feedback and availability • Create standard data definitions and business rules for interpretation		structure for sharing diagnostic codes (e.g., 701/501) • Recommend/develop bundling for inpt/outpt/amb surg/other • Formalize process and controls on data and information management • Identify/recommend an effective measure of data validation • Recognize that data standardization will become VA policy and will be assessed through audits and performance measures

TABLE 15.3. Data quality journey workgroups: high-priority action items.

Council/leadership	Employee education, training, and communication	Local accountabilities	Patient access	Standards process
Establish management board that defines data standards	Create availability/accessibility of information management tool sets, ensuring ease of use	In coordination with non-VA care task group, ensures all data is captured and available for non-VA care	Develop patient focus groups to assist in the development of a standardized patient health summary	Compile and synopsize data standards efforts, post information on the Data Quality web page, ensure that efforts are cohesive, minimize redundant data initiatives
Charter high-level action group as a review board for data quality issues to oversee work done by the Data Consortium, the Standards Process workgroup, and other VHA groups	Adapt educational solutions from existing sources (i.e., learning maps)	Determine areas where trust of the data is most vital to the business and improve at least one of these areas at the local level	Allow patients access to their own data by multiple methods	Develop a VHA-wide business practice that ad hoc and canned reports include specific details about the data contained therein
Establish National Data Validation Task Force to deal with local, VISN and national levels	Optimize and improve understanding of existing systems (VistA/DSS, etc.)	Manage business processes that capture data	Provide patients and their families with information about appointments, preventive care, and medication	Provide VHA field elements with national guidance on compliance with national healthcare industry standards for patient care data
Create Data Registration Authority (meta data, ISO/IEC 1179)				

- Create availability/accessibility of information management tool sets, ensuring ease of use to improve understanding of data quality for the end users (i.e., consideration of the human factor involved in use of tools)
- Adapt educational solutions from existing sources (e.g., learning maps)
- Optimize and improve understanding of existing systems

Local Accountabilities Workgroup

The Local Accountabilities workgroup was made responsible for ensuring that data quality initiatives were brought to the local levels, which own most of the business processes that generate data quality problems (e.g., patient registration, coding). This team would work closely with the Standards Process and Employee Education, Training, and Communications groups. The group would report to the Council after the first phase of the project was completed.

This workgroup would:

- Ensure, in coordination with non-VA care task group, that all data are captured and available for non-VA care.
- Determine areas where trust in the data was most vital to the business and improve at least one of these areas at the local level.
- Manage business processes that capture data.

Patient Access Workgroup

The Under Secretary for Health was charged with providing veterans with access to their health information. The Patient Access group would be responsible for addressing this charge. They collaborated with other project groups at the VHA to assess veterans' needs for access to their own healthcare information and to general healthcare information like educational materials on preventive care. After the first phase of the project, this group may become an advisory committee for all VHA projects focusing on veterans' access to information.

This workgroup would:

- Develop patient focus groups to assist in the development of a standardized patient health summary.
- Allow patients access to their own data (electronic medical record, progress notes, treatment plans) by multiple methods.
- Provide patients and their families with information regarding appointments, preventive care, health maintenance, and medication.

Plans to Accomplish the Action Items

Each team developed its own specific workplan, all of which were tracked and reviewed at the monthly meetings. Each plan included a task to assess the current environment. In doing so, the groups discovered that some of their efforts were similar to work being done by other groups. For example, the Standards Process workgroup had action items similar to those of the Data Consortium, and both groups were working on a task to develop/recommend standard report legends. They are now working together to accomplish this task.

The Patient Access workgroup had similar goals to those of two Internet project groups, the Veterans Focused Internet Redesign Project (VFIRP) and Health eVet. The Patient Access group developed a list of questions to assess veterans' needs for access to healthcare information and determine what they wanted to see on a health summary. The VFIRP group conducted veterans' focus groups in the summer of 1999 and distributed the questions to the participants.

The workgroups developed ways to facilitate communication between the groups during the first phase of the project. Some members belonged to more than one data quality workgroup; others were participants on related projects. These individuals volunteered to be liaisons between the data quality workgroups and the other project teams. For example, a member of the Patient Access workgroup also belonged to the Health eVet project team and kept both groups apprised of progress and issues. The key was to recognize and leverage the information, knowledge, and learning from the other teams to create synergies, *not* duplication of efforts or differences in results.

Developing Policies: Data Quality Council and Data Standards Guidance Documents

The Council/Leadership and Standards Process workgroups developed and reviewed existing VHA policies related to data quality. The Council/Leadership group then provided feedback and recommendations on the VHA directives and guidance documents dealing with data collection and systems.

Data Quality Council Guidance Document

The Council/Leadership workgroup developed a Data Quality Council guidance document. The purpose of the document is to form a Data Quality Council at the VHA and set its charge. Submitted through the formal concurrence process at the VHA, this document describes the structure of the council, including reporting relationships, membership, and frequency of the meetings. At this writing, the document is being evaluated for final approval.

Data Standards Guidance Document

The Standards Process workgroup is developing a Data Standards guidance document. This document, which establishes a policy to assist any office in the VHA in determining their data needs, assigns responsibility to the Office of the CIO. Included are:

- Procedures for adding, changing, inactivating, or deleting a data element
- Procedures to be followed to ensure data elements are consistent with recognized healthcare standards
- Communication and documentation processes to ensure data quality

At this writing, stakeholders are providing inputs concerning these guidance documents.

Evaluating Progress: Lessons Learned

During the first few months of the data quality project, the VHA learned a number of lessons that organizations should consider before embarking on a journey of this type. Key lessons included:

- Choose one central theme on which all teams can focus at the very beginning. The central theme must be an important business issue for the organization. Stovepipes or vertical silos will result unless groups work together on a common goal.
- Communication is critical for an organization the size of the VHA, especially when team members are located all over the country. In the VHA, workgroup chairpersons were brought together for a face-to-face meeting 3 months into the project to facilitate communication between the workgroups. Tools like websites and e-mail also can be used to facilitate communication.
- Support, dedication, and commitment are indispensable. In the VHA, all workgroup members and chairpersons were volunteers. Turnover and attendance were issues for some of the teams.
- Organizational commitment and sponsorship from the highest levels in the organization is critical to a project's ultimate success.
- Data quality is not an information systems department issue. It must be incorporated into the daily work of all employees. Stakeholders from all sectors of the business must be actively involved in data quality initiatives.

Looking Ahead: Future Development

This chapter has covered only the first phase of the VHA's Data Quality Journey. In truth, the journey has just begun. The VHA must navigate a long, difficult path to the ultimate goal: improving the quality of the data used to support decision making and patient care at the national, regional, and local levels. Implementing these programs takes time and persistence.

As the journey continues, the VHA will engage in the following activities:

- Procedure development. The VHA plans to develop procedures to support the Data Quality Program. The Data Quality Council will oversee this task. Procedures slated for development are data quality, inventory, sharing, availability, architecture, privacy, and rules of use.
- Education/orientation of staff. Thomas Redman and Ken Orr stress the need and importance of education and training as components of successful data quality programs (Redman 1998; Orr 1998). The efforts of the Local Accountabilities and Employee Education, Training, and Communications workgroups will focus on communicating data quality initiatives to employees at all levels in the organization. Websites and learning maps will likely be used as tools.
- Implementation of the data quality program. The VHA is currently developing plans to address such questions as where the data quality function belongs in the organizational structure, what the program should look like, and what will be the staffing needs and roles.
- Evaluation of the data quality program. The VHA will consider questions like how and how often the program will be evaluated, which measures define success, and whether the return on investment will be measured.
- Planning for continuous quality improvement. Laura Baviello, Director of IS Planning and Data Management at the Hospital of St. Raphael, New Haven, Connecticut, has implemented a data quality program on the belief that an organization must incorporate data quality into the daily work of all employees to be successful (Baviello 1998). Ken Orr states that continuous measurement and feedback is critical for success (Orr 1998). For a successful data quality journey, the VHA must allocate resources for ongoing education, training, and communication.

Other Data Quality Efforts at the VHA

The Data Quality Journey project is one of several data quality efforts at the VHA. The following groups are also working on initiatives to improve the quality of the organization's data:

- Health Information Management Systems
- The Data Consortium
- Corporate Compliance
- The Data Management Program

Health Information Management Systems

The Health Information Management Systems (HIMS) department reports to the Office of the CIO. The department is responsible for medical records coding and documentation and for the National Patient Care Database Systems. The group is working on several initiatives to improve data quality at the VHA. Starting in July 1999, the VHA provided a series of weekly satellite broadcasts on medical records coding and documentation for Compliance. Quadramed and the Profile Group were among the presenters, and the broadcasts included training on data validation, medical necessity, modifiers, coding and documentation of evaluation and management, surgery, anesthesia, physician extenders, mental health, and ancillary services. The broadcasts were so popular that, after 2 months, the sessions were extended through December 1999.

The HIMS department also developed coding resources for the organization. Many resources are available to all VHA staff, including a coding resources toolkit on the VHA's intranet, a phone number for coding questions, a video education series on fraud and abuse, surgical coding, and modifiers (from American Health Information Management Association), and *Coding Clinic*, published by the American Hospital Association.

Finally, to support the VHA's Compliance initiatives, the HIMS department is developing education and training mechanisms. Under development are a coding expert panel, a coding handbook, and a web-based coding training program (in collaboration with the American Health Information Management Association).

Corporate Compliance Efforts

In 1998, the Department of Justice identified healthcare fraud and abuse as second only to crimes of violence to target for prosecution. The Office of the Inspector General, Department of Health and Human Services (HHS OIG) has identified 119 projects in their FY 1999 work plan. The Inspector General of the Department of Health and Human Services found that in FY 1997, the Medicare program alone overpaid hospitals, doctors, and other healthcare providers more than $20 billion, or 11% of Medicare payments to providers. The HHS OIG seven elements of a model hospital compliance plan were not formally issued until 1998.

The healthcare environment characterized by an aging population, increase in patient acuity, decreased inpatient hospitalization or length of stay, transition to outpatient care, alternate levels of care, and managed care have had a tremendous impact from a clinical and financial perspective.

In efforts to compete for patients and practitioners, the private sector has been focused on demonstrating that they provide high-quality care and service, effectively recruit and retain employees, and operate efficiently under various laws and regulations. Specific examples of this include the increased national attention given to healthcare costs and the attention given to cases with significant financial and criminal penalties, as evidenced through the PATH audits at the University of Pennsylvania and the pending criminal actions against officials at Columbia/HCA.

The VHA has an active plan with critical events identified. The program is based on the industry standard criteria of the seven elements of the Health and Human Services, Office of Inspector Generals Model Hospital Compliance Plan. At this writing, the final objective was to complete all training and have all compliance program elements in place by October 2000.

The Compliance Office has been formally created within the organization, and the National Policy Board has approved funding. Recruitment for an Associate Chief Financial Officer for Compliance is under way, a national Compliance Advisory Board has been created, and a meeting is scheduled for November.

The Data Management Program

The Corporate Data Registry project falls under the Data Management Program in the Office of Information. The Corporate Data Registry project group is developing centralized documentation of metadata (data about data) in the VHA systems, including sources, standards, points of contact, and definitions. The project group is developing a web-based tool to enable access to the registry.

Conclusion

Based on lessons learned, feedback from the workgroups, and information gleaned from the literature, future phases of the Data Quality Journey project will focus on one important business issue facing the organization: the improvement of ambulatory care data. The five workgroups will consolidate into one workgroup and focus on this issue. This approach will enhance communication and provide a more efficient and cost-effective structure for completing tasks. The workgroup will collaborate with the Office of Compliance, the HIMS department, and the Ambulatory Care Collaborative group on these efforts.

References

Baviello, L.E. 1998. *Enterprise-wide Data Management Strategies*. Annual HIMSS Conference, February 23, Orlando, FL.
Department of Veterans Affairs. *Journey for Change*. VHA strategic plan. Department of Veterans Affairs website, *www.va.gov*.

English, L.P. 1999. *Improving Data Warehouse and Business Information Quality*. New York: Wiley.

Johns, M.L. 1997. *Information Management for Health Professions, The Health Information Management Series*. Albany, NY: Delmar.

Orr, K. 1998. "Data Quality and Systems." *Communications of the ACM* 41(2):66–71.

Redman, T.C. 1996. *Data Quality for the Information Age*. Norwood, MA: Artech House, Inc.

Redman, T.C. 1998. "The Impact of Poor Data Quality on the Typical Enterprise." *Communications of the ACM* 41(2):79–82.

Rosenthal, S.P. 1999. "Quality Data is Essential to Preserving Quality Care." *National Association of VA Physician and Dentists Newsletter* Feb/March.

Tayi, G.K., Ballou, D.P. "Examining Data Quality." *Communications of the ACM* 41(2):54–57.

16
Resource Allocation Dilemmas in Large Federal Healthcare Systems

W. Paul Kearns III, Maj. Julie Hall, W. Todd Grams, and Gina Barhoumy

Achieving equitable allocation of financial resources within health pro-grams is a continuing challenge within large federal healthcare systems. In the latter half of the 1990s, the public sector's two largest healthcare systems—the Department of Defense's Military Health System (MHS) and The Veterans Department's Veterans Health Administration (VHA)—both faced this daunting task. The DoD's MHS and the VHA both have large but constrained budgets that must meet growing beneficiary needs: the MHS has an annual budget of $16 billion, and the VHA's annual budget is $18 billion. Not only were these systems confronted with the difficulty of distributing health resources across complex, bureaucratic organizations, they also faced the obstacle of changing years of financial allocation tradi-tion. The old system, based on rewarding workload production, strongly emphasized high utilization of costly inpatient services. This approach clashed with the healthcare industry's new focus on shifting as much inpa-tient care as is clinically appropriate to the ambulatory setting to increase healthcare quality and cost-effectiveness and improve consumer access to care.

This chapter describes how each system addressed the challenge of equi-table resource allocation by linking financial data and utilization data. The common threads running through each section suggest that many of the financial management challenges in public sector health care are similar to those encountered in the private sector.

The MHS Experience

Fiscal year (FY) 1998 was a successful "transition year" for the MHS. Their Enrollment-Based Capitation (EBC) methodology was set to cover 112 military treatment facilities, and the necessary EBC automated reports were designed and deployed. Education of medical facility managers was accomplished through several initiatives: presentations at conferences, medical financial management training programs, and a World Wide Web home page. As of October 1, 1998, the methodology and the information system infrastructure were fully implemented and deployed.

The development of the EBC model, which is continuously revised, represents the most advanced version of the MHS's capitation methodology. The first capitation model, introduced in FY 1994 and developed to allocate medical funds to the Army, Navy, and Air Force medical facilities, provided the foundation for EBC. However, while the 1994 model allocated funds based on estimated user population, EBC has the potential to allocate funds down to the facility level based on actual enrollees.

The evolution of the EBC model has been much more complex than this thumbnail sketch indicates. Here, we provide some background on the MHS, describe early methodologies that preceded EBC, and trace EBC's eventual emergence.

Composition of the MHS

The MHS, which cost $16.3 billion in FY 1999, employs approximately 99,500 military medical personnel and 39,600 civilian employees, serves a population of 8.2 million eligible beneficiaries, and has an annual budget comparable to that of such companies as Electronic Data Systems and Archer Daniels Midland. Approximately 5.9 million (72%) of these are regular users of the system. The remaining 28% do not currently use the Military Health System because they either have access to other commercial health insurance or are covered by Medicare. Of the 5.9 million users, 52% are enrolled with the military treatment facilities, 7% are enrolled with the managed care support contractor's civilian network, and 41% are not enrolled.

Most other large employers act as healthcare purchaser and payor while the selected health plan provides the benefits. This situation is different within the DoD. For its civil service civilian employees (32% of the workforce), the DoD acts like any other large employer, offering various coverage options under the Federal Employee Health Benefits Program (FEHBP). Civilian employees make an annual choice of the health plan and coverage option that meets their needs. The DoD's employer health benefit for active duty military employees (68% of the workforce) is more complicated, because the Department functions as provider, purchaser, and payor of the health benefit through the MHS.

To understand why such a complicated system is maintained to provide health benefits for military employees, we must first understand the basic mission and structure of the Department of Defense (DoD), one of the country's largest employers. To fulfill its mission of protecting and defending the United States, the DoD has evolved into a single Department that includes three separate and distinct Military Departments (the Army, Navy, and Air Force) and four distinct military services (the Army, Navy, Marines, and Air Force). Because each of these Departments developed its own medical service and mission support functions, each military installation usually had its own hospital or medical clinic where active duty military members could obtain employer-provided healthcare services. These military treatment facilities (MTFs) were originally designed to support active duty military personnel and, on a "space-available" basis only, active duty families and the retirees and their families.

The CHAMPUS Program

During the Korean War era, the demands on MTF capacity were such that approximately 40% of active duty families did not have access to "space-available" care. This situation led to the enactment of the Dependents' Medical Care Act of 1956 (P.L. 84-569) and the Military Medical Benefits Amendments of 1966 (P.L. 89-614), which entitled active duty families, retirees, and their families to limited medical and dental care from civilian sources at government expense. This was the beginning of the Department's Civilian Health and Medical Program of the Uniformed Services (CHAMPUS), intended to supplement space-available care for authorized beneficiaries. Funding for both the CHAMPUS program and the MTFs was provided by the medical budgets of the three Military Departments until FY 1975, when Congress transferred CHAMPUS funding to a central budget account in the Operation and Maintenance appropriation.

In FY 1988, as a response to the rapid cost growth of the CHAMPUS program, the Department initiated the CHAMPUS Reform Initiative (CRI). CRI, which awarded a fixed-price, at-risk contract for all CHAMPUS costs in California and Hawaii, marked the Department's introduction of managed care principles into its medical program. The experience gained from the CRI and the Military Departments' Catchment Area Management (CAM) demonstration projects served as the basis for the Department's current TRICARE program.

The TRICARE Program

The TRICARE program, begun in 1995 in Oregon and Washington, is the Department's response to rapidly rising healthcare costs and the impact of military base and hospital closures. The TRICARE program is for active duty military members, their qualified family members, eligible retirees, and their family members and survivors under age 65. It is designed to expand access to care, ensure high-quality care, control healthcare costs for patients and taxpayers, and improve medical readiness. The program is a regional partnership of civilian contractors and military hospitals and clinics. The continental United States is divided into 10 regions, each with a Lead Agent who is a commander of a military treatment facility. This agent oversees the integration of healthcare services between military medical facilities and the civilian contractor in that region.

The TRICARE program offers eligible beneficiaries three choices:

- TRICARE Standard, a fee-for-service equivalent of CHAMPUS
- TRICARE Extra, a preferred provider option that saves money over Standard
- TRICARE Prime, an option in which military treatment facilities are the principal source of care and the civilian contractor's network of hospitals and providers offers an alternate source

The Defense Health Program

In 1991, the Deputy Secretary of Defense created the Defense Health Program (DHP) under the direction of the Assistant Secretary of Defense (Health Affairs). By consolidating the medical budgets of CHAMPUS and the three Military Departments into a single program and budget, the DHP would strengthen the DoD's medical functions and establish one manager for its medical program. The only exceptions to the consolidation were military personnel funds and resources to support medical readiness functions (e.g., deployable medical systems, shipboard medical operations, and medical evacuation helicopters). These were retained in the budgets of the three Military Departments.

The initial consolidation included five separate appropriations, for a total of $15.3 billion (Figure 16.1).

- Operation and maintenance (O&M) appropriation available for 1 year to pay civilian salaries, supplies, contracts, equipment, utilities, and maintenance
- Procurement appropriation available for 3 years to acquire capital equipment items
- Military Personnel appropriation available for 1 year to pay the salaries of the Army, Navy, and Air Force medical personnel
- Medical military construction appropriation available for 5 years to build and modify medical facilities
- Medical research, development, test, and evaluation (RDT&E) appropriation available for 2 years

In February 1992, the Department's FY 1993 budget submission to Congress included the first consolidated DoD medical budget. Congress did not agree with the proposed consolidation of medical RDT&E funds in the

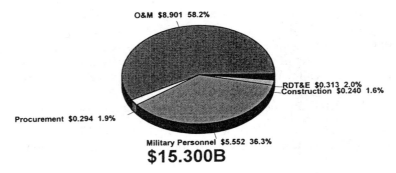

O&M $8.901 58.2%

RDT&E $0.313 2.0%
Construction $0.240 1.6%

Procurement $0.294 1.9%

Military Personnel $5.552 36.3%

$15.300B

FIGURE 16.1. FY 93 Medical program (in billions). Note: The FY 93 DHP President's Budget included $0.313B for RDT&E per PBD No. 742, December 14, 1991; however, Congress subsequently disapproved the inclusion of RDT&E in the DHP appropriation.

DHP and advised that these funds be retained in the Military Departments' budgets.

In FY 1994, the DoD Medical Program was $15.057 billion, a figure that included $9.6 billion in the DHP appropriation ($0.3 billion for capital equipment and $9.3 billion for O&M). Figure 16.2 shows the distribution of the $9.3 billion in O&M funds to the three Military Departments and three field activities. All but 4% of the DHP appropriation is allocated to the three Military Departments.

In FY 1994, approximately 40% of the O&M budget was allocated to purchase healthcare services from the private sector. The balance, 60%, was for operating Army, Navy, and Air Force MTFs and their related education and training programs (Figure 16.3). Before FY 1994, the Military Departments were funded on the basis of past inpatient and ambulatory workload

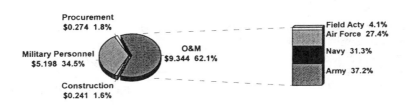

Procurement
$0.274 1.8%

Military Personnel
$5.198 34.5%

O&M
$9.344 62.1%

Construction
$0.241 1.6%

Field Acty 4.1%
Air Force 27.4%

Navy 31.3%

Army 37.2%

$15.057B

FIGURE 16.2. FY 1994 DHP O&M distribution. Field Activities include: Defense Medical Program Activity (DMPA), OCHAMPUS, & Uniformed Services University of the Health Sciences (USUHS).

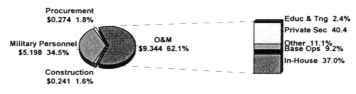

Procurement
$0.274 1.8%

Military Personnel
$5.198 34.5%

O&M
$9.344 62.1%

Construction
$0.241 1.6%

Educ & Tng 2.4%
Private Sec 40.4
Other 11.1%
Base Ops 9.2%
In-House 37.0%

$15.057B

FIGURE 16.3. DHP O&M composition. Other includes: Central Information Management ($0.248), Consolidate Health Support ($0.684), and Management Activities ($0.101).

produced in their MTFs. This funding policy provided strong incentives to increase utilization of healthcare services, especially the more expensive inpatient care. The more inpatient and ambulatory care a facility produced, the larger was its budget allocation.

Introduction of Capitation Financing

FY 1994 marked a crucial turning point: the introduction of a DHP capitation financing and resource allocation model. The historical financial incentives of MTFs—that is, the more services an MTF produced, the larger its budget grew—had been recognized as contrary to the incentives needed to support managed care operations. The concept of capitation financing had been percolating since 1975, when a major Presidential report recommended that "resource programming and budgeting for the MHSS in CONUS should be done on a capitation basis." Nineteen years later, this farsighted recommendation was becoming an established component of the civilian managed care industry.

A July 1993 policy memorandum by the Acting Assistant Secretary of Defense (Health Affairs) directed the implementation of the TRICARE capitation financing methodology. It would serve as the basis for programming future long-range budget requirements and for allocating budget resources in an objective and equitable manner among the Army, Navy, and Air Force medical components of the Department.

One of the basic purposes of capitation is to empower an entity with a predetermined level of financial resources to provide a defined population with healthcare services. The entity then determines how to allocate the funds across the spectrum of healthcare services to meet the health and wellness needs of the supported population. The first capitation model was designed to include funding from both the military personnel and the operation and maintenance (O&M) appropriations that had been the main focus in budget development and allocation.

After an initial analysis of elements of the DHP operation with the closest ties to the population served, there emerged a capitation model with three separate resource categories, further divided into subcategories. Categorizing resources helped identify and fund the medical readiness mission, enabled the application of appropriate population-based cost drivers, and facilitated comparisons between the cost-effectiveness of DoD health care and that of civilian health care. A more detailed description of each category is presented next.

Category 1: Overseas and Military Unique Noncapitated Functions

- Overseas Activities: includes all resources necessary to support the DHP's overseas medical presence. Resources are estimated on a capitation basis using active duty members and dependents as a cost driver.
- Other Military Unique Noncapitated Functions: includes all resources for Aeromedical Evacuation, the Armed Forces Institute of Pathology (AFIP), and the Military Entrance and Processing Command (MEPCOM). This subcategory is programmed on a noncapitated, level-of-effort basis.

Category 2: Military Unique Capitated and Education and Training

- Military Unique Capitated Functions: includes Public and Occupational Health, Blood, Dental, Veterinary Medicine, Optical, and Readiness Exercises. Resources are estimated using the active duty military population as a cost driver.
- Education and Training: includes the medical technical schools operated by the three Military Departments, the Health Professions Scholarship Program (HPSP), and Graduate Medical Education (GME) programs. The driver for this subcategory is the active duty military medical population.

Category 3: Capitated Medical Care

This category contains approximately three-fourths of DHP resources and is divided into these areas:

- Inhouse Direct Care
- Purchased Civilian Care (CHAMPUS)
- Other Support

These three subcategories are further divided for the 6-year long-range programming model by beneficiary category: active duty military members, CHAMPUS users, and eligible Medicare users. The purpose of the programming model was to determine what portion of the DoD budget should be earmarked for the medical program. The schematic in Figure 16.4 shows

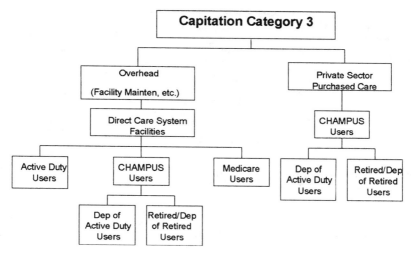

FIGURE 16.4. Capitation category 3.

the relationships of the funding subcategories and the population drivers used to program category 3 resources for the long-range budget. The allocation model identifies resources required by the Army, Navy, and Air Force.

Although this model was the initial step in defining and aligning resources, it was not a true capitation model because its basis of programming and allocation was an estimated user population, not actual enrollment. The modified methodology represented a valuable transitional approach until an actual enrollment system was fully implemented throughout the MHS. The denominator for this modified capitation formula was the number of eligible beneficiaries reported to reside within each MTF's 40-mile catchment area, modified by the rate of estimated MHS usage by those beneficiaries as determined through a semiannual user survey. The numerator of the modified formula was the historical cost of healthcare services each MTF provided to all eligible beneficiaries, plus the cost of all civilian care provided to eligible beneficiaries under the private sector care program (i.e., CHAMPUS and Managed Care Support Contracts).

Figure 16.5 shows the framework of the three-category capitation model. The computation of the category 3 allocation is linked to base year per capita costs that are adjusted to the target year and applied to the target year population. There are three types of adjustments: mission changes, management initiatives, and notional adjustments. The notional adjustments maintain equity among the three DHP components for structural dif-

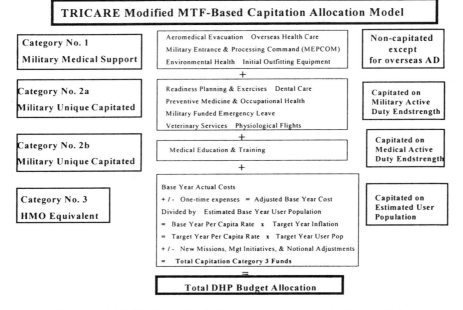

FIGURE 16.5. Framework of the three-category capitation model.

ferences not related to population. Examples of these notional adjustments are differences in funding responsibility for management headquarters, differences in facility maintenance funding responsibility, and differences in the levels of borrowed military labor received.

Figure 16.6 shows the basic capitation formula for FY 1999 that was used to determine the amount of the DHP O&M fund allocation to the three Military Departments.

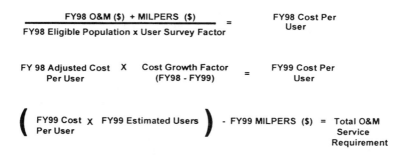

FIGURE 16.6. Basic capitation equation for FY 1999.

TABLE 16.1. Comparison of capitation allocation distribution, FY 1994 and FY 1999.

	FY 1994	FY 1999
Total HDP Distribution	$15.057	$16.309
Noncapitated	1.033 (6.9%)	1.403 (8.6%)
Capitated	14.024 (93.1%)	14.906 (91.4%)
Breakdown of Capitated		
By service		
Air Force	4.544 (32.4%)	4.755 (31.9%)
Navy	4.446 (31.7%)	4.576 (30.7%)
Army	5.035 (35.9%)	5.560 (37.3%)
By category		
Category 1	1.641 (11.7%)	1.655 (11.1%)
Category 2	1.599 (11.4%)	2.251 (15.1%)
Category 3	10.770 (76.8%)	10.986 (73.7%)

More than 90% of the Department's medical resources were covered by the modification capitation model. Table 16.1 shows a comparison of the capitation allocation distribution for the first year, FY 1994, and the most recent year, FY 1999. A comparison of the composition of the allocation by category reflects a decrease in the category 3 allocation between FY 1994 and FY 1999 and a comparable increase in category 2, while category 1 remained relatively consistent.

Six-Year Results of the Modified Capitation Allocation Model

For the 6-year period from FY 1994 to FY 1999, the modified capitation allocation model produced the following results:

- The category 3 DoD capitation rate increased at an average annual growth rate of 1.9% from $1,865 in FY 1994 to $2,051 in FY 1999.
- The combined DoD capitation rate for all three categories increased at an average annual growth rate of 3.4% from $2,161 in FY 1994 to $2,555 in FY 1999.
- The worldwide beneficiary user population decreased at an average rate of 2.1% from 6.5 million in FY 1994 to 5.8 million in FY 1999.

From FY 1994 to FY 1999, the modified capitation allocation model was the basic method of allocating the DHP budget. During that same period, the Military Departments were encouraged to use the same basic three-category model for allocating funding to their respective MTFs. However, this financing model still did not adequately address the priority of enrollment versus nonenrollment of the beneficiary population, and the model also was unresponsive to any changes in health delivery patterns that occurred after the fund allocation was decided.

Enrollment-Based Capitation

In May 1995, the Assistant Secretary of Defense (Health Affairs) issued a Transfer Payment Policy as the next step in the evolutionary development of the FY 1994 modified capitation. The purpose of this transfer payment policy was to provide a framework and identify the resource impacts related to shifting referral workload patterns caused by the new incentives of the modified capitation methodology. The metric selected to monitor shifts in referral workload patterns was inpatient diagnostic-related groups (DRGs) aggregated into base relative weighted products (RWPs) for each MTF. Although the conceptual objective of the transfer payment policy was laudable, it was never fully implemented by the Military Departments because of the burden of data accumulation, the lack of timeliness of the underlying data, and the processes involved. The transfer payment policy was subsequently superseded by the new enrollment-based capitation (EBC) policy.

In January 1997, the acting Assistant Secretary of Defense (Health Affairs) decided to proceed with the next evolutionary development of the capitation methodology with the introduction of EBC. The new EBC allocation methodology represented the third step in the evolutionary development of capitation within the Department's DHP. A 40-person, multidisciplinary workgroup was formed with representatives from the three Military Departments and from the office of the Assistant Secretary of Defense (Health Affairs) to develop and implement an EBC methodology for FY 1998. This group was tasked with developing the first version of the EBC methodology, programming this methodology into an automated model, and designing automated systems support to run the model and generate automated reports available to managers at each organizational level within the MHS.

The EBC methodology was designed to focus on the basic category three healthcare delivery costs of the modified three-category capitation model. There are essentially three primary features of EBC. The first is that a per-member, per-month (PMPM) premium is earned by the MTF for each TRICARE Prime patient enrolled. Next, additional revenues are earned by the MTF for providing care to external customers if the MTF's capacity permits. Finally, care for TRICARE Prime enrollees that is referred out by a primary care manager (PCM) is billed to the "owning" MTF, that is, the MTF where the beneficiary is enrolled. The "earned revenue" and the "cost of purchased care" are computed and reported on a monthly basis at all levels of the MHS. This information is intended to assist decision makers in making adjustments to their initial fund allocation decisions.

Basically, the EBC model is a further refinement of capitation category 3 at the MTF level, as is shown in Figure 16.7, which highlights the emphasis on Prime enrollment.

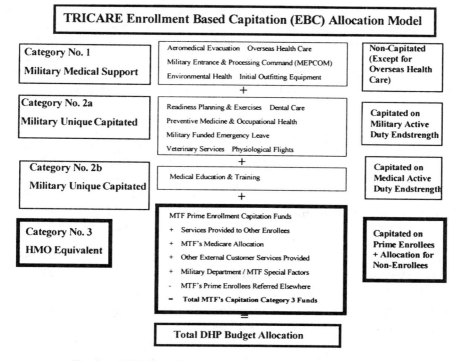

FIGURE 16.7. Enrollment-based capitation alocation model.

Success and Refinement of EBC

FY 1998 was designated as the "EBC transition year" with four main objectives:

- Implementation of the new EBC methodology
- Development and deployment of the automated EBC reports for MHS managers
- Education of MHS managers on the new EBC methodology
- Identification of data quality issues to be resolved and methodology enhancements to be implemented

During this successful transition year, the Department continued its efforts to refine EBC based on actual data analysis, encourage enrollment in TRICARE Prime, focus on delivering quality health care, and improve the quality of data collection and reporting processes that supported EBC. This phased implementation of the EBC methodology gave the Department an excellent opportunity and incentive to take an "integrated" view of its data collection and reporting processes, including data from financial accounting systems, demographic data collection and analyses, and healthcare services workload data reporting systems. Enabling this assessment process were monthly EBC scorecards that examined the targeted or budget enrollment, care to external customers, and care referred outside the facility, and then compared them with actual experience. These reports were distributed via regional servers accessible to all levels of MHS management and all MTFs.

This approach uncovered areas that could be improved; for example, numerous data quality issues were identified. Correct and complete patient encounter data was needed from the Composite Health Care System (CHCS) and the Ambulatory Data System (ADS), and the three Military Departments in the DoD Medical Expense and Performance Reporting System (MEPRS) needed to implement more uniform procedures. In addition to the data quality issues, the EBC experience in FY 1998 highlighted some necessary improvements for the next year. In FY 1999, major revisions were made and management reports were revised and improved to assist managers at all organizational levels throughout the MHS. The following is a summary of these major enhancements to the EBC methodology:

- Per capita costs were based on actual enrollee cost data from FY 1998 experience, not estimated based on full-time equivalent (FTE) users.
- Enrollment targets based on conversion of excess space available care to Prime enrollees (the previous year, targets were based on survey data about primary care visit production and utilization).
- Regions 1, 2, 5, and Alaska were fully incorporated into EBC.
- The Equivalent Lives Factor for weighting enrollees was based on actual FY 1998 costs, not survey data.
- MTFs' fixed costs were fully allocated among their own enrollees *and* other Prime enrollees.
- Based on an empirical study, labor and certain contract costs were allocated as 20% fixed and 80% variable (in FY 1998, they were 70% fixed and 30% variable).
- A "budget neutral" adjustment factor was included to reconcile EBC results with actual budget funds available.
- Ambulatory visits were converted to a "DRG-like" classification of visits for cost allocation.
- Stand-alone ancillary services were separately identified for cost allocation.
- TRICARE Senior Prime enrollees were separately identified in EBC reports.

Future Challenges for EBC

The EBC program faces several challenges in the future. Although the program does provide an objective measure of the peacetime mission performance of military facilities in terms of efficiency of operations, it does not address the effectiveness of operations in maintaining a healthy user population—a primary tenet of managed care. In addition, because the EBC program provides data-driven support for resource allocation and midyear reallocation decisions, it relies on accurate, fully developed, and timely data systems and processes. Data integrity, therefore, is a top priority. Linking occasions of service to the patient's enrollment status and accurately determining costs are crucial to the program's success. The local facility manager has always been accountable for the data generated by his or her facility, but now the visibility of EBC scorecards and MTF "price lists" will make it much easier to assess the level of attention to these information systems and the data they report.

The success of EBC may require technical skills like data analysis and data input personnel as well as new systems requirements that facilities do not have the funds to absorb. The administrative resources for daily operations and compliance requirements at the facilities are already taxed, and the commitment to EBC at the local level will be ranked with the other priorities of that facility. With no movement of dollars or realignment of resources to good performers, there may be little incentive to redirect critical resources to improve current data collection processes.

As with any major initiative in a large organization, there are those who welcome the change eagerly, and there are some that are very uncomfortable with using new management information tools. As more managers are educated in the use of this new tool and as the data become more readily available, the quality and timeliness of the data will improve. In FY 2000, we are still seeking to improve financial incentives throughout the system in ways that encourage and reward enrollment and develop financial allocation mechanisms that complement high-quality, clinically appropriate, cost-effective healthcare services for all our beneficiaries.

The VHA Experience

The VHA is the United States' healthcare system for veterans and their dependents. Through the years, the VHA has been challenged to develop a means of equitably distributing the funds assigned to the department in a way that would promote both high-quality healthcare services and appropriate utilization. The VHA system, like the MHS, requires accurate data to monitor reimbursement and has explored various methodologies for allocating financial resources throughout a large and complex delivery system. Unlike the MHS EBC efforts, which have resulted in no actual movement of DoD medical dollars or budget action taken, the VHA does have some experience with the impact of shifting dollars based on a new resource allocation methodology. To date, this experience has been a mostly positive one.

Composition of the VHA

As an operation with $18 billion a year in revenue and a patient load of 3.5 million veterans and their dependents seeking care on an annual basis, the VHA is the largest integrated healthcare system in the country. The combined populations of the states of Montana, North Dakota, South Dakota, Vermont, and Wyoming would fall 200,000 persons short of the annual patient care responsibility of the VHA system. The staff to support this system exceeds the combined federal staffs of the departments of Commerce, Education, Energy, Housing and Urban Development, Labor, State, Health and Human Services, National Aeronautics and Space Administration, and the Nuclear Regulatory Commission. The annual revenue of VHA is equal to that of such powerhouse industry-leading companies as Coca-Cola, Dow Chemical, Dell Computer, Bristol-Myers Squibb, RJR Nabisco, and for-profit peer Columbia/HCA Healthcare Corporation.

If the size of the VHA system is not enough to impress the most ambitious managed care executive in the private sector, the characteristics of the population served create a significant challenge for administrators and caregivers alike. Veterans and their dependents tend to be older, less financially stable, and more likely to suffer from social problems and physical and mental illnesses than are the recipients of private health insurance.

In addition to managing the complexity of physical, mental, and social problems, the VHA system offers a slate of benefits unheard of in most private healthcare plans. Veterans and their eligible dependents can receive everything from primary care to transplants, eyeglasses to pacemakers, office visits to extended nursing home care, surgery, mental health services, prescriptions, and prosthetics, all provided by the VHA benefits system. This spectrum of services must be coordinated and paid for within the VHA system or through services contracted with the VHA.

The VHA administers this comprehensive slate of benefits to a complex population via a continuum of providers organized into 22 veteran integrated service networks (VISNs). Similar to integrated delivery networks (IDNs) in the private sector, VISNs provide a broad spectrum of inpatient, outpatient, pharmacy, and other healthcare services within an organized network. As of October 1998, these VISNs contained 171 inpatient facilities with more than 25,000 acute care beds, 133 nursing homes, 600 ambulatory clinics, 40 domiciliaries, 206 counseling centers, and 73 home health programs. These services are distributed across the 48 contiguous states, Alaska, Hawaii, Guam, the Virgin Islands, the Philippines, and Puerto Rico (http://www.va.gov/vhareorg/reeng10-98.doc, July, 1999). Veterans can move from VISN to VISN and may seek care in different parts of the country at different times of the year when traveling.

Early Methodologies

The VHA's major task is determining how to equitably distribute $18 billion dollars in congressionally appropriated funds for medical care among the 22 VISNs. Historically, a variety of funding allocations had been attempted, all with significant disadvantages. Generally speaking, the systems were too complex to be comprehended by stakeholders and did not allocate funds in an equitable manner. As a result, the previous systems lacked credibility. Some field units were provided with too much money, which perpetuated inefficiencies, while other field units were not provided with enough money, which limited care and access to veterans who were ill.

Early methodologies (1985 through 1990) allocated funds to facilities based on the number of inpatients admitted. If it was possible to perform a procedure on an outpatient basis, providers were discouraged from doing so because of the higher reimbursement allocated to inpatient care. As the private sector moved toward more ambulatory care, the VHA's old system was mired in a complex allocation mechanism that rewarded inefficiency. Because more rewards were issued for inpatient care, facilities could develop more inpatient beds, allow longer lengths of stay, and promote the resulting increases in staffing levels and costs. VISNs in one part of the country used more than twice the funds of other low-cost VISNs that could not be entirely accounted for by patient workload or geographic differences in labor costs. Regardless of the allocation method, financially struggling VISNs came to rely on fiscal rescues from VHA headquarters.

Need for Change

From 1990 to 1996, the VA migrated to a prospective payment system similar to that of the private sector. The complexity of the model and the difficulty of the final budget allocation negotiations made for a largely negative experience. Because the system did not fund all facilities at a nationally adjusted average price, the funding, efficiency, and access disparities remained.

In 1994, to address the suspicions about funding inequities across the networks, the VHA began to examine and document resource consumption (e.g., per-patient costs, per-patient staffing levels, bed days of care, and lengths of stay) within the VISNs. Documenting the differences was the first task; developing a new allocation strategy was a greater challenge. Over the next few years, the need for a new strategy was underscored by several developments:

- In 1995, the VHA's Under Secretary for Health called for a "fundamental change in the way VHA allocates its healthcare resources" (Department of Veterans Affairs 1998)

- In February of 1996, the General Accounting Office echoed this call for change
- The VA's FY 1997 Appropriation Act instructed the VHA to create a plan to equitably allocate funds and submit that plan to Congress
- The VHA's Chief Financial Officer conducted an analysis that uncovered the extent of the historical inconsistencies in resource utilization among networks

Under the leadership of the VHA's Chief Financial Officer, a task force comprised of healthcare and administrative professionals from various VISNs met in 1996 to collaborate on a new allocation system. The chief design principles, as championed by the Chief Financial Officer, aimed to ensure that the new system would be simple, easy to administer, and focused on actual patient demands, not on increasing the previous year's budget on an annual basis. In addition, the VHA clarified their expectation to only fund cost overruns that were quantifiable, significant, and based on factors outside the control of local management.

In summary, the goals for the new allocation methodology were to:

- Equitably reallocate funds
- Reduce costs by 30%
- Increase patients treated by 20%
- Reduce unnecessary hospital care
- Increase outpatient care
- Increase access to the system
- Enhance quality

Veterans Equitable Resource Allocation

By 1997, the new allocation system, backed by a 1996 General Accounting Office (GAO) report and the United States Congress (Public Law 104-204), became the new method of distributing funds to the VISNs. Known as the Veterans Equitable Resource Allocation (VERA), the new system revealed that VISNs in the northeast and central areas of the country were significantly overfunded, whereas VISNs in the south and southwest were significantly underfunded. VERA called for a shift of over $500 million across VISNs. To ensure that no VISN facing a funding reduction was suddenly and dramatically affected, potential reductions were capped at 5% in FY 1997, 1998, and 1999; this gave local management time to plan for the reductions in an orderly fashion.

Linking financial and utilization data under VERA effected dramatic results. Sample indicators of the program's effectiveness from 1996 through 1998 include the following:

- 13% reduction in costs
- 13% increase in patients treated

- 16% less staff
- 47% less bed days of care
- 17% more outpatient visits

Through 1999, functioning as a prospective, capitated financial system, VERA moved $581 million away from the higher-cost, inefficient VISNs to those that were historically underfunded.

In the subsections that follow, we offer a closer look at VERA's effects since the new system's inception. We include proposed refinements and speculation on future directions.

VERA in FY 1997

(The following subsections extract information from the 1999 edition of the VERA book, published by the Department of Veterans Affairs.)

Although it was a relatively simple system to understand, VERA also acknowledged and addressed the complexities inherent in the veterans healthcare system. In FY 1997, VERA began by assigning a national price for each unit of workload for "basic care" ($2,857) and "complex care" ($36,955). Basic care would include veterans with healthcare needs relatively low in intensity and cost. Complex care would include veterans with more intensive service needs, such as those with spinal cord injury, traumatic brain injury, end-stage renal disease, and nursing home care needs.

VERA was composed of two funding components: General Purpose Funds, distributed to the networks at the start of the fiscal year, and Specific Purpose Funds, distributed during the year for special activities and programs. The amount of funding each VISN received for basic and complex care was calculated by multiplying their prospective workloads in each care component by the price of each care component; this ensured that all VISNs were funded equally for their projected patient workload. As Figure 16.8 indicates, VERA's shifting of funds among the networks resulted in budget increases for most VISNs.

To summarize:

- 16 networks received more funding than they did in FY 1996
- No network's funding level was reduced below 1.26% of its FY 1996 level
- For 55% of the networks, funding increases were greater than the total rate of increase in the system's funding from FY 1996 to FY 1997 (2.75%)

Because VERA accounted for the networks' varying mixes of patients, labor costs, research, and education activities, networks that had been underfunded could now operate closer to the national average cost

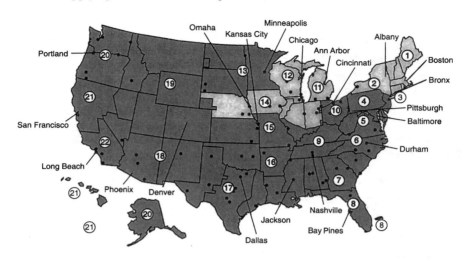

Legend

■ VISN budget increase from 1996

□ VISN budget decrease from 1996

FIGURE 16.8. FY 1997 budget allocations.

per patient. For those networks, this change would increase access to care, enhance the quality and timeliness of service, and ensure that each network has the resources to provide the same quality of care to veterans regardless of where they live. For a closer look at these changes in network budgets in the year following VERA implementation, see Table 16.2.

VERA reaped praise for the changes it effected. In spring of 1997, the chairman of the HUD Senate Appropriations Subcommittee, Senator "Kit" Bond, stated that "... VA has overhauled its allocation methodology, vastly improving fairness and appropriateness with which resources are allocated to facilities ... the new system is a tremendous step forward." A GAO report agreed that VERA was "making resource allocation more equitable than previous allocation systems."

Still, the new system was not without its flaws. The GAO report indicated that VERA required better oversight and made two recommendations for change. First, the GAO suggested the VHA track changes in key VERA workload measures and medical care practices by creating more timely and detailed indicators. To do this, the VHA implemented a tracking system to monitor the Complex Care workload relative to funding allocations and conducted a review of Basic Care workload for each network. The VHA also brought in a contractor to evaluate such factors as the accuracy of

TABLE 16.2. Change in network budgets for 1996 and 1997 with phase-in implementation ($ in millions).

	Network	FY 96	FY 97	Difference ($)	Difference (%)
1	Boston	822	811	−10	−1.26
2	Albany	421	416	−5	−1.17
3	Bronx	988	976	−11	−1.16
4	Pittsburgh	744	746	2	0.22
5	Baltimore	408	425	17	4.07
6	Durham	656	681	25	3.76
7	Atlanta	748	785	37	4.93
8	Bay Pines	928	985	57	6.15
9	Nashville	662	671	10	1.46
10	Cincinnati	489	508	19	3.84
11	Ann Arbor	633	631	−1	−0.23
12	Chicago	801	793	−8	−1.05
13	Minneapolis	400	406	6	1.51
14	Omaha	277	276	−1	−0.42
15	Kansas City	560	590	30	5.31
16	Jackson	1,032	1,090	58	5.58
17	Dallas	566	601	35	6.14
18	Phoenix	466	498	32	6.90
19	Denver	353	369	17	4.70
20	Portland	561	595	34	6.09
21	San Francisco	665	696	31	4.71
22	Long Beach	868	884	17	1.91
VHA	**National Data**	**$14,048**	**$14,434**	**$386**	**2.75**

VERA's secondary data, methods of data collection and analysis, and the timeliness of work processes.

The GAO's second recommendation was that the VHA improve the way the VISNs allocated resources to their facilities. To do this, the VHA would have to develop criteria for the VISNs to follow when creating their allocation methodologies, review and improve the methodologies on a regular basis, and monitor the impact of the methodologies on veteran care. In October 1997, the Under Secretary for Health issued a VHA Directive stating that resource allocation should be guided by certain principles that advance systemwide objectives. According to these guiding principles, network allocation systems must meet several criteria:

- Be understandable and produce predictable allocations
- Support integrated patient-centered operations
- Provide incentives to deliver appropriate care
- Support research and education missions
- Be consistent with eligibility requirements/priorities

- Encourage innovation, managerial flexibility, and increases in alternative revenue collections

Another VERA limitation was that some factors affecting the cost of patient care were not under the control of local VISN management. To make VERA truly equitable, these factors had to be determined, quantified, and used to make adjustments to the VISNs' basic and complex allocations. The factors that passed the test and became part of the VERA model included labor costs, research support, academic program support, nonrecurring maintenance, and equipment. Funds for each of these components would be added or subtracted from the basic and complex care allocations to develop the VISNs' total annual budgets.

VERA in FY 1998

FY 1998 was the VHA's first full year with VERA. During this year, significant funds were relocated to underfunded networks: 13 networks received funding increases over their FY 1997 allocations and 9 received less. To make sure VERA continued to meet its objectives, the VHA decided to engage an independent consulting firm, PricewaterhouseCoopers LLP, to evaluate VERA.

In a March 1998 report, PricewaterhouseCoopers concluded that VERA was ahead of other global budgeting systems across the world. The report called VERA a "well designed system that met VHA's goals of simplicity, equity and fairness" with its "sound" "conceptual and methodological underpinnings." (PricewaterhouseCoopers 1998). However, the firm also had some specific immediate and long-term recommendations for further improvement (Table 16.3).

VERA in FY 1999

In FY 1999, 15 networks received increased funding over their FY 1998 levels and 7 networks received less. VERA now included three levels of pricing based on patient care. The first level, for single outpatient visits (also known as "non-vested" care), would be funded at the rate of $66. The next

TABLE 16.3. Recommendations for improving VERA.

Immediate recommendations	Long-term recommendations
Simplify data inputs	Implement a strategic enrollment system
Revise patient classifications and budget split	Revise patient classes
Strengthen data accuracy and accountability	Tie performance measures to budget
Clarify and improve process	

Adapted from PriceWaterhouseCoopers (1998).

level of basic care, referred to as "vested basic" (for noncomplex recurring care), would be funded at $2,857. The highest level of funding is reserved for heavy-dependency patients ("vested complex") and will be reimbursed at $36,955 annually.

Several other changes took hold in FY 1999:

- The data integrity workgroup implemented a standardized procedure for field review of data outputs.
- The VA planned to implement a strategy-based enrollment system, as required by law.
- The VA began to implement new policies for equipment allocations and nonrecurring maintenance allocations. The equipment allocations would be based solely on patient workload, and the nonrecurring maintenance allocations would be based on patient workload but modified according to regional differences in construction costs.

According to the 1999 Department of Veterans Affairs publication on VERA, the VHA recognizes that the ongoing "development and implementation of VERA are dynamic processes" (iv). As the VHA moves forward, their challenge will be ensuring that the funding methodology that supports the care delivery system for veterans and their eligible dependents successfully balances the twin goals of simplicity and sensitivity.

VERA in FY 2000 and Beyond

In 2000, VERA will further evolve to redefine vested patients in a manner that continues to promote preventive care and health improvement. For a VISN to earn credit for a vested patient and receive the higher vested basic reimbursement, the providers must ensure that the patient enters into the system and has, over a 3-year period, at least one physical exam and various age- and gender-appropriate preventive healthcare measures.

For FY 2000 and beyond, proposed VERA refinements under development include the following:

- Establishing a transfer pricing mechanism to account for veterans/dependents who seek care in networks outside their home area
- Reviewing the patient classification system, perhaps to include functional status assessment as a way to more accurately align allocations with resources required
- Considering updating the budget split between basic and complex care categories to reflect recent actual expenditures
- Evaluating the labor index
- Reviewing "specific purpose" accounts to minimize the "earmarking" of funds and to allow for managerial flexibility

Despite continuation of the 5% lid on reductions over previous FY allocations, special interest groups continue to pressure congressional leaders to fight VERA. Typically, these constituencies are representatives of states in the northeast and north central United States. However, ongoing refinement of VERA, along with solid data supporting the methodology, continues to make VERA the logical choice for allocation distribution.

Through VERA, the VHA proved that it could do more with fewer funds, and even do it better than ever before. This triumph came about largely because VERA struck an appropriate balance between recognizing the system's complexities and remaining understandable to employees and stakeholders.

VERA dramatically demonstrates the positive results that can be achieved when financial data and utilization data are linked for the common good. According to a document on the VA website (http://www.va.gov/vhareorg/reeng10-98.doc), implementing VERA has helped the VHA increase patient satisfaction, initiate a primary care model, and garner positive comparisons to benchmarks in several preventive health and chronic disease management programs.

Conclusion

The experiences of the DoD's MHS and the VHA demonstrate how large, complex organizations with constrained budgets and increasing beneficiary needs can achieve equitable allocation of financial resources within their health programs. As public sector health care faces similar challenges, organizations can use these experiences as valuable financial management models. In the new century, as the emphasis on inpatient care becomes increasingly pronounced, such models for equitable resource allocation will help improve healthcare quality, cost-effectiveness, access to care, and consumer satisfaction.

Acknowledgment. The authors thank Bruce Hallowell for his assistance in facilitating this chapter.

References

Department of Veterans Affairs. 1998. *Veterans Equitable Resource Allocation: VERA.* Brochure, Veterans Health Administration Office of Finance.
Department of Veterans Affairs. 1999. *Veterans Equitable Resource Allocation 1999.* Publication of the Veterans Health Administration.
PricewaterhouseCoopers. 1998. Report: Veterans Equitable Resource Allocation Assessment.

Preparing the Military Health Services System (MHSS) for Capitation-based Resource Allocation. Acting Assistant Secretary of Defense (Health Affairs) policy memorandum, July 23, 1993.

TRICARE Marketing Office. 1998. *TRICARE Introduction,* OASD(HA), (*http://www.ha.osd.mil*).

VA website, http://www.va.gov/vhareorg/reeng10-98.doc

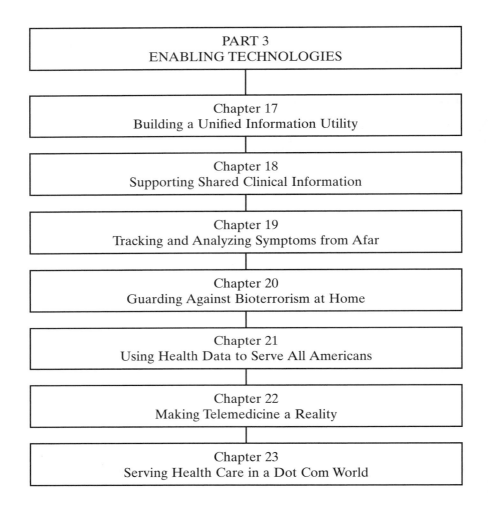

PART 3
ENABLING TECHNOLOGIES

Chapter 17
Building a Unified Information Utility

Chapter 18
Supporting Shared Clinical Information

Chapter 19
Tracking and Analyzing Symptoms from Afar

Chapter 20
Guarding Against Bioterrorism at Home

Chapter 21
Using Health Data to Serve All Americans

Chapter 22
Making Telemedicine a Reality

Chapter 23
Serving Health Care in a Dot Com World

Part 3
Enabling Technologies

17
Infrastructure and Architecture

Lt. Col. Edward Kline, Jim Demetriades, and John Manson

As healthcare organizations have begun recognizing the need to develop information technology (IT) to either become or remain competitive, sound infrastructure implementation has become a paramount strategic goal. There are countless aspects to infrastructure in this new information age, and even the most casual reviewer can quickly become engulfed in a sea of infrastructure information. When faced with such complex issues as the Internet, intranets, architectural designs, security, and various topologies, we can easily begin sinking and not know where or when to send out an S.O.S. However, rising above the waves of information need not be overwhelming. The key is to set a course determined by fundamental strategic principles, sound enterprise architectural precepts, and implementation built on a foundation of standards.

We believe the first crucial step is learning to view IT infrastructure as a twenty-first century utility. When facility planners support a decision to either acquire or build facilities, which issues do they consider first? Obviously, the location, structural integrity, and architectural issues of the facility and the surrounding grounds are notable, and utilities like heating and cooling systems, the electrical system, and plumbing have all become second nature in facilities planning. However, in this information age, how much consideration is given to the information infrastructure of the building? As we move quickly into an information-dominated environment, it is imperative that a new utility be added: IT infrastructure and enterprise designs.

Before we understand what IT infrastructure is, we must be able to describe it. Although there is much room for debate in this area, we believe that IT infrastructure includes any element that supports the transmission of voice, video, or data. As we describe later in this chapter, an ideal IT infrastructure is an integrated capability that can support all three types of transmissions. Just as all home appliances ultimately run from the same electrical distribution box in the home, so should all types of information technology be consolidated to the greatest degree possible. Today, this is most often not the case. In most government facilities, telephones still belong to the facility manager and computers belong to the Chief Information Officer (CIO). In this new century, integrated infrastructure that supports each of these communication modalities will become a critical success factor for our healthcare delivery systems.

In this chapter, we examine some business cases and case studies and look at the key principles associated with integrated IT infrastructure. These include the following points:

- Where to start
- How to approach requirements
- How to develop enterprise architectural designs that integrate and can be used as a foundation on which to build methodically
- Why infrastructure needs to be part of the enterprise's strategic game plan and addressed in an integrated fashion

Project Definition and Preparation

Defining IT Architecture

Precisely defining what the term "architecture" means within an information technology context is nearly impossible. In recent years, the computer industry has widely embraced the term architecture and applied it to so many contexts that it has become one of the most loosely used terms. Several respected definitions do exist.

- The Institute for Electrical and Electronics Engineers (IEEE) defines the term architecture as IT structures or components, their relationships, and the principles and guidelines governing their design and evolution over time (IEEE 1990).
- According to the Gartner Group, architecture has two definitions. In reference to computers, software or networks, it is the overall design of a computing system and the logical and physical interrelationships between its components. Architecture is also a series of principles, guidelines, or rules used by an enterprise to direct the process of acquiring, building, modifying, and interfacing IT resources throughout the enterprise.
- The Open Group defines information technology architecture as a detailed plan from which a system can be implemented.
- Within the Information Technology Management Reform Act of 1996 (the Clinger–Cohen Act), information technology architecture is broadly defined as an integrated framework for evolving or maintaining existing information technology and acquiring new information technology to achieve the agency's strategic goals and information resources management goals (Section 5125 [d]).

TABLE 17.1. Supporting Principles of Department of Energy: Los Alamos.

Customer	Customer focus is most important.
Shared information	• Shared information is the foundation of a unified Laboratory.
	• Access to information is the rule, not the exception.
	• Security is designed into our data, products, and services.
Stewardship	• Laboratory information and data are corporate assets and are managed accordingly.
	• Identified stewards are responsible for data, applications, and the infrastructure.
	• Data is gathered once at the source.
User	• We use digital communication tools to accomplish our work.
	• Proficiency in the use of information tools is a shared responsibility.
	• User interfaces are intuitive, consistent, flexible, and secure.
Infrastructure	• The Laboratory provides a common suite of desktop tools.
	• Direct access to the infrastructure is provided throughout the Laboratory.
	• The infrastructure is based upon interoperability and standards, supporting the sharing of resources.
	• Levels of support are defined and provided for services and products.
Provider	• Information solutions add value to the Laboratory and enhance our competitive position.
	• Information solutions are deployed quickly in usable components.
	• We reuse before we buy and buy before we build.
Responsibility	We conduct computing and information activities in a responsible manner, complying with applicable laws, orders, and regulations.
Evolution	• We seek and influence cost-effective technologies that facilitate science and research activities at the Laboratory.
	• The Information Architecture continues to evolve.

Source: http://www.lanl.gov/projects/ia/library/foundation/fnd-html/4prin/400summa.html.

Establishing Supporting Principles

Articulating the key principles of an organization serves to keep its main beliefs more visible and less prone to be cast aside. Having a well-published set of principles can help the organization remain mindful of long-term core beliefs and philosophy as more urgent day-to-day pressures tempt decision makers to settle for shortcuts. An example, taken from the Los Alamos Department of Energy, is shown in Table 17.1.

Defining Critical Attributes

Defining the desirable attributes of an enterprise architecture, as with principles, helps diverse business units and individuals focus on the big picture when solving specific problems. As this occurs, the organizational architecture begins to self-converge and benefits from a more cooperative harmonization, lessening the requirement for legislated change.

TABLE 17.2. Critical attributes of the VHA.

Interoperability	VHA's architecture provides a framework that facilitates reliable and seamless data exchange between heterogeneous applications throughout the business enterprise in a consistent manner.
Connectivity	The architecture promotes membership of VHA's information systems (and consequently our users) into a much larger community.
Security	The security architecture preserves and protects against unwanted loss, damage, or disclosure of data.
Maintainability	The architecture uses highly leveraged technologies that are cost-effective, modular, and readily available.
Standards-based	The architecture makes extensive use of standards.

The Veterans Health Administration (VHA) provides a good example (Table 17.2).

Using Performance Measures

An organization's critical attributes can be adapted to serve as performance measures, which can be particularly helpful when evaluating specific projects or systems. For new initiatives, these can serve to appraise various approaches and their level of conformance. A sample list of performance measures from the VHA information technology architecture (ITA) is shown in Table 17.3.

Selection of Architecture Models

Information architecture models, the blueprints of any ITA, depict various information, data, systems, infrastructure, and standards. There is a vast range of models, typically biased to solve an equally large number of specific needs. Unpopulated models serve to classify questions within a framework, whereas populated models serve to answer them in a structured

TABLE 17.3. Example of VHA ITA performance measures.

Does the architecture employ standards-based data interchange methods that maintain data integrity and provide for multipoint sharing?

Does the architecture enable data interchange with external knowledge sources (e.g., via the Internet), alliances, partners, administrations, and agencies?

Does the architecture widely employ the standards identified in the VHA Standards Profile?

Are documented breaches and the results of planned penetration studies within acceptable limits? Are continuous architectural improvements being made in *anticipation* of future needs?

Does the architecture avoid unnecessary complexity, tightly coupled systems, native interfaces, and proprietary solutions where reasonably avoidable?

manner. Any ITA is composed of a smaller subset of available models, several of which are listed here and described in the sections that follow:

- Reference Architecture Model
- Technical Reference Model/Standards Profile
- Operational Architecture Model
- Data Architecture Model
- Systems Architecture Model
- Security Architecture Model
- Telecommunications Architecture Model

Reference Architecture Model

A Reference Architecture model can be thought of as a high-level abstraction or depiction. Within an enterprise context, many if not most of the popular reference models trace their roots back to one produced by the National Institute of Standards and Technology (NIST). This model was developed in a consensus meeting of leading industry authorities. It contains five major components that frame the relationships among business processes, information needs, application systems, data definitions, and delivery systems or infrastructure.

The Reference Architecture model acknowledges standards and security profiles and how they logically interconnect through business, information, and technology. It is fully described in the NIST Special Publication 500–167, "Information Management Directions: The Integration Challenge," published in September 1989. The model (Figure 17.1) has grown increasingly popular; among the many groups that have embraced it or some variant include X/Open, the U.S. Federal Government's Chief Information Officers (CIO) Council, and major U.S. departments like the Department of Defense, NASA, the Department of Energy, and the VA.

The model serves as a general technical framework useful in understanding how current systems operate and how the evolution of systems may proceed. It is a management tool that can help organize relationships among business, information, and systems technology and evaluate enterprise initiatives against business needs. An organization may use the levels of the reference architecture to identify the following components:

- **Business:** Policies and procedures that identify the business aspects of the architecture and strategic objectives of the organization.
- **Information:** Information flow throughout the organization, defining what, when, where, and how information is captured from or presented to the user.
- **Applications:** Responsibilities and functions of the applications used by the organization. The applications level helps ensure that application

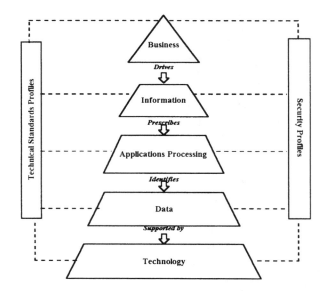

FIGURE 17.1. NIST reference architecture model.

functionality aligns with and supports the information flow and business strategies and objectives.

- **Data:** Standard methods of data storage and utilization that support the accuracy, interoperability, and processing of data throughout the organization. It further defines the type of data and the authoritative source.
- **Infrastructure:** Includes the policies, procedures, and standards governing the framework of the organization. It describes, including graphics, the systems and interconnections supporting data, applications, information, and business functions.

Technical Reference Model (TRM)

A technical reference model (TRM) identifies IT services, interfaces, standards, and the relationships among them. It provides a technically descriptive framework of information systems upon which standards and engineering specifications are based, shared building blocks are constructed, and product lines are developed. Most importantly, it also defines a common taxonomy.

One leading TRM is published by IEEE in their 1003.2 Guide to the POSIX Open System Environment (OSE) (IEEE 1995). Other well-established reference models, many of which are based on the IEEE model, include these:

- DoD Technical Architecture Framework for Information Management (TAFIM)
- National Institute of Standards and Technology (NIST) Application Portability Profile (APP)
- USPTO Technical Reference Model
- Open Group X/Open Technical Reference Model

Application of a technical reference model can result in improvements to user productivity, development efficiency, portability, scalability, interoperability, security, and manageability. It also promotes vendor independence and can reduce life cycle costs.

Standards Profile

The standards profile identifies the set of IT standards that specifically support services corresponding to those outlined in the TRM. The profile is a key component of a strong, flexible architecture. According to the International Standards Organization (ISO), standards are defined as:

"... documented agreements containing technical specifications or other precise criteria to be used consistently as rules, guidelines, or definitions of characteristics, to ensure that materials, products, processes and services are fit for their purpose."

The standards profile applies to the information, applications, data, and infrastructure layers of the reference architecture. It is not uncommon to use (reuse) the same classification scheme as within a TRM to organize standards within a standards profile.

Security standards are a special item that may be referenced from within a standards profile to a separate Security Architecture Framework document. Within a standards profile, security standards may be divided into four areas: administrative, personnel, physical, and technical. The standards identify both physical and logical security; they further provide methods to audit security information, rectify security breaches, and address unauthorized use of the system.

Benefits of adherence to standards include the following:

- Greater interoperability within systems
- Lower system life cycle cost
- Higher quality assurance
- Increased protection of the confidentiality and integrity of systems and data
- Increased reuse of existing infrastructure and automated solutions
- Provision of a more consistent and integrated view of applications and information
- Positioning of the enterprise to use open and vendor-independent technologies

- Provision of a framework for IT application and infrastructure development

Operational Architecture Model

An operational architecture model or view captures the business drivers, tasks, activities, and information flows used to accomplish or support business functions. It models the actual enterprise assets, processes, and interconnections, essentially depicting the what, how, and where of the business view. This procedure is done at a relatively high level of abstraction independent from any system or implementation-specific restrictions.

By contrast, information flow particulars like the types of information exchanged, the frequency of exchange, and the nature of these exchanges are captured in detail and permit the extraction of specific interoperability requirements. The result is a uniform set of enterprise-wide definitions and diagrams used to facilitate understanding of crosscutting business functions, information flows, and work products.

Systems Architecture Model

The systems architecture view is a description of supporting hardware, software, and communications technologies. These descriptions are typically design-style views that indicate how multiple systems and applications link and interoperate. The designs, which may be very richly detailed, capture the internal construction and operations of individual systems within the architecture. Actual hardware circuits, software, and middleware components with specific nodes may be described.

These design models are principally used for implementation, maintenance, and change management; they allow an enterprise to respond more rapidly to changing business needs.

Data Architecture Model

An organization's data architecture and its data models are at ground zero in terms of their importance as a corporate asset. Business processes, reporting needs, applications, and systems all change at a much greater rate than do the kinds of data surrounding an organization. A robust data architecture serves as a solid anchor for ever-changing business needs and virtually all information technology activities.

Central to data architecture is the need to collect metadata, or "data about data." A more primitive form of data collection is the use of a data dictionary that may describe the more technical attributes of an element, such as length, type, encoding, or transform rules. Dictionaries have evolved into data encyclopedias and, more recently, into metadata registries. Rapidly rising in popularity, the use of metadata registries is instrumental in the emerging discipline of business intelligence. Metadata registries go well beyond dictionaries and include such data as authoritative source, traceability, currency, and custody.

In addition to metadata, data models are a key component of any data architecture and a feasible means of classification. Data models can vary greatly in terms of their level of abstraction, and many different notation methods exist. One of the more common forms of data modeling involves the identification of data entities and the relationship that exists between entities. This is known as entity–relationship diagramming, or ERD. Some common forms of modeling notation are IDEF1X, which is in the public domain, and those of Chen and Martin.

Security Architecture

A Security Architecture Framework (SAF) is an integral component or extension of an enterprise ITA and is rarely developed independent of it. In part, it abstracts portions of ITA subordinate architectures to form a collage in which the constant thread is security. Security considerations permeate every level of the reference model and are a component of all subordinate architectures. The creation of a unified security view positions relevant security architecture concerns in a single place.

The goal of the SAF is to present a framework for the development of a comprehensive, measurable, cost-effective IT security architecture program. This step directly supports information security, the primary objective of which is to protect information and system assets through confidentiality, integrity, and system availability. The SAF does not develop new policies or requirements, nor does it identify new threats or risks.

Components of a Security Architecture Framework may include the following:

- **Principles:** A description of security-related principles necessary to provide confidentiality, integrity, and availability of information.
- **Standards:** A description of security standards needed to support an accessible and interoperable environment.
- **Models:** An organized structure of components, methods, boundaries, and rules for creating technical security architectures harmonized with the enterprise ITA.
- **Process:** A complete process component would allow for the consistent integration of security requirements, policies, and standards into the model. Associated with process would be an evaluation methodology component for the assessment of state information and other findings. Architecture processes may or may not be included as an integral component; they may instead be a companion document that complements the ITA and is part of a larger portfolio of architecture products.

Telecommunications Architecture

Telecommunications Architecture models deal with aspects of managing data, video, and voice transport over distance. The models help frame a variety of telecommunication components, including logical network interfaces, physical interfaces, network services, signaling protocols, addressing plans, bandwidth, and security.

By helping to answer both business and technical questions, the telecommunications architecture models help an organization evaluate new initiatives and navigate change management efforts. Good telecommunications architectures will be cost-effective, scalable, and flexible. They will resolve a variety of crucial issues, including efficient domain interconnection, multienvironment usage, accommodation of mixed media, and traffic delay reductions.

Major Model Classes Summary

Table 17.4 encapsulates the general objective of each architecture model.

Establishing a Business Case

As is the case for any strategic initiative, a strong business case must be made for the establishment of an IT infrastructure. However, most organizations do not currently approach IT infrastructure in the same

TABLE 17.4. Objectives of architecture models.

Model	Purpose
Reference architecture	Evaluate initiatives against business needs, current environment, information sources, requirements, collection, standards, and infrastructure to ensure that these initiatives align with VHA business requirements.
Technical reference	Evaluate initiatives against technical standards, services, protocols, and products.
Standards profile	Evaluate initiatives against standards and rules.
Operational architecture	Evaluate initiatives against information flows, operational elements, assigned tasks, and applications required to support existing business functions.
Systems architecture	Evaluate initiatives against systems and interconnections between systems.
Data architecture	Evaluate initiatives for data classes, type, methods of capture, extraction, use, access, management, security, and other attributes.
Security architecture	Evaluate initiatives against established security standards and practices.
Telecommunications architecture	Evaluate initiatives against systems, services, interconnections, and protocols.

strategic manner. Planning activities are common for financial resources, strategic program implementations, and other enterprise-wide activities, but IT infrastructure planning traditionally has been viewed as an IT-specific initiative. This point of view has led to the design and implementation of infrastructure components that are neither adaptable nor interoperable and often are more costly than necessary. The fundamental reason for this practice is that many organizations neglect to establish a strong business case for the development and maintenance of an enterprise architectural strategy and plan. IT infrastructure needs to be institutionalized in the same manner as budgeting, strategic planning, and other enterprise activities, with time, personnel, and dollars allocated to support its mission-critical activities.

For the information technology infrastructure to provide value in a healthcare organization, the organization as a whole must be committed to a strong information technology vision. Many healthcare organizations focus on improving their departmental systems through a financial IT focus rather than concentrating on information technology that supports clinical infrastructure. Organizations need to identify the processes, technology, and standards to be implemented at an enterprise level and maximize use of supportable, commercially available technologies in widespread use in the marketplace. Most importantly, information technology should support the changing business needs of the organization.

Understanding Trends and Drivers

Many business trends and drivers existing in today's healthcare environment are influencing the manner in which government organizations are delivering and managing care. These drivers help shape a business case for the implementation and establishment of an IT infrastructure, significantly impact the future of healthcare delivery, and require a technological framework to support current and future organizational strategic objectives. Table 17.5 lists some of the drivers, separated into several general categories.

Planning the Architecture

For the healthcare enterprise to be successful in the future, its business and clinical requirements must be clearly defined, and the technology necessary to meet those requirements must be functional and consistent across the organization. Government healthcare institutions can no longer survive on very large, mostly medical center-focused applications that yield more compact information models and increasingly pervasive data exchanges between integrated information systems. There must be a consistent architecture model that meets the current and future goals of the organization

TABLE 17.5. Healthcare business trends and drivers.

Government	• Health Information Portability and Accountability Act (HIPAA) of 1996 • Information Technology Management and Responsibility Act of 1996 (Clinger-Cohen)
Healthcare technologies	• Computer-based medical records • Telemedicine
Information technology	• Web-enabled and client–server applications • N-tier technology • Decision support • OLAP tools • Telecommunications
Standards development organizations	• International Standards Organization Technical Committee • American National Standards Institute • Health Level 7 • ANSI X12 • American Society for Testing and Materials • Digital Imaging and Communications in Medicine • Department of Health and Human Services
General	• Managed care • Shift from inpatient to outpatient care • Outsourcing • Quality organizations • Aging U.S. population

and functions as the accepted structure for providing effective technology solutions.

The design and implementation of an infrastructure/architecture is a strategic initiative that will facilitate and support the direction of the entire enterprise. Therefore, the architecture must be well planned and integrated into the strategic plans of the organization. Like a strategic initiative, the architecture plan is created by tapping into the strategy of the organization, assessing the current environment, developing a vision, analyzing gaps between the current environment and vision, and generating appropriate action plans to reach the envisioned architecture.

Tapping into the Strategy

The first step in developing an effective architecture plan is tapping into the strategy of the organization. Does the organization have a mission statement and objectives? What are the strategic and financial goals of the organization for the next 1 to 5 years? What major business or clinical initiatives are being undertaken by the department for the next year? The answers to these questions provide insight into the strategic direction of the typical government healthcare organization.

Strategic objectives of a healthcare organization are not always easy to find. Documented strategies are often missing, hidden, outdated, or even conflicting. During the initiation of the architecture planning process, the strategic objectives of the organization must be clearly documented as part of the plan. More importantly, the strategic objectives should tie directly to persons, documents, or strategic planning processes in the healthcare organization, so that as those plans change, the architecture plan can be updated accordingly.

There are many good sources for uncovering strategic information in healthcare organizations:

- Mission statements
- Enterprise strategic plans
- Budgets
- Departmental objectives
- Inventory of special projects
- Organizational metrics
- Interviews with organizational leaders
- Operating strategies

The information from these sources should be referenced and documented into a clear and concise set of strategies that can be used as a foundation for the architecture plan. In addition, senior management responsible for these planning activities should be consulted and included in the architecture planning effort. This step will ensure that the architecture plan not only reflects the strategic activities of the organization but also is a critical component of these activities.

Assessing the Current Environment

Only in rare instances does an architecture plan begin in a new organization with no preexisting infrastructure, building, technology, or processes. Typically, an organization begins its architecture planning process with inconsistent or outdated technologies, the need to connect new remote business units that have different operational and technological processes, and myriad other challenges and issues.

Documentation of the current environment, often referred to as the "as-is" environment, should include details on the business, information, applications, data, and infrastructure components of the organization. Whenever possible, these should be the actual documents used by the network administrators, database administrators, applications managers, and other operations personnel. Besides saving time, this approach ensures that the architecture plan is a living document that will change as the current environment of the organization changes.

The main purpose of assessing the current environment is to establish a baseline for the architectural planning and subsequent actions. Typical components include identification of business requirements, business drivers, and information technology trends and drivers. Detailed listings of applications, organization charts, data models, data flow diagrams, and network architecture schematics are often helpful in presenting a "layered" view of the organization's current environment. The assessment should contain components that provide a clear and comprehensive picture of the current state of the organization, including a reference architecture model like NIST to classify and organize information. The assessment should be documented so that it is understandable to senior management but detailed enough to provide technical and operational personnel with the information they need.

Developing a Vision

The future business needs of government healthcare organizations are no more predictable than today's complex needs were in the past. However, documenting a clear vision of the future is an important cornerstone in the architectural planning process. How will health care be delivered in the year 2000? 2005? 2010? How will the "futuristic" technologies of today be integrated into the everyday delivery of care? The purpose of developing a vision is to document and communicate the organization's best guess at what the future will look like. This vision provides a target for the organization, identifying the attributes and (where possible) the specifics of the future environment.

Healthcare organizations have approached architectural visioning in many different ways, some of them disastrous. Some organizations, particularly those heavily invested in single vendor or single technology solutions, have accepted "the future" as described to them by their primary technology vendors. Unfortunately, such visions often did not allow for flexibility or change outside the proprietary vision. Other healthcare institutions assigned the tasks to a single technical visionary armed with extensive knowledge of the latest hardware, software, and networking technologies. This visionary would replace every "obsolete" component of the architecture with the latest technology, often resulting in an architectural vision that was neither accepted by the majority of the organization's personnel nor supportive of strategic goals.

The key to developing an effective and workable vision is to combine people, current processes, and technology to create a practical yet effective picture of the new architecture. A well-developed architectural vision, like the other components of the architecture plan, is best developed with the full participation of strategic, technical, and clinical leadership. The vision should contain both general and specific characteristics and components of the future environment. For example, the architecture could be described as being patient health centered, accessible, and secure at a high level. Detailed information on these characteristics could include compliance with HIPAA regulations, encryption, and firewall descriptions. The main objective of the vision is to describe exactly what the organization is aiming for architecturally.

Analyzing Gaps

The next step in the architectural planning process is to determine the "why." Why is the organization not able to compare data from one facility to another? Why do interfaces take so long to develop in the current environment? A gap analysis asks these types of questions and illustrates the differences between the architectural vision and the current environment. Each architectural vision component is evaluated against the current environment. Deficiencies or missing components of the current environment are then identified as gaps.

Generating Action Plans

The final step in the architectural planning process is describing how the organization will reach its destination. Action plans are the series of steps and projects that map out how to get from the current environment to the vision. These action plans represent a high-level profile of the projects and initiatives required to achieve the architectural vision.

For example, the Veterans Health Administration's Information Technology Architecture summarized its 1999 vision, gaps, and action plans using a single grid. This document was an effective tool for referencing and highlighting the most important plan components in a concise and powerful manner. Table 17.6 illustrates how the vision components related to the

TABLE 17.6. Action plans for cross business line integration.

Vision component	Gaps	Plan to bridge gap
• Computer-based patient record	• Inconsistent hardware platforms	• Address hygiene
• Corporate data sharing	• Insufficient WAN/LAN performance	• Application messaging
• Data cleansing functions	• Nonstandard interfaces	• Corporate data registry
• Data quality functions	• Nonstandard reference data	• Lexical services
• Data roles/registry/ standards	• Poor quality patient data	• National provider identification
• Extramural information exchange	• Poor quality provider data	• Person name standardization
• GCPR	• Proprietary application messaging	• Standards tables
• Global interconnectivity	• Vocabulary differences	• WAN backbone
• HL7 standards for messaging		• Wintel/NT common platform

business objective of Cross Business Line Integration were translated into action plans.

After this step, the VHA provided high-level descriptions of each of the action plans, detailing the following components:

- Description of the problem (gap)
- Description of the solution (vision component)
- Sponsorship
- Development resource
- Financial investment
- Business requirements met by plan
- Plan dependencies
- Scope
- References or additional information sources

These plans provided VHA with a roadmap for taking them from their current environment to their envisioned architecture.

Case Study: Goals of Air Force Medical Service's Medical Systems Infrastructure Modernization Program

In 1994, a group from the Air Force's Air Mobility Command (a Regional Headquarters responsible for 12 medical centers and hospitals) embarked on a project known as the Medical Systems Infrastructure Modernization (MSIM). The objective of this effort was to develop a comprehensive and enduring communications architecture that would support the needs of the Air Force medical services community through the year 2010. To accomplish this task, the physical and information infrastructure of the various Medical Treatment Facilities (MTFs) had to be baselined and modeled. The future information flows and physical architectures then had to be modeled and designed, and an integration/acquisition plan had to be developed as a roadmap for the implementation of a standard, high-performance, integrated tele- and data communications infrastructure for each facility.

As this group established a timeless methodology that now has unique applications to the medical community, its detailed objectives are interesting to revisit. The main objectives were to provide the technical expertise required to determine existing and required architectures for voice, data, and imaging communications and to engineer and identify a standard, high-performance/intelligent, fully integrated network at each site. The group would begin with a survey that would document an as-is model by developing highly detailed schematics (in digital format). The model would also include documentation that represented a picture of each MTF and described what exists and what is planned in the near term for data and telecommunications requirements.

The team used systematic design tools using IDEF 0 and 1 to develop baseline information flows and models of data architecture in support of the "as-is" and "to-be" models. Close coordination with the Defense Medical Systems Support Center (DMSSC) and the Defense Information Infrastructure (DII) of the Defense Information Systems Agency (DISA) were required to ensure that they integrated at the community and national level. The team also set out to determine the "delta" between site, command headquarters, and regional and national requirements. Their to-be models would be designed and engineered to be state of the art and to endure for years to come. With this came key high-level architectural requirements:

- Reliability
- Zero downtime networking
- Central control of network assets
- Distributed automated network management services
- Support for many classes of services
- Network security
- Network usage accountability
- High capacity
- Upgradable and scalable

To our knowledge, this was the first DoD medical communications architecture project that was accomplished in such an exhaustive manner and incorporated the three key services—voice, data, and imagery—in an integrated fashion. For example, the system they designed was to be open and interoperable, and it would provide all corporate and regional applications with a standard data communication infrastructure to support shared services at each of their facilities. Each site's to-be model would incorporate existing and planned technology targeted for implementation from medical community headquarters and commercial and other governmental sources. All sites needed to thoroughly evaluate the functional and technical aspects of their systems implementation plans, the integrated ancillary support system Composite Health Care System (CHCS), the MDIS, the Military Health Information Computer System (MHICMS), the Medical Telephone Appointing System (MTAS), and many other DoD and/or Air Force systems.

Their goals for technical design were also thoroughly thought out, and they demonstrate many of today's challenges. For example, the to-be model was to incorporate automated enterprise management services, asynchronous transfer mode switching, connection-based secure fast packet switching, full-duplex switched Ethernet, and LAN packet to ATM cell conversion. DECNET's TCP/IP would be converted to Open LAN, and remote-user and built-in network diagnostics were to be supported. The to-be model would also design a network system compliant with the DoD's

Medical Hospital Systems Standard (MHSS) and emerging civilian standards such as HL-7.

To prepare each facility for digital imagery, the design included data/voice jacks in each room of the MTF served by intelligent communication hubs (upgradable to Asynchronous Transfer Mode), a fiber optic backbone that supported bandwidth greater than 100 MB, and a common data and telecommunication backbone that supported Ethernet, Token Ring, FDDI, High Speed Optical, and Wide Area Networking. Because their medical facilities were located on Air Force bases, much as commercial hospitals are located in communities, their infrastructure was to interface to the base infrastructure and integrate with future plans for the Air Force's Base Level Systems Modernization Plan and the Defense Information Infrastructure. The building codes being developed by DISA's DII and the AF would also have to be adhered to in all designs. The bases that had satellite buildings would also have to be surveyed, and an interface between the main building and their satellite buildings (sometimes located off the base) would have to be established.

Regional support issues demanded that each facility be surveyed and have a plan for development. This plan would allow for data communication within and between DoD Medical Regions and their commercial medical partners in the communities where the Air Force base was located. Therefore, various long-haul communication protocols would be reviewed to provide the following:

- Shared file capability
- Client access to typical server functions
- Electronic mail (e-mail) using Defense Message Service (DMS) compliant message handling (x.400) and directory services (x.500) protocols with access to the Defense Data Network (DDN)
- Capability to move advanced medical imaging packages regionally
- Wide Area Network connections
- Enterprise Network management
- Other regional communication requirements

Regional support considerations were a crucial component of each facility survey. For example, Travis AFB would have to support all DoD facilities in North Central California (DoD Region 10). In the Region 10 example, close coordination between corporate headquarters (DMSSC) engineering teams, the Veterans Administration, and the contractor were required to ensure standardization, compatibility, and integration with the Veterans Administration facility architectures and existing infrastructures.

The Air Mobility Team began by performing a site survey at each of their facilities to accomplish an as-is model. The as-is model would include documentation of existing tele- and data communications capabilities, legacy systems, common and specific requirements (hardware/software/applications), and the formulation of a list of required hardware/

software/applications, labor, implementation, training, and maintenance to achieve an integrated architectural design. One goal was to provide a minimum standard architecture that would map functional requirements and position the MTF for integration with upcoming technologies and systems, thus supporting all their anticipated future medical data, voice, and image requirements. The ultimate goal was to transform infrastructure from a labor-intensive, costly, and constraining factor (in terms of information growth) to a standard utility that would support a cost shift and help them move quickly into a ubiquitous information enterprise.

To give a high-level review of this project, we must present the key attributes of its methodology. Most if not all these steps can be applied in any infrastructure setting today—large or small—and can easily serve as a baseline to nearly any communications project.

Establishing Minimal Essential Design Criteria

Looking across the project steps, the MSIM program team would first establish their as-is model and use this to design the to-be model, which would incorporate several minimum essential requirements. From a vertical infrastructure perspective, a Collapsed Fiber Backbone would be the minimum standard because of its inherent reliability, expandability, and scalability. The horizontal wiring would include the addition of drops to support all existing data, voice, and imagery requirements and, most importantly, future deployment of systems like electronic medical records and/or digital radiological capabilities. As described earlier, connectivity to both the medical campus and their host Air Force base would be established through their existing local area networks and their connections with office automation and other community local area networks.

The medical treatment facilities' most significant integrated ancillary support systems, the Composite Health Care System, was now a legacy system that ran on DEC LAT and would require a migration to TCP/IP. From a LAN perspective, a subsequent migration from Routed Network Architecture to Switched Network Architecture was seen as critical to success.

Facility CIO Responsibilities

As with any project of this magnitude, the facility would become an integral part of the implementation team. The team's many responsibilities included accomplishing all coordination with their host Air Force base communications experts to integrate the medical campus with the base communities systems. Because of the need for core drilling, ceiling cable runs, upgrades, and security to communication closets, the facility needed to work to coordinate efforts with civil engineering and facilities management. The CIO of the facility would also accept ultimate responsibility for the work so that the CIO staff would actively participate in design reviews and coordinate with the base communications squadron and base civil engineering. The CIO would also have to manage the deluge of site preparation requirements, such as storage space, scheduling communication outages during cutover, ventilation, power, and testing and acceptance.

During the first 2 weeks the MSIM team would be on site, work began on generating the as-is model and matching these to the overall requirements, both known and anticipated over the course of the next several years. The team would provide more details concerning information required to complete the implementation, and further functional and physical data would be gathered. The existing network would be baselined to fundamentally support the as-is model, and most importantly, the implementation would determine the maximum amount of reuse potential for existing horizontal and vertical infrastructure. The as-is model would also determined the civil engineering requirements to include asbestos abatement and other requirements associated with the physical plant.

To ensure that the team would not miss any area of a facility, the CIO and his/her staff would cover several prearrival issues. For example, security issues associated with the team's ability to access all computer and communication rooms and permission to photograph and/or videotape would be resolved. As the architectural team was less familiar with the medical facility campus, documentation (floor plans, facility drawings, etc.), computer maintenance, and scheduled downtime would be planned well before arrival. The CIO also would arrange for workspace for the survey team and safe storage space for large volumes of communications gear and wiring and other products during implementation.

Engineering Design Team

Critical to the ultimate design would be the engineering site survey team. The engineers would begin their work through a series of data collection tasks. For example, the inventory of each computer room, satellite communication closet or area, and total client systems (both in use and projected) would have to be determined to support a fully integrated architectural design. The team conducted an inspection of existing cable plant for reuse potential. If a 5% random sample of all network drops tested satisfactorily, the plant was deemed capable of supporting the goals over the course of several implementations. Network interconnections and topology via equipment lists, photographs, and drawings would be needed to establish as much clarity as possible.

There were often several network protocols running simultaneously, and software revisions would be needed for the integrated solution. The engineering team would complete software revisions needed for network switches and concentrators, Inter-network Operating System (IOS) upgrades needed for network routers, network router interior gateway protocol and exterior gateway protocol configurations used at the facility, and identification of any additional network services or capacity that would be required.

Designing the Solution

Following the as-is model, the design process would begin. To ensure that a robust engineering LAN design was developed, several iterations of design review and approval were needed. This step would serve as the blueprint for the actual implementation and was seen as a critical success factor in the overall implementation.

To begin, at least two major design reviews were planned: the preliminary design review and the final design review. These major reviews consist of a series of components, including several representations of the overall architecture. For example, the technical data package consisted of the network survey report outlining the as-is model and its design and a plan for the new network installation, which would also accommodate a phased installation plan.

Contributing to the overall plan for installations were several sections associated with new infrastructure design. The design guidelines specified the interbuilding backbone, the collapsed fiber backbone between the computer room, communications rooms, and all satellite buildings. For scalability, a minimum standard of 24 strands of 62.5/125-micron (micrometer, μm) multimode fiber to all communications rooms was part of the design plans.

Most facilities had satellite buildings, which called for a separate section of the plan. The interbuilding backbone would use as much of the existing capability as possible with upgrades. Wherever possible, multimode fiber would be installed, and when distances exceeded the capability of multimode fiber, single-mode fiber would be used. Because of the inherent costs and relative immaturity of the product, wireless technology was reserved for only those situations that absolutely required this technical solution.

The design specified plenum-rated Category-5 Un-shielded twisted Par (UPT) copper cabling to be used for the desktop. Scalability, reliability, costs, and several other factors drove this design standard. Drop densities were determined using the functional IDEF portion of the as-is model; however, room capacities were almost always maximized to support future expansions and greater user reliance on the infrastructure. For the most part, triple or quad drops every 100 square feet were installed, but each functional area—for example, inpatient versus outpatient area—may drive increases to the drop density.

Later installations layered in design requirements (including Y2K compliance) into all network components. In addition, leasing of the network components was established to offset the costs of technology refresh.

Because of the inherent costs of multiple vendor sustainment, the number of vendors was minimized to support enterprise sustainment and reduce overall costs of the program.

The Network survey reports were used as the benchmark for the overall design process. Presite survey data provided the CIO's staff with network configuration and performance measurements, which the engineering team used as an as-is model to develop the to-be plan. This network configuration plan had several overarching minimal essential elements and used several specific technologies to establish a robust, scalable support system. For example, a fast Ethernet core backbone was chosen for its price per performance. In addition, in areas or satellite buildings that might demand greater capability, an ATM core backbone was designed. For the desktop, the MSIM team developed switched 10/100Mbit Ethernet for connectivity. In all areas, redundancy was considered and maximum fault tolerance was developed within the overall plans.

Approving the Solution

Network design reports and overviews would serve as the entry point to a series of design reviews. The network design included cable plan design, network configuration designs, drawing packages, estimated installation bill of materials, and an electronic bill of materials covering all components to be used for the installation. Approximately 8 weeks after the site survey team completed their work, the Preliminary Design review was held with the CIO and members such as facilities management, corporate headquarters, and base communications engineers. The beginning of vital dialogue between all parties would ensure that the overall design would not only meet the needs of the facility, but also integrate into the overall Internet and intranet strategies of all the associated communities. To ensure that the greatest possible amount of communication was established, the preliminary design review also included installation plans and checklists, a plan for testing and acceptance, and, most importantly, plans for cutover from the old infrastructure to the newly installed.

Depending on the number of changes and additional research required, the final design review would be presented approximately 4 weeks from the date of the preliminary design review. Once again, all key organizational representatives would attend and a final blessing would be sought so that installation could begin.

Installing the New Network

With a certified plan and design, the deployment phase of the Medical Systems Infrastructure Modernization could now begin. Several key issues, many learned by trial and error, led to an extremely successful implementation over the course of the program.

Logistical issues like lead times associated with network components, bulk cable orders, and secure temporary storage on site were extremely important to the timeliness and cost overrun avoidance portion of the program. Access support, security, and minimizing critical information system downtime within a facility all contributed to the overall need for highly detailed and thorough logistical planning.

Before cutover to the newly installed architecture, quality assurance was accomplished through independent validation and verification of the installed network as conducted. In the experience of the MSIM team, this needed to be handled by a third-party vendor to ensure the high level of scrutiny and maximizing reliability following cutover. During this phase, three critical reports were generated: the physical configuration audit (PCA), the functional configuration audit (FCA), and the testing and acceptance plan. Once all three reports were completed and the installing contracting team resolved discrepancies, the final stage of the MSIM implementation began.

From the CIO's perspective, cutover was the most anxiety-laden portion of the entire project. Here, the CIO would have to schedule relatively short but potentially devastating disruptions to both information and voice communications services. Would the newly installed network perform as it should? Would there be unforeseen incompatibilities between the critical clinical and appointment and scheduling systems and the new network design? Would the newly integrated network architecture fail to support actual peak loads? Although these were all worrisome questions, there usually were only minor incidences of service outages during the cutover phase. Because of early morning scheduling, they were of minimal impact. As the program progressed and experience grew, cutover became a relatively painless portion of the overall installation.

Once cutover was complete and all problems resolved, the final digital as-built drawings were delivered to the CIO. Now the entire voice, data, and imagery network was integrated, which greatly reduced overall sustainment costs inherent to previously disparate networks. New services no longer required facility disruptions, new cable installations, and delays; rather, simple software changes in communications areas would "turn on" new services in just a few minutes, a process that previously might have taken weeks or months. Remote management was now possible, and the integration to the community and corporate headquarters streamlined business processes.

Overall, the CIO was allowed to shift more focus on new services and less on burdensome sustainment issues. Costs could be shifted from maintenance to moving the facility forward, and customers saw faster turnaround through MSIM infrastructure. The entire facility was transformed from an old factory fighting to sustain itself to a center of excellence with an information-dominant position.

The Air Force Medical Service MSIM infrastructure design and implementation methodology was adopted across the military services in 1995 and 1996. It was so robust and so well accepted that DoD established a new Tri-Service medical organization called the Tri-Service Infrastructure Management Program Office (TIMPO). This group adopted the MSIM principles, continued to advance the standards and architectural design elements established by it, and continued the effort with more than $120M in infrastructure capabilities. Today, TIMPO has fully equipped many of its medical centers and clinics with robust architecture and will continue to deploy for the next few years. The facilities that have received this capability truly stand ready to meet the cutting-edge technology demands of data, voice, and video well into the twenty-first century.

References

Fong, E.N., Goldfine, A.H. 1989. Information Management Directions: The Integration Challenge. Gaithersburg, MO: U.S. Department of Commerce.

IEEE (Institute of Electrical and Electronics Engineers). 1995. *IEEE Guide to the POSIX Open System Environment (OSE)*, Std. 1003.0. IEEE, New York.

IEEE (Institute of Electrical and Electronics Engineers). 1990. IEEE Standard Glossary of Software Engineering Terminology, Std. 610. 12-1990. IEEE, New York.

The Information Technology Management Reform Act of 1996 (Clinger-Cohen Act). Section 5125 [d]. Can be accessed at http://wwwoirm.nih.gov/policy/itmra.html; last accessed August 2000.

Websites

http://gartner11.gartnerweb.com/gg/static/itjournal/itglossary/gloscov.html
http://www.lanl.gov/projects/ia/library/foundation/fnd-html/4prin/400summa.html
http://www.opengroup.org/public/tech/mg-1095.htm
http://www.va.gov/vha-ita

18
The Future of GCPR: A Hybrid Approach

PETER GROEN, CAPT JAMES McCAIN, ROBERT KOLODNER,
CAPT JAMES GARVIE, LT. COL. JANET MARTINO,
AND GINNY HOUGHTON

"... I am directing the Departments of Defense and Veterans Affairs to create a new Force Health Protection Program. Every soldier, sailor, airman and marine will have a comprehensive, lifelong medical record of all illnesses and injuries they suffer, the care and inoculations they receive and their exposure to different hazards. These records will help us prevent illness and identify and cure those that occur . . ."

—President Clinton

On November 8, 1997, in response to the December 1996 Final Report of the Presidential Advisory Committee on Gulf War Veterans' Illnesses, President Clinton charged the Department of Veterans Affairs (VA) and the Department of Defense (DoD) with creating a lifelong medical record for servicemen and servicewomen. His directive reinforced initiatives already undertaken in August 1997 by the VA/DoD Executive Council, led by co-chairs Dr. Kenneth Kizer, the Under Secretary for Health in VA, and Dr. Edward Martin, the Acting Assistant Secretary for Health in the DoD. Drs. Kizer and Martin instructed the CIOs of their respective organizations to identify potential information technology-sharing opportunities. In December 1997, the Council endorsed the recommendation that the two agencies join together in the development of a "common medical record."

Together, these two events catalyzed the formation of the Government Computer-based Patient Record (GCPR) Program. In December 1997, staff from the VA and DoD joined with colleagues from the Indian Health Service (IHS) and the Louisiana State University Medical Center to define the best method for achieving a "common medical record." The result was not only the GCPR Program, but also the outline of the first collaborative project, the GCPR Framework. The two additional members of the GCPR Program contributed broader input into requirements definition.

The GCPR governing bodies firmly believe that broad participation by both state and private facilities will prevent the development of a government-specific medical record concept that would isolate federal healthcare organizations from their counterparts in the private sector. In this way, the perspective, outcome, and long-term benefits of the GCPR Framework Project will be enhanced. This intention has been delayed by the absence of authority-fostering collaboration and shared funding between state and federal entities, leading to the postponement of Louisiana State University Medical Center's participation. Legislation to enable such collaboration is currently being considered in Congress, and it may be in law by the time this book is published.

Vision, Goals, and Guiding Principles

As the first undertaking of the GCPR Program, the GCPR Framework Project aligns closely with the GCPR vision and goals. At the initial meeting of the participating agencies in January 1998, program participants drafted a vision statement and identified high-level goals for the GCPR organization (Table 18.1).

The GCPR Executive Committee recently has assumed the task of revising and updating the goals of the collaboration, as well as documenting a draft set of guiding principles. Although the principles are under review and have not been finalized as of this writing, the drafted list is shown in Table 18.2. These principles will be reviewed and finalized in the coming months by the GCPR Executive Committee before final action by the GCPR Board of Directors.

The identification of the vision, goals, and guiding principles of the project, as well as conceptual views of the objectives, took place in an open, collaborative forum. The willingness of staff from each agency to candidly share their perceptions, requirements, issues, and concerns brought the project to its current state—on track, on time, and designed to incorporate individual agency healthcare missions and technology migration plans. The continued success of the program and its first project will rest on good faith and trust.

TABLE 18.1. Vision and high-level goals of GCPR organization.

Vision:
Improve public and individual health status by sharing appropriate clinical information.

Goals:
1. Create a collaborative effort to appropriately share clinical information via a standards-based, comprehensive, lifelong medical record.
2. Where no standards exist, the agencies will seek to advance the development, establishment, and adherence to standards.

TABLE 18.2. Draft of guiding principles for GCPR organization.

1. Protect and respect the privacy and confidentiality of each person's health information.
2. Support the improvement of lifelong health and well-being by providing appropriate and secure access to individual and population health information.
3. Support creativity that allows for clinical innovation and discovery.
4. Support the decision-making process to improve individual health status and public health status of populations.
5. Create solutions that:
   • Incorporate flexibility in the design of solutions to support health information needs
   • Preserve the integrity and the context of health data
   • Are based on common information and medical terminology models
   • Accommodate a process that supports clinical needs and practice patterns while allowing for the use of various technical solutions
   • Accommodate different timelines and multiple migration paths
   • Are unobtrusive to the provider and the patient/provider relationship

GCPR Governance Structure

The GCPR organization's role is to identify projects that enhance appropriate clinical information sharing among participating groups. The GCPR Framework project was the organization's initial project, and currently it is their only one. Because of the impact of the project on participating agency planning activities and the size of the project's resource and capital requirements, the Board of Directors decided to focus the organization solely on this effort. As the project progresses, the Board may choose to initiate additional projects that further the vision of improving health through appropriate information sharing.

The following organizational chart (Figure 18.1) illustrates the GCPR structure. Organizational entities depicted in the gray boxes belong to the umbrella GCPR Organization, while those in the white boxes belong specifically to the GCPR Framework project. The Board of Directors for the GCPR Organization includes one member from each of the participating agencies (Department of Defense, Indian Health Service, and Department of Veterans Affairs), one of whom acts as the Board Chairperson. The Executive Committee includes two members from each of the participating agencies. The GCPR Framework Project is managed by a Project Team consisting of a Project Manager (VA), Deputy Project Manager (DoD), Chief Clinical Officer (VA), and Chief Technical Officer (IHS).

Project Definition and Vendor Selection

In a departure from many Government Information System procurement projects, in which detailed functional, technical, and program requirements are determined and included in a Request for Proposal, the GCPR project

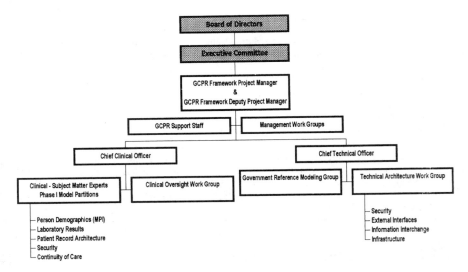

FIGURE 18.1. GCPR structure.

defined requirements using a Statement of Objectives (SOO) Request for Proposal document. The SOO, developed as an interagency effort, articulated the problems associated with sharing clinical information and caring for shared populations of patients across the three agencies. Additionally, the GCPR project leadership developed a set of minimum technical and functional requirements and illustrated the purpose of the GCPR Framework through real-life scenarios, which described the flow of patients across agency boundaries.

Potential vendors for the GCPR Framework Project were invited to respond to the SOO with a technical solution, and again, in an interagency forum, the proposals were reviewed and scored. The outcome of this process was the selection of Litton PRC as the prime vendor for the project. Though the Litton PRC proposal included many products to be procured from a host of vendors, Litton would act as the prime integrator and retain responsibility for building the GCPR Framework prototype.

Key Components and Functions of the GCPR Framework Project

The baseline architecture of the GCPR Framework consists of four major components that are scalable and extensible to accommodate future growth and enhancements (Figure 18.2 illustrates these components). The Framework provides fundamental interoperability based on open technology adaptive interfaces, multiple communication paradigms,

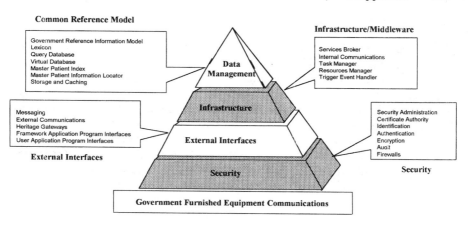

FIGURE 18.2. GCPR framework components.

decentralized information management, and an integrated information model, captured within a dynamic design. A consolidated functional concept, the Framework clearly expresses all of the significant functional features.

The Framework's functions are divided into layers that represent both their structural dependencies and their visibility outside the Framework itself: security, external interfaces, infrastructure/middleware, and data management/common reference models. These functions must be as transparent as possible and visible only when necessary. The Framework exists as a central hub, supporting detailed interactions between the participating agencies.

Security

Security is one of the most visible functions in the GCPR Framework. All access to Framework information will be through secure gateways that identify and authenticate all Framework "users," whether they are people, existing and future systems, or medical devices. Highly visible as the first point of integration within the GCPR Framework, these functions also permeate all the other functional layers. The security requirements, which will be supported by mature technologies, include the following:

- Single sign-on and role-based security
- C2 compliance
- Mechanisms that are transparent and unobtrusive
- Medical Information Privacy and Security Act and HIPAA
- Certificate-based data encryption that is DoD/GSA/PKI-compliant
- Rigorous identification and authentication at all interface points

External Interfaces

Interfaces are defined in terms of services provided by the Framework. Thus, a web browser application that retrieves patient records could access a query service that communicates with Data Management, as well as a display service that would format the results into HTML or XML for viewing. Most users of the Framework will understand it by its interfaces to the outside world: existing and future systems, web browsers, messaging, and any applications the agencies may develop in the future to exploit the strength of the GCPR Framework. While all these interfaces serve dramatically different functions, they share many basic similarities, because they are conduits by which different systems and organizations interact with the Framework.

Infrastructure/Middleware

This component provides the ties necessary to connect the external interfaces to the Data Management Region. It is concerned with low-level processing activities like internal communications, message handling, dispatching trigger events, and higher-level brokering services and resources. Most users will never be aware of this component.

Data Management/Common Reference Models

Data management is the element of the GCPR Framework architecture that provides users and applications with distributed access to data throughout the GCPR partner systems. This access is generally in the form of queries executed by a user or an application (e.g., a doctor's request to retrieve a patient's medical records, or an application developed to conduct population studies or retrospective analysis). The data management element also provides the implementing mechanisms to model and transform information across the GCPR enterprise. It is here that the GCPR Reference Models for information and terminology are used.

The primary components of the data management architecture are these:

- Query Services
- Common Data Representation
- Master Patient Information Locator
- Virtual Database
- Cache/Storage Management

The Common Data Representation in the GCPR Framework depends on semantic mediation, which in turn relies on a coded, concept-based vocabulary. Each concept in the Common Data Representation is assigned a unique identifier, enabling the Framework to deal with the semantics or meaning of a piece of data, not its linguistic representation. The mediation services assist in transforming the syntax and semantics of the source system data to that of the target systems. Additional detail on the technical architecture is included later in the chapter.

Project Scope

The scope of the GCPR Framework project includes a dynamic, real-time transfer of information across multiple, disparate systems, as well as the ability to support retrospective analyses of population health. To satisfy these objectives, a standards-based, distributed object architecture has been proposed. As the prime contractor, Litton PRC is building the Framework using the Common Object Request Broker Architecture (CORBA) standard put forth by the Object Management Group (OMG) as the backbone of the GCPR architecture. The conceptual model in Figure 18.3, provided by Litton PRC, illustrates the broad architecture of the Framework. The architecture is described in detail later in the chapter.

Early conceptual models for the GCPR define crucial elements of the Framework, including common data representation, a common data model, event triggers, security, and communications. Accurate translation of information from one agency system to another depends on the accurate transfer of the clinical context. The GCPR Framework will include the mechanisms to define data content and data transport from existing heritage systems and provide for the integration of new systems; this

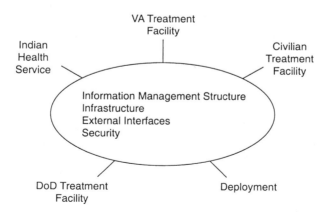

FIGURE 18.3. GCPR framework architecture. (Source: Litton PRC.)

provides a seamless "plug-and-play" environment for access to and sharing of patient information. The user, which might even be an application like an expert system, will be able to access and manipulate patient information independent of any specific system or application, data source, or location.

Technology and Architecture

The GCPR Executive Committee does not visualize the Framework as simply another computer-based patient record system. Rather, the cooperating agencies conceive of the Framework as a collection of interoperable enabling technologies that do the following:

- Share information from heterogeneous existing systems
- Access multiple levels of data
- Use common information and medical terminology models

The Framework is intended to be open, adhering to broadly supported standards in security, data transmission, message handling, and health information-related areas. Additionally, it is intended to have an evolutionary capability that can respond to the expected ongoing revolutions in information technology. The architecture and chosen technologies would have to support these long-term goals.

Framework Architecture

Accessing the "virtual" longitudinal patient record is the fundamental operation of the Framework. To the user, it is a unified, complete set of data that is readily retrieved based on the patient's name and identification as though from a single online database. The GCPR Coordinating Committee has chosen an object-oriented components approach to provide maximum interoperability during longitudinal access to patient records. Object technologies and frameworks deliver enterprise-wide deployability, reduced duplication of functionality, and a simpler maintenance and evolution path.

The primary technical aim of the Framework architecture is to present a seamless interface to the existing heritage systems of the cooperating agencies, including the DoD's Composite Health Care System (CHCS), IHS's Resource and Patient Management System (RPMS), and VA's Veterans Health Information Systems and Technology Architecture system (V*IST*A). Interfaces to newly developed healthcare systems and to emerging technologies also must be accommodated. The Framework must do the following:

- Support a common viewpoint for retrieving data distributed over a variety of sources (common reference models)
- Provide any transformations necessary to ensure common understanding (data management)
- Ensure the security and integrity of patient data
- Provide the services necessary for healthcare professionals to interact with the data and each other (external interfaces)
- Conform to appropriate standards and guidelines governing privacy, data, and messaging required for communication between government and civilian healthcare providers

Technology

As the aim of the Framework is to enable the cooperating agencies to access longitudinal patient records, share clinical information, and perform retrospective analysis, the diverse agency computer systems (CHCS, RPMS, VISTA) must achieve interoperability. They must be able to (1) share patient data with no loss of meaning or usefulness, and (2) cooperate in the joint execution of tasks. Multiple levels of data obtained from the different heritage systems must be translated and transformed into the representation expected by the other systems, applications, and care providers sharing data, and these functions must be as transparent as possible. The Framework technical solution provides this fundamental interoperability based on open technology adaptive interfaces, multiple communication paradigms, decentralized information management, and an integrated information model, captured within a dynamic design.

The proposed Framework technology will be a hybrid, integrating several standards-based, commercial off-the-shelf (COTS) and government off-the-shelf (GOTS) products. This approach places each technology where it functions the best and relies on proven bridging technologies to join them. Using standards-based components provides the advantage of replacing any component seamlessly and inexpensively with an improved component, while allowing the other processes and technologies to remain intact.

The planned architecture fuses the best attributes of several elements:

- **CORBA:** The core technology of the hybrid architecture is the underlying backbone provided by Common Object Request Broker Architecture/Object Management Architecture (CORBA/OMA) distributed object standard, developed by the Object Management Group (OMG).
- **Web technology:** The web acts as the general-purpose front end. Technologies include a combination of web browsers, Hypertext Markup Language (HTML), Extensible Markup Language (XML), JAVA, and Remote Method Invocation (RMI).

- **COM-based desktop applications:** These are supplied by the Distributed Compound Object Model (DCOM) and ActiveX component technology developed by the Microsoft Corporation.
- **EnterWorks Virtual DB data integration product:** This product implements a powerful and flexible virtual database engine that supports the other elements.

Initial Project Phases

On April 15, 1999, Litton PRC was awarded the task delivery order for the first phase of the GCPR Framework Project. Phase I of the Framework Project addresses the design and initial development of the Framework, the initial proof-of-concept demonstration, and the final prototype demonstration. Additional phases for GCPR Framework, including pilot installation, testing, and deployment at multiple agency sites, is planned pending successful delivery of the prototype.

The nature of the planned distributed database approach lends itself to distributed interfaces, and the design of mediation services and gateways allows for connection to a wide variety of heritage systems. These combine to provide integration and growth potential to each of the cooperating agencies, while providing a simple query approach to obtaining the medical information needed on patients.

Features of the Framework system include these:

- **Virtual database approach:** Simplifies access to data in a variety of databases.
- **Object-oriented approach to databases:** Can access data on different types of databases without different user actions.
- **Open system architecture:** Components of the system can be updated without significant effort; no single-vendor lock-in.
- **Web-enabled interface:** Easy access to information from various locations and platforms.
- **Data security levels up to smart cards and certificates:** Partners can establish data security levels as needed, by workstation location or other criteria.
- **Common Information Model and Common Data Representation:** Allows integration of all cooperating agency information systems.
- **Master Patient Information Locator (MPIL):** Contains pointers to medical record segments in each agency's systems. Only those heritage systems that contain data are accessed, and each agency can determine the business rules for accessing data.
- **User terminology interfaces:** Users do not need to learn a new interface or procedures as the system is upgraded; authorized care-

givers/users can access multiple levels of data using their own consistent interface.

How the System Will Work

The Framework must present a different face to nearly every person or process that views it. To a healthcare provider, it should provide access to an online database containing all the electronic patient data stored for any individual covered by the system. To a heritage system, the Framework provides a mechanism to exchange messages in standard healthcare messaging formats and to support event triggers across system, site, and agency boundaries.

Common Object Request Broker Architecture/Object Management Architecture (CORBA/OMA)

CORBA/OMA was developed by the Object Management Group (OMG), a not-for-profit international organization that develops standards for system integration using object technology. It is a standard architecture that provides common interfaces and descriptions for objects, which are pieces of code that each represent a discrete operation and together make up programs. CORBA allows applications to communicate with one another no matter where they are located or who has designed them, and regardless of programming languages or operating systems.

The Object Request Broker (ORB) is the middleware that establishes the client–server relationship between objects. When a client sends out a request invoking a method on a server, the ORB intercepts the request and looks for the object that can implement the request, either on the same machine or across a network, and returns the results.

OMA objects are described using Interface Definition Language (IDL), which provides the traditional benefits of object orientation to the interfaces of all elements, regardless of their implementation strategy. In an ORB-based solution, developers simply model the heritage system component using the same IDL they use for creating new objects. Heritage systems will have their interfaces to the system disguised via CORBA "wrappers" so that they resemble CORBA service objects to the Framework.

Virtual Database

The data management element running under CORBA contains a virtual database engine, the Enterworks Virtual DB, that will perform the data retrieval tasks. The virtual database will provide the schema, transformation rules, logical to physical mapping information, gateways to remote systems, and the workspace to provide a single interface to a variety of distributed, heterogeneous data sources. Because a virtual database does not itself contain any data, it is inherently scalable. Within the Framework architecture, the virtual database will be a CORBA-wrapped object, ensuring that client applications remain encapsulated and that the Framework is vendor independent.

The Virtual DB architecture consists of three primary components: object server, data server, and API server. Its object-oriented MetaCatalog, which defines the Common Information Model for the Framework, maps enterprise data to semantically meaningful terms for rapidly prototyping, building, and modifying business views without impacting existing systems. The virtual database can be installed on as many servers as necessary to balance the load organizationally, geographically, and with respect to the number of simultaneous users. A virtual database solution can also minimize organizational impacts, eliminating the need to reprogram or modify existing systems.

Web-Enabled Front End

End users will see the data from the Framework within the system specific to their organization. For those organizations that do not choose or are not able to integrate the data in their existing computer-based patient record systems, the GCPR Framework will provide two alternatives for viewing the data: a Java-equipped browser that runs on all workstations, or a COM-based Microsoft Windows workstation that allows integration of the Framework with desktop applications. The COM workstations will not be included in the first phase of the project.

Security

The GCPR Framework performs the critical function of preserving the confidentiality and security of the information. Confidentiality of clinical patient information is of the utmost importance; one of the biggest concerns in moving from paper-based patient records to electronic records is the potential for breaches in patient privacy. The Framework must adhere to all security, privacy, and confidentiality legislation, regulations, and policies. The security element of the Framework is responsible for physical authentication devices, secure communications and encryption, access control, web security, and firewalls.

All access to Framework information will be through secure gateways that identify and authenticate all Framework "users," whether they are people, existing and future systems, or medical devices. The security requirements will be supported by mature technologies. The technical solution contains several additional functions that work in concert with message passing to ensure that information is available to those who should have it but is withheld and protected from others.

Physical authentication, coupled with the LDAP Directory Server and a secure web server, provide a rigorous foundation for identification and authentication. The servers will support a standard set of roles and associated permissions to adjudicate requests for access to patient record information. Users will be limited to the functions they are authorized to perform and the data they are allowed to access. Data access restrictions may also be encoded in the business rules of the Common Information Model (CIM); this allows the host system to impose a further set of business rules for access.

Workstations will be configured with a physical authentication mechanism in addition to native Windows NT security features. Heritage systems will have gateway software, referred to as object wrappers, acting on requests for desired information from the GCPR. Interactions between the gateway software and the Framework are carried out using software encryption enabled by digital certificates. Each object mediator, web server, and user will have a digital certificate to enable identification, authentication, and data protection. Communication through firewalls is only allowed to and from certified devices.

Data also must be protected from unauthorized disclosure or modification during communications or storage. The approach to data encryption is certificate based, provides 128-bit encryption, and is DoD/GSA Public Key Infrastructure (PKI) compliant.

Data Management

Data management is the element of the GCPR Framework architecture that provides users and applications with distributed access to data throughout the GCPR cooperating agencies' systems, the hub where the virtual computer-based patient record exists. Access generally takes the form of queries that are executed by a user or an application (e.g., a doctor's request to retrieve a patient's medical records or an application developed to conduct population studies or retrospective analysis).

The GCPR Framework must support several types of access, including:

- Access through an organization's computer-based patient record system or through the supplied web-based front end by which healthcare professionals can access patient data
- Incoming and outgoing healthcare message traffic in accepted formats, such as HL7 and DICOM
- A query mechanism to retrieve electronic patient data from heritage systems

- Support for new external applications for workflow, trigger event responses, resource sharing, decision aids, etc.

The Framework will support the development of query services based on a multitiered architecture consisting of high-end services, cache services, and client applications. This architecture will support both event-based object messaging and request–response style data sharing. The distributed objects can include messaging broadcast services, study/query services, and a caching service, all available using distributed object servers within the Framework.

In response to client requests, the query service finds and activates various component objects to facilitate query processing, including:

- Lexical Mediation Service
- Transaction Management
- Master Patient Information Locator (MPIL)
- Distributed Cache

The basic GCPR Framework will allow the user to access all or selected parts of a longitudinal patient record using a browser-based GUI to initiate the request, select the information to be displayed, and display the record itself. Each agency will select the business rules that will determine which patient information is available.

The Framework's architecture will facilitate data sharing:

- On a short-term basis in conjunction with the clinical, administrative, and research tasks carried out while providing health care
- Between facilities when a longitudinal patient record is required
- Among the cooperating agencies for research and trending analysis

The Framework query servers serving specific facilities or groups of facilities (e.g., a facility with supporting clinics) will cache data requested by users at those facilities. The capability to share information locally will facilitate trending of short-term information. Also, data already retrieved can be delivered rapidly without the additional overhead in time and communications traffic to retrieve the data again. When systems are temporarily unavailable, the Framework will queue queries and responses and deliver them when the systems do become available. The user will be notified when queries are queued, informed of the reason(s) for queuing, and updated on the status of the queue.

By supporting the distribution of query services as objects via an object server architecture, the Framework's query services isolate client systems and applications from data sources (storage), while providing reusable objects to application developers throughout the enterprise. This mode enables the development of retrospective and trending analysis applications, which can provide desired domain-specific functionality at the client layer as required by the partners.

In the future, as the agencies' systems are integrated with the GCPR Framework, the systems themselves will be able to access data from other agency systems. The GCPR Framework will, in concert with existing systems, keep track of the locations where the data is stored and provide it to the requesting system in the expected format, structure, and terminology.

Because CORBA, Java, and COM encapsulate the back-end database structure from the client code, the client applications' access to the database can remain constant even though the underlying data model and back-end databases will change over time. This approach provides an added degree of "openness" to the cooperating agency systems by immediately providing an alternative to vendor-specific solutions for accessing and updating databases. An added benefit of the IDL hierarchy is that back-end database systems can be migrated to newer technology or replaced with a different vendor database product without impacting the Framework client applications.

Contribution to the Healthcare Sector

The Federal agencies involved believe that the processes, tools, models, and lessons learned in this project should be made available to the healthcare sector at large. The agencies have solicited industry and academic input into key project components and have identified specific benefits they would like to see achieved through the GCPR Framework project. They have sponsored seminars and initiated discussions with leading authorities in the private sector, public sector, standards organizations, and the academic community to obtain expertise on key issues for the Framework. Some of these involve clinical lexicons, reference information models, terminology models, and associated design considerations. The interaction with experts in these subject areas has been invaluable in broadening the agency's knowledge of the issues, as well as communicating the GCPR Framework project design objectives and requirements to a broad public and private sector audience.

The following is an initial set of benefits to be derived from the GCPR Framework project:

- Improved health encounters for patients and their families, including enhanced information access and availability and increased patient involvement
- Reference information and terminology models to facilitate interoperability between disparate systems
- Enhanced healthcare information standards

These benefits will have a large and lasting impact on healthcare delivery, information access and exchange, and the quality of the patient–provider encounter. As we look to the future of health record ownership, protection, maintenance, and availability, the GCPR Framework project is one of a handful of technology efforts that has the potential to substantially improve the lives of healthcare consumers.

19
Force Health Protection Through Global Medical Surveillance

BRIG. GEN. KLAUS SCHAFER, LT. COL. EDWARD KLINE,
COL. ROBERT L. WILLIAMS, CAPT. ROBERT HARDIE, MAJ. DAVID PARKER,
MSGT. JAMES MENDES, TODD A. RITTER, AND DAVID BEAULIEU

The Desert Storm conflict of 1991 and 1992 was a strategic military victory for the United States, but in its wake came reports of medical ailments that became known as "Gulf War Syndrome" or "Persian Gulf Illness." Like the post-Vietnam era, when many veterans complained that exposure to Agent Orange left them debilitated, Desert Storm raised critical issues for the Military Health System (MHS) and the United States Military. Thousands of American service personnel reported ailments following the conflict, and headlines told of birth defects found in Gulf War babies. Multiple theories were advanced, including oil-fume inhalation, exposure to chemical weapons, and delayed reactions to vaccines, but the cause proved elusive.

The overall lack of medical and environmental information on individuals led to these uncertainties. Throughout the Desert Storm conflict, many pieces of medical and bioenvironmental information that could have proved helpful in finding possible causes were missing. For example, tracking an individual in terms of location, environmental exposure, and general healthcare status was done using paper-based records. Because the logistics of maintaining, forwarding, and tracking paper-based medical records was very difficult, an individual record had many missing episodes and medical events. From an epidemiological perspective, analyzing overall health status from a population perspective was very difficult.

Although much consideration was given to the possibility of overt biological or chemical attacks upon U.S. and allied forces, little consideration was focused on the possibility of covert biological attacks that might manifest chronic results over the course of months or years. In the future, we need to consider the latter a distinct possibility and develop a plan to manage it. This chapter describes the development and deployment of the military's first system designed to take corrective measures through use of multifaceted technologies. These technologies were combined to provide a sophisticated web of capabilities aimed first at protecting the individual and then at supporting large numbers of individuals through early warning. The steps taken have produced the nation's first Force Health Protection and Global Medical Surveillance System.

Project Background

Following Desert Storm, U.S. forces maintained a significant presence in southwest Asia, the same location that gave us Gulf War Syndrome. The question was inevitable: Could the unknown causes of this syndrome still be present as an unsuspected biological agent? Could governments hostile to allied nations support in southwest Asia contaminate food, air, or water or use inaudible germ warfare? Weapons like these could have a far greater impact than the kamikaze bombing we had come to expect.

The problem was not confined to southwest Asia. Since 1992 there had been Air Expeditionary Forces to the Pacific and Europe, more than 500 humanitarian missions around the world, including the former Soviet Union, and some 100 deployments to Africa. Yet with all these deployments, the process of collecting medical and environmental data on individuals had not changed. The basis of global disease reporting in the Department of Defense (DoD) primarily consisted of daily casualty reports and a general disease grouping called Disease Non-Battle Injury (DNBI). The DNBI groupings, separated into such categories as Respiratory, Gastrointestinal, and Musculoskeletal, offered little detailed information about the symptoms, specific diagnosis, and medical procedures rendered. Because a diverse, highly mobile population makes linkages to exposures nearly impossible to draw, diagnostic trends among large numbers of airmen could not be studied. Not only does this make it difficult to substantiate or refute an individual claim of ill health, it also precludes early warning of disease trends to diminish the effects of a covert biological attack.

Simply put, the situation was grim: "one service person's ailment would be just an isolated symptom in the middle of nowhere. The ailment would be dosed with medicine, recorded on a paper-based system, and forgotten." (Gates 1999, p. 350). Unless the patient's paper medical record was available, which was unlikely, it was extremely difficult to track the health of troops in hostile environments or their exposure histories, link ailments back to preexisting medical conditions, or trend "at risk" data for populations. No existing methodology would systematically and efficiently collect and trend crucial medical data in the field. The need for Global Medical Surveillance was urgent.

With 28,000 Air Force members deployed to southwest Asia each year since the end of the Gulf War, the likelihood and potential consequence of a biological attack became increasingly worrisome. We had to take steps to collect more detailed health information on our deployed airmen and secure the data that might link environmental exposure to a medical visit.

First, automation technology would have to be applied to capture standardized electronic medical data and store them in a database that would undergo regular analysis. Data collected had to include symptoms, laboratory data, workplace chemical exposure histories, background air sampling for potential toxins, and chemical or biological agents. The authors of this chapter initially turned to existing MHS information systems and quickly found that the system would not support this project's requirements (or, if there was a program aimed at solving the problem, solution delivery was too far in the future). What we needed to support a theater clinical encounter was not available in the MHS, nor was it readily available in the commercial marketplace.

Because of the lack of government solutions, we launched a project called Desert Care in late 1996. Desert Care was aimed at fully supporting the healthcare information needs of the individual, the medical provider, the epidemiologist, and the medical intelligence expert. The project, launched in several phases, emphasized continuous improvement through direct user input. It would use the tenant's sound life cycle management while remaining free of traditional MHS processes that were cumbersome and costly in terms of delivering product to users. We were able to work around the formal MHS acquisitions processes through a program called the Medical Defense Performance Review, created under Vice President Al Gore's Reinventing Government initiative. This program allowed the project to move quickly from requirements to development, testing, and fielding in just a few months.

Data Capture Requirements

To define the requirements of data capture in Desert Care, the overarching goals of the project were identified and the critical success factors were carefully considered. High-level goals were grouped into three major categories: Standardized Data Capture, Secure Data Analysis/Distribution, and Identification/Knowledge Distribution. Each of these areas contained a complex set of requirements supported by underlying technologies that had never before been woven into a sophisticated tool set that specialists in different fields could use.

Ideally, the technology used in this project would capitalize on new concepts of operations and supporting technologies. For example, the Air Force line components like intelligence and command and control were moving toward new concepts of operations that would dramatically decrease the numbers of forward-deployed individuals but greatly increase deployed technology supported by bases in the United States. Their "reach back" concepts garnered the latest in technology, decreased the overall threat to human life, and significantly increased theater presence through virtual mechanics. These concepts could be applied to the medical presence through the use of similar technologies.

Building toward the future would also require a strong commitment to Internet and World Wide Web integration. This need proved to be especially important in establishing data analysis objectives like "real time epidemiology." To our knowledge, this was the first instance of real-time analysis applied to the field of epidemiology.

From a sustainment perspective, the remote environment raised many fresh challenges. Traditional application support for computerized patient records is challenging enough in the most sophisticated technological environments in the United States, but it was unheard of to support these applications (under huge time differences) from the United States in locations like Kuwait, Saudi Arabia, and other countries in southwest Asia. We established objectives like maintaining support 24 hours a day, 7 days a week from the United States (even within the limitations of time and distance) and made the most of technology to ensure that users would be supported and data would flow consistently.

The overall goal of the team's design was to build a means of collecting point-of-care healthcare information in dispersed locations and support requirements. The team knew that any solution would have to be reliable and intuitive, and because training would have to occur before individuals left for theater deployments, training labs with realistic scenarios would be required to ensure success.

Although the theater environment is austere, the military is often in certain locations for extended periods of time where buildups over the course of years can be expected. The capability would have to be scalable—upward to larger facility support, and downward to the single user. One of the project's fundamental objectives was to collect standardized healthcare information each time an airman saw a healthcare provider for any reason. Patient data needed to be captured wherever patients might present in a remote theater of operations, and those data had to be simple for the clinicians to collect and record. All the supporting hardware/software and data transfer requirements would have to remain constant whether the environment was relatively robust or extremely austere. The scalability of the application, therefore, was a required technical goal to support data capture, transfer, and analysis across a continuum of users.

Development Methodology

After an initial meeting with the Air Combat Command (ACC) team to review the problem and brainstorm potential solutions, representatives from Microsoft, Sun Microsystems, and AT&T agreed to donate support in such areas as architectural design, technical services, and communications. Working with an integrator hired by the ACC and committed to completing the project in a short timeframe, a cadre of experts met virtually to build a solution that would be:

- Detailed in its documentation of each clinical encounter
- Scalable (from medical technician operating alone to bedded facility)
- Sustainable from the continental United States
- Fault tolerant (able to work if some components failed)

Using a modified structured development methodology, the team took the user-supplied critical success factors and documented the requirements. Mapping these requirements to process/data models in existing healthcare information systems defined the foundation for the project and prioritized requirements. Each data element was evaluated on three dimensions of support: patient record, epidemiology, and early warning biothreat (Figure 19.1). Priority was given to those elements that served all three dimensions.

Functionally, Desert Care had to be intuitive for end users. Each data element, as shown in Figure 19.1, would have to be carefully selected and planned to garner as much return on investment as possible. Desert Care would use two powerful yet simple tools: laptop computers and easy-to-use commercial off-the-shelf software with database capabilities and intuitive user interfaces. This plan was the first step toward the goal of institutionalizing support using multitiered client architectures.

The team's user-driven requirement approach and rapid development methodology was deliberate and low in cost. Before Desert Care, projects were built on traditional military models for weapon systems acquisition that proved to be expensive, time-consuming, and often obsolete by the time they were fielded. By approaching the development differently, the team overcame limited funding and short timelines and was able to capture the necessary end user support.

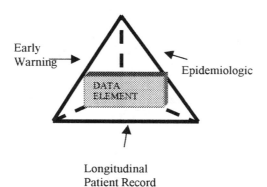

FIGURE 19.1. Three dimensions of support for Desert Care data elements.

To create a reliable and intuitive system, we decided early in the process on a multitiered, web-enabled topology. We assumed that the limited communications capability would improve annually with the release of new long-haul communications capabilities like Iridium, Globalstar, and Teledesic. For example, globally available "Web Tone"—akin to the global dial tone we have today with voice communications—would continue to mature rapidly to support worldwide operational deployment.

Working within the conceptual framework, Schafer took steps to refine and increase standard data capture using ICD-9 codes. A standardized clinical note was added, including Common Procedural Terminology (CPT), to ensure data capture for symptom analysis. Data collection occurred at multiple locations via web-based forms on personal computers. These computers were linked to a central server in the military theater that encrypted the data and forwarded it to Langley Air Force Base in Virginia, where it was analyzed within 24 hours. From collection to analysis, data flow from the theater was performed in real time, building the foundation for early warning capabilities.

Initial efforts produced an electronic medical record that included patient past history, vital signs, clinical notes (based on the standard DoD form 600s), patient problem lists, patient disposition information, drug lists, and ICD-9 and CPT-4 codes. Because system interfaces like voice recognition and handheld point-and-click devices were not mature enough for deployment, we relied on notebook computers and mouse pointers for the applications interface. Because patient visits require a team approach, we also had to support the technician recording vital signs, the nurse performing disposition instructions, and administrators responsible for supplies, visit rates, etc.

This application was designed to support data capture with a simple, intuitive user interface. As seen in Figure 19.2, we used tabs down the left side of the screen, each of which had several subaction capabilities. The tabs represented major functions recorded during patient visits and presented as much information as possible pertaining to each tab. Subactions for each would allow further information and updates, and most of the subtasks could be displayed without additional clicks from the end user. Summary information was presented whenever possible so that the applications maintained an intuitive, uncomplicated look and feel.

At the same time, our goal was to present and capture just as much information as was recorded on standard medical forms. A critical success factor was the integration of the chores performed by the technician and physician. This procedure would eliminate duplicate efforts and ensure that the process of a patient visit was streamlined through use of the automated system.

In terms of remote support, the team agreed that web technologies could meet their most crucial requirements. Web users share administrative responsibility; when they need help, they turn to electronic portals, e-mail,

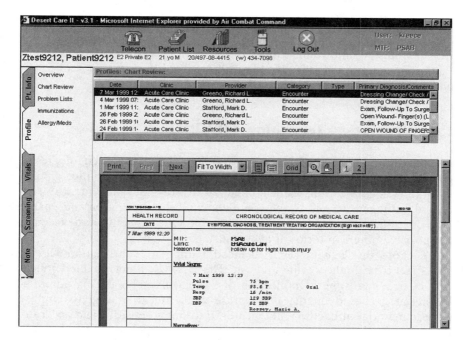

FIGURE 19.2. Web browser version of DC II.

and web-based features like frequently asked questions (FAQs) as their first line of defense. The team would have to devise unique ways of supporting users using a similar model, because a help line often is *not* "just a phone call away" in remote locations. Help routines and troubleshooting would have to be "pushed forward" to users.

Air Force fighting forces are given priority for communication lines back to the States, making electronic access for medical personnel very limited and potentially unreliable. Functionality for these users must be highly intuitive. In the event of a "communications out" situation, the database and communications software have to work in harmony to support the end user and determine when best to send data to the States. The database must be ready to handle partial updates and reconciliation with the database at Langley Air Force Base in Virginia, and the various databases located throughout theaters of operation would have to work in concert with one another.

The impact of the project was greatly dependent on initial implementation. The team deployed a product that provided a snapshot of requirements and then sought end user evaluation and feedback. Because of the distances involved, the team had to address implementation challenges like remote application deployment.

Web technologies were employed to support both the downloading of applications and remote training requirements. Because of the relative maturity of infrastructure in the theater, 12 locations could download appropriate files through web services and communicate through e-mail. Implementation and training using these modalities were conducted from January through April 1997. By May 1997, all 12 locations were collecting and appropriately coding 99% of their visits electronically.

Complementary Technology: RAPID

As we built automation technology, we searched for other technologies to complement our computerized patient record by adding frontier clinical laboratory identification. We searched for a tool that could identify suspected pathogens to add to the complete clinical presentation and enable early identification in a terrorist environment. One capability far exceeded the possible others in terms of availability.

We chose the Ruggedized Advanced Pathogen Identification Device (RAPID) from Idaho Technology Inc. The RAPID, which enabled collection of near real time identification of biological agents posing potential biothreats, is based on the polymerase chain reaction used to amplify genetic material of bacteria and viruses. Extremely sensitive and accurate, this device had the power to make data incredibly powerful. The RAPID strengthened individual diagnosis capabilities, armed the epidemiologist with crucial early warning information, moved past traditional data based purely on history and symptoms, and integrated those data into the electronic patient record. This technology also worked quickly; in less than 2 hours, the testing process could do what used to take 2 to 3 days.

RAPID connectivity would route the lab data from the encounter along two paths. The first path supported the needs of the provider caring for the patient. The second path was to ACC for the trend analysis reported by the Global Epidemiology Tracking System. From here, the data would pass to the U.S. Army Medical Research Institute for Infectious Disease or the Armed Forces Institute of Pathology. In the event that the data might indicate a biological attack, the second path provided a crucial path to authorities and specialized medical experts. By structuring the data flow in this way, we were able to both support routine care and address potential biothreats.

Used at the point of care, the RAPID was integrated into our network and allowed us to see epidemiological laboratory results across an entire theater made up of multiple locations. To further integrate the capability of the RAPID, we provided its output through the Internet using highly secure services, which allowed authorized personnel located anywhere in the nation to review the laboratory output of the device. This service provided medical personnel in the field with invaluable support that would be needed, for example, to determine whether a particular organism was natural or bio-manufactured. While in the past it would take up to 2 weeks to send a clinical sample of blood, urine, or saliva to the United States to make a definitive decision, this device would identify a pathogen, on location, within 20 minutes. It also worked with such nonclinical samples as food, water, and soil, other potential areas of contamination.

Data Analysis

Desert Care expanded the patient record to include vital signs, immunizations, medications, and details on any current or past exposures. Standardized and electronic real-time data supported detection and surveillance in two key areas. First, population medicine used the data for traditional analysis, including endemic disease rates and baseline. Then, early warning systems analyzed the data to identify biowarfare symptoms, mitigate them, and initiate counter-measures. In essence, Desert Care was beginning to meet the fuller spectrum of force health protection and generate DNBI reports with greater depth of analysis and detail—in short, increased granularity.

Once the application was mature and coding of outpatient visits reached a baseline state, the team added functionality that "rolled up" each day's visits by location and by patient. These data were encrypted and e-mailed to a central location in southwest Asia. This hub aggregated data from the entire theater of operations and, through encrypted e-mail, sent the data to Langley, where daily reports by theater, individual sites, disease, and individual patient record were stored securely in a central database. Individual patient visits were now available electronically and could be used later to support retrospective healthcare analysis of individual military personnel.

Seeing that we could move data securely and almost immediately, we began taking further steps to develop data distribution capability. The RAPID capability was the first step that led to the development of the Global Epidemiology Tracking System. Here, turning on an automated service would statistically analyze all the data returning from southwest Asia, marking the first real-time epidemiology in the DoD.

The next step was to build an infrastructure and capitalize newer database technologies. Each location would be networked to view trends across the entire enterprise (for us on this project, that meant the entire theater of operation). For example, multiple locations across Saudi Arabia, Kuwait, Bahrain, and any other location to which we might deploy would have to be supported. The data had to be captured whether or not the long-haul communications were available; fortunately, the replication features of Microsoft SQL could serve both communications on and off situations. The database offered features that would send when communications were in place and hold for a later send when communications where temporarily down.

To analyze the data, we applied standard statistical run charts with upper and lower control limits to determine trends. The goal was to track the data across the entire theater and drill down to individual locations, even to specific events, and eventually link directly to the original electronic clinical record of the patient encounter. This model for moving data proved successful.

Available through the Global Epidemiology Tracking System (GETS), the weekly DNBI reports are organized by military diagnostic code (MDC), based on the International Classification of Diseases (ICD) and categorized by level. Level 0 provides an Alert Selection listing of all MDC categories by region and installation. Drilling down to a particular theater, Level 1 displays epidemiological data and plots statistical patterns for a specific diagnosis, listing the number of alerts, cases, and total population within a particular theater over a 30-week period. Going deeper, Level 2 presents MDC-specific data by installation for a given week. Level 3 displays the same data as Level 1, but it drills down to the individual installation. For force health protection, these reports provided a level of granularity that was previously unavailable.

Integrating Desert Care into Analysis, Identification, and Reaction

The next step for the ACC was to integrate the work toward establishing a standard patient record and communicate it stateside with work done by other agencies, notably the Defense Applied Research Projects Agency (DARPA), in the area of disaster management. Two critical steps were added to the original three requirements of data capture, distribution, and analysis: these new steps were Knowledge Distribution and Command and Control.

With the addition of the RAPID, data distribution and analysis now required us to address the aspects of command and control. What would happen if a case of anthrax or tularemia were identified? Who needs to be notified? Are the data accurate? What if the technician made a mistake? What does it mean if positive results are found across several sites? When is it a naturally occurring disease, and when is it an induced epidemic?

DARPA had been working on consequence management for about a year and had already developed a number of tools to make our work quicker and easier. These new tools—ENCOMPASS, BASIS, and Care Central—help build more capability into what we now call the Global Expeditionary Medical System (GEMS), which stemmed from the Air Force's new expeditionary concept. The concept provides global disease surveillance, early warning of epidemics, command and control, and the ability to provide knowledge at the point of care.

Enhanced Consequence Management Planning and Support System (ENCOMPASS)

ENCOMPASS is a tool developed by the Defense Advanced Research Programs Agency that tracks and reports events using sophisticated computerized tools. An example is electronic "watchboards," which allow on-scene commanders to keep track of multiple events in an organized fashion and make quicker and more informed decisions. Electronic watchboards with views that can be customized automatically share information with all appropriate responders and agencies. Patient tracking at a casualty scene with multiple patients might be an example of how this is used.

The capabilities developed by ACC are complemented by the Enhanced Consequence Management Planning and Support System (ENCOMPASS), also developed by DARPA. Designed to enhance incident planning and management, ENCOMPASS provides state-of-the-art electronic tools for those who respond on the scene and personnel who respond from remote locations. These "command and control" capabilities enable military authorities to mount aggressive, effective, and coordinated responses to natural disasters or attacks.

Among the components ENCOMPASS provides are templates to create electronic "playbooks." Based on a wide variety of incident models, the playbooks prescribe effective responses and generate electronic checklists for those responding to a given type of incident. An incident repository stores data for use "on demand" at the time of the incident and afterward for review and analysis. Multiple web-based tools provide real-time patient/casualty tracking from the "hot zone" through triage transport to definitive care (e.g., a field hospital). A responder can locate an individual or identify the current state of care facilities with a simple mouse click. ENCOMPASS components support effective collaboration by presenting an accurate real-time view of operations to all respondents simultaneously, regardless of their locations.

The distribution of knowledge deals not only with the initial capture of clinical data but also the new collection of RAPID data. It includes the ability to tap into specialized medical experts in infectious diseases at the Centers for Disease Control and the U.S. Army Research Institute of Infectious Disease (USAMRIID). Artificial intelligence tools like BASIS (following) and web-based resources provide clinical treatment protocols not normally known to most providers.

Biological Agent Symptomatology Information System (BASIS)

For covert biological warfare events, BASIS enhances situational awareness by supporting the detection and identification of biological agents via analysis of electronic casualty medical records from the affected area. BASIS enables rapid determination of the most probable agent or agents and supports identification of the most effective response approach. Easy "drill-down" capabilities into medical records circumvent time-consuming research during critical medical emergencies. BASIS can be used for nearly any infectious disease agent.

BASIS, for instance, shows settings for High Fever that are set to check for activity every 15 minutes across the entire database. The tool displays all the cases of flulike symptoms (bottom lines) over a 1-year period relative to the total "sick call" cases and indicates what a "normal" epidemiological pattern of events would be. Deviations from this pattern would indicate unusual activity.

Care Central

For ACC, the Care Central concept encapsulates the concept of force health protection through global surveillance and detection; it integrates efforts developed under Desert Care with work done by DARPA. Here, the final circle of activity is culminated in support of the system user. When providers in a forward remote location see a disease they have never confronted before, they can receive care plans for the condition on location through the network established by Desert Care. For the first time, teams located in the United States can push vital information almost instantaneously to a physician on the ground and give detailed instructions on how to handle the medical condition.

Through these initiatives, Air Combat Command has provided a tool that can coordinate treatment plans for all regions of the world from one location. It provides chronic and acute disease management to the theater, as well as coordinated biowarfare treatment guidelines based on the USAMRIID's Blue Book. These data are available on the Web, courtesy of DARPA.

Beyond Desert Care

As data and information become more and more integrated, organizations will increase their dependence on information systems. Desert Care effectively used an integrated network, designed using commercially available technologies, to support the health of individuals and the force as a whole in some of the most remote and physically hostile areas of the globe.

Desert Care was a successful model for many reasons. This project:

- Was implemented at a low cost and with unusual speed
- Tested architecture
- Used multitiered architectures and communications capabilities

- Improved data capture solutions
- Transmitted data stateside in real time for unique analysis

Desert Care created the basis for protecting the health of American forces through ongoing surveillance and detection. In terms of technological integration, it is the first of its kind, tightly integrating computerized patient record technologies with sophisticated laboratory identification, real-time epidemiology analysis, situational awareness, and other referential knowledge bases.

To date, more than 100,000 patient visits have been recorded using Desert Care, which is already serving as a model for other branches of the military. A Presidential memorandum signed in November 1998 directs the Departments of Defense and Veterans Affairs to create a new Force Health Protection Program: "Every soldier, sailor, airman and marine will have a comprehensive, lifelong medical record of all illnesses and injuries they suffer, the care and inoculations they receive and their exposure to different hazards. These records will help us prevent illness and identify and cure those that occur." In addition, the Center for Disease Control has recently established their Health Alert Network and partnered with Brig. Gen. Klaus Schafer and his team to begin implementing a similar network in the continental United States to guard urban areas against covert biological attack.

As population health becomes the focus of both private and public sectors, the lessons learned in Desert Care will prove instructive. Perhaps these lessons will not completely eliminate the threats posed by biological and chemical agents, but they can provide a model for understanding the epidemiology of diseases in a population where symptoms are correlated with specific incidents and exposures. We hope this methodology will serve as a model to others as health care continues to grow from a cottage industry of medicine into an information-dominated sector.

Reference

Gates, B. 1999. *Business @ the Speed of Thought: Using a Digital Nervous System.* New York: Warner Books.

20
Global Expeditionary Medical Surveillance (GEMS) Support of Domestic Preparedness

Col. John S. Silva

After the World Trade Organization (WTO) announced that its annual meeting for 1999 would be in Seattle, Washington, the Seattle-King County (SKC) Department of Public Health considered the potential impact. It was estimated that 15,000 foreign visitors would enter Seattle during the WTO meeting, and many of these attendees would be coming from underdeveloped countries where serious infectious diseases were known to exist. In addition, the event would attract up to 40,000 protesters from other countries and the United States, many of whom could have close contact with the WTO attendees.

In view of the high risk for entry and dissemination of an infectious agent, the Department of Public Health invited the Centers for Disease Control (CDC) to provide surveillance support before, during, and for a week after the WTO meeting. This chapter describes the activities, methods, and organizations involved in developing and deploying the suite of tools that provided syndromic surveillance.

Part One: Defining the System

As a first step, SKC and CDC established principal goals for this effort:

- Data would be collected in participating hospitals by CDC personnel
- Technical direction and architecture would be provided jointly by CDC and Defense Advanced Research Projects Agency (DARPA)
- Applications would be developed based on a formal process of knowledge acquisition (understanding what the user really wants) and rapid prototyping within an architecture (DARPA)

In late October, DARPA and CDC's Bioterrorism Preparedness and Response Division met to discuss WTO surveillance requirements and the feasibility of developing and deploying a syndromic surveillance system within extraordinarily tight timelines (2 weeks). DARPA had already begun to develop the Global Expeditionary Medical System (GEMS) with the Air

316

RAPID DEVELOPMENT AND DEPLOYMENT

ID	🛈	Task Name	November 27 30 02 05 08 11 14 17 20 23 26 29	December 02 05 08 11 14 17 20 23 26 29	January 01 04 07
1		Gems design and Deployment - WTO Seattle			
2		Initial Meeting with CDC in Atlantic			
3		Initial Meeting with CDC in Atlantic	10/29		
4		Application Design and Initial Build	11/08 ▮▮▮ 11/12		
5		Ship Lap Tops and Server to Seatle	11/15 ▮▮▮ 11/19		
6		Begin Data Collection and Medical Surveillance			
7		Site Visits to 8 Hospitals	11/15 ▮ 11/15		
8		Complete Lap Top and Server Configuration	11/16 ▮ 11/16		
9		Install Lap Tops in 8 Local Hospitals	11/17 ▮ 11/17		
10		Train Users in Hospitals	11/18 ▮▮ 11/19		
11		Install and Configure Medview	11/22 ▮ 11/22		
12		Install and Configure Basis	11/22 ▮ 11/22		
13		Begin Data Collection for Baseline	▾ 11/23		
14		Gems - Go Live			
15		WTO Surveillance	11/30 ▮▮▮ 12/05		
16		Post Surveillance		12/06 ▮▮▮▮ 12/13	
17		Gems - WTO - Completed		◆ 12/14	

FIGURE 20.1. WTO—GEMS program schedule.

Combat Command as a part of the Enhanced Consequence Management Planning and Support System (ENCOMPASS). The October meeting determined that several components of the GEMS-ENCOMPASS could be extended rapidly. These components and the resulting flexible architecture would meet the needs for data collection and analysis. Figure 20.1 depicts the actual program plan for this effort.

Establishing Team Members and Duties

In addition to the conceptual design, establishment of the CDC, DARPA, and SKC team members was a crucial early step. CDC personnel, participating hospitals, and local health department officials would specify the requirements for the system and evaluate all prototypes with fast feedback to the development team. The DARPA team would then construct the data collection system, a monitoring system to review these data, and a visual display of the data. Figure 20.2 shows the sequence of knowledge acquisition (KA), development activities, and system delivery. As members of the DARPA team had already established working relationships and excellent rapport, close collaboration among KA analysts and developers facilitated rapid analysis, design, development, and deployment activities.

Knowledge Acquisition

The process of extending the GEMS-ENCOMPASS applications began with a number of Knowledge Acquisition (KA) sessions with members of the Biological Surveillance Unit. During these sessions, the KA efforts

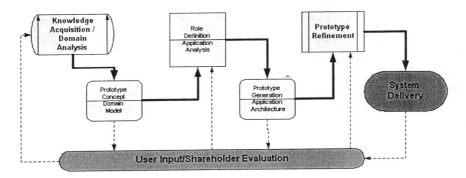

FIGURE 20.2. Developmental process.

defined user needs, captured the operational environment, and focused on the overall goal of the CDC. The symptoms to be monitored were identified, as well as what area hospitals would be involved in the effort. In addition, a sample patient information form to be used by the hospitals was obtained. This form further defined what information would be collected and entered into the database, giving additional perspective to the program. Once all this information was gathered and processed, work began on conceptualizing how the prototype would function to meet the user needs.

For the WTO meeting, the CDC concentrated on syndromic surveillance rather than attempting to collect detailed medical data for each patient. CDC personnel defined eight disease syndromes:

1. Unexplained death with history of fever (not including trauma, surgery, or cardiac cases)
2. Meningitis, encephalitis, or unexplained acute encephalopathy/delirium
3. Botulism-like syndrome (cranial nerve impairment and weakness)
4. Rash and fever
5. Nonpneumonia respiratory tract infection with fever
6. Pneumonia
7. Sepsis or nontraumatic shock
8. Diarrhea/gastroenteritis

Medical care providers would be asked to classify each emergency room patient as one of these syndromes or "none of the above." An ENCOM-PASS component called BASIS, which provides surveillance monitoring using field medical record data, was selected for the WTO monitoring application. BASIS was modified to provide syndromic surveillance and filtering, monitor each syndrome at each hospital as well as countywide, and provide graphical drill-down capabilities on case-by-case data (by gender, age, hospital, syndrome, and race).

In addition to the data collection and surveillance applications, the CDC defined a need to visualize the information collected at each hospital. The MedView component was conceived as an extension to an existing ENCOMPASS component with the following features in mind:

- Visual representation of the hospital locations in the Seattle area via an imported map
- Retrieval/display of each symptom (nine total) being monitored by the CDC and stored in a database
- Display of admission totals
- A timeline and playback function relating to the data displayed
- Color-changing hospital icons combined with spatial locations to highlight possible outbreak patterns
- Capability for user to set individual threshold limits for the color change effect
- Quick retrieval of hospital contact information for callback/verification purposes should a pattern be identified

Application Development

For this project, application development refers to three major tasks: BASIS extensions and integration, development of the data collection application, and MedView development. Given the short timeline, extensions to and integration of BASIS began 2 weeks before the start of the WTO meeting and continued into the event. (The application, built by PSR, is discussed further in Part 2 of this chapter.) Development of the data collection application was started on a parallel course with the KA sessions. Figures 20.3 and 20.4 show the actual forms that were developed over a 2-week period by Oracle consultants, based on the KA sessions and iterative refinement of prototypes.

Because of the quick turnaround time required, ViewPort, an ENCOM-PASS component based on Visio™, was evaluated and selected as the option best suited for the software requirements. The MedView application emerged over a 2-week back-and-forth effort between the KA team and the developer, ScenPro. Following approval of the prototype, the map of the Seattle area was introduced and geo-referenced, hospitals were placed on the map, and MedView was connected to the Oracle-built syndromic surveillance database.

In Seattle, MedView was introduced to the CDC personnel, who were able to use it with minimal guidance or training. During the week before the WTO event, CDC users worked with developers to add further capa-

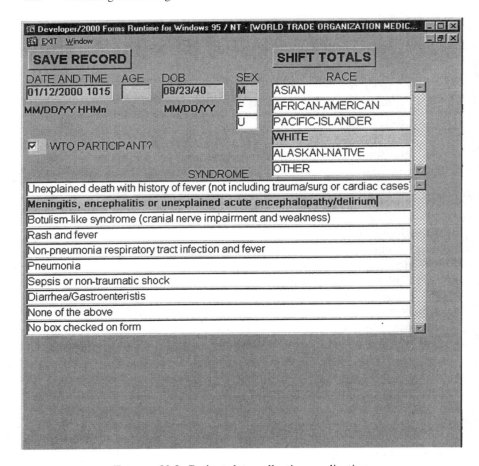

FIGURE 20.3. Patient data collection application.

bilities (e.g., total admissions/symptom ratio display, ability to "hide" hospital names, ability to pause/stop the timeline function). Figure 20.5 shows the application as used during the WTO meetings.

Project Architecture

Early in the project, several potential configurations of the components were discussed; these were all driven by the communications availability. Segments of the communications network consisted of the following:

- Hospital accessibility to the SKC Wide Area Network (WAN)
- Location of the data server on the SKC WAN (inside or outside the firewall)
- Availability of dedicated telephone lines at the hospitals

SHIFT **1**

DAY   = 1
EVE   = 2
NIGHT = 3

TOTAL FOR SHIFT [   ]
ADMITTED TO HOSPITAL [   ]
ADMITTED TO ICU [   ]

SAVE TOTALS

FIGURE 20.4. "Shift totals" box. The blank space at the bottom of the screen in Figure 22.3 is where this "shift totals" box was displayed.

It was not known if all hospitals could access either the Internet or the SKC WAN. In addition, it was not known if the local computer system administrators would be willing or able, because of the short notice, to permit installation of an application on their systems. Although an Internet solution would have eliminated the latter requirement, other availability and permission questions remained unanswered. After considering the known and unknown communication factors as well as the short time period, the team established the following architecture (shown in Figure 20.6):

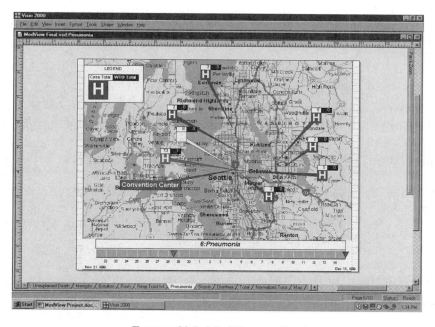

FIGURE 20.5. MedView application.

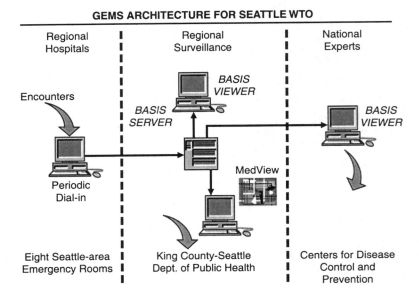

FIGURE 20.6. Project architecture.

- A central data server running Windows NT and Oracle 8i repository for surveillance data
- Notebook computer running Windows 95 or 98, the Oracle 8i database, and the data collection application that was stationed in participating hospitals
- Periodic telephone connection from the hospital to the central data server, during which data collected would be uploaded
- Telephone lines used by hospital fax machines, which would serve double duty as both the fax line and the workstation dial-in

Part Two: Deploying the Application and Results

The teams deployed to the Seattle area 10 days before the WTO event. Although several minor hardware and communication problems emerged, the teams were able to work around them and began collecting baseline data 1 week before the start of the event.

Monitoring Syndromes

There were nine monitoring combinations for the WTO activity, one for each of the eight hospitals and a countywide combination that included data from all eight hospitals. As each monitoring combination assessed nine syndromic conditions, a total of 81 BASIS monitoring streams were implemented on a single notebook computer. The BASIS system interrogated the database server every 15 minutes. Immediate feedback from the on-site CDC surveillance team introduced a steady stream of new requirements and problems. Changes to the software were sometimes accomplished locally in Seattle and other times remotely from the Washington, D.C. area, permitting continuous improvement of the BASIS software according to the needs of the surveillance team.

Because baseline data collection is an essential requirement of epidemiological monitoring, the CDC team had arranged to begin data collection 10 days in advance of the opening of the WTO meeting. By the opening of the WTO meeting, data collection, data logging, and BASIS monitoring were operating smoothly with sufficient baseline data for effective surveillance.

The BASIS Client/Server application successfully provided automated statistical analysis of disease syndromes during the Seattle WTO. In one instance, data led to a BASIS alarm for pneumonia at a single hospital following a 5-day baseline period, and a lag period of 1 day. The alert for this data had a threshold corresponding to a 5% probability of being exceeded at random. A brief inquiry confirmed nothing unusual about these four cases.

Evaluating Results

The goal, articulated as "using technology, design a system that will provide medical surveillance and early detection of covert biowarfare events," was accomplished in an unprecedented timeline to support the 1999 WTO Meeting in Seattle, Washington. The results were invaluable to the public health officers monitoring the event. Although no biological encounters were observed, monitoring the medical emergencies proved pivotal to uncovering serious communicable diseases.

During the data collection period, 10,577 total Emergency Department visits were recorded. The distribution of these by syndromic indicator is shown in Table 20.1.

In the case of meningitis, the BASIS alarm alerted SKC officials that a potentially serious event was occurring. Subsequent discussions with the hospital confirmed that this was the case, and the hospital was able to take appropriate actions to contain the situation.

Conclusion

This syndromic surveillance project proved invaluable to the public health officials at Seattle, King County, CDC, and the development team. Each party gained substantial experience, as they were able to see firsthand what

TABLE 20.1. Distribution of emergency department visits by syndromic indicator.

Syndromic indicator	Number
Botulism-like syndrome (cranial nerve impairment and weakness)	2
Diarrhea/gastroenteritis	156
Meningitis, encephalitis, or unexplained acute encephalopathy/delirium	7
Nonpneumonia respiratory tract infection and fever	123
Pneumonia	128
Rash and fever	38
Sepsis or nontraumatic shock	20
Unexplained death with history of fever (not including trauma/surgery or cardiac cases)	17
None of the above	8,856
No box checked on form	1,230

the operation entailed. All participants praised the common picture the tools gave to the local epidemiologists and to the remote experts. This project also marked several firsts (or near-firsts) for CDC: this was one of the first times CDC deployed an automated data collection facility to the field with real-time links to CDC headquarters in Atlanta, Georgia, and it was the first time they deployed in advance of a major event.

Perhaps the most remarkable story to come from the WTO meeting will not be the protesters who received front page and national TV news coverage, but the men and women of the joint team discussed in this chapter. Government, state, local, and contractor staff worked together literally day and night to build and implement a surveillance system in just under 3 weeks. The product of their efforts will be a crucial weapon in the fight against bioterrorism. It is an essential prototype of the automated surveillance system the United States needs to protect its borders and port cities against an influx of serious infectious disease.

Acknowledgments. The author wishes to thank the following individuals for their contributions to this chapter: at Oracle, Ruth Ann Nelson and William Heney; at PSR, Gene McClelland and Ed Pratt; and at Scen Pro, Bob Williams and Jim Mantock.

21
Eliminating Disparities in Minority Health

Selina Smith and Mary Walker

The health promotion campaigns and research efforts of the past two decades have clearly impacted the health of this nation: as recent trends in morbidity and mortality data indicate, Americans are living longer, more productive lives. However, despite overall improvements in health status, there are continuing disparities in the burden of illness and death experienced by some groups of Americans. Compared to the U.S. population as a whole, African Americans, Hispanics, Native Americans/Alaska Natives, and Pacific Islanders are more likely to be victims of the leading causes of death, including coronary heart disease and cancer.

Future health care for America as a whole will be influenced by the way this disparity issue is addressed. New approaches are needed to align the health profiles of minorities with those of the general population. Because these disparities concern us all, it is to everybody's benefit to address them. This chapter aims to do so by these points:

- Clarifying the critical nature of health disparities through statistics
- Discussing general information technology solutions to the problem
- Offering a brief overview of state initiatives working toward positive change
- Examining the specific steps the Department of Health and Human Services (HHS) is taking to reduce the economic and social burden of health disparities

Health Disparities: Statistical Evidence

Although the death rate associated with many major diseases may be decreasing in the United States, these encouraging signs are not yet applicable to all racial and ethnic groups. For example, the age-adjusted death rate for coronary heart disease, which is the leading cause of death for all racial and ethnic groups, declined by 20% for the total population from 1987 to 1995. For African Americans, however, the overall decrease was only

13%; African American men alone suffer from heart disease at nearly twice the rates of whites. Compared with rates for whites, coronary heart disease mortality was 40% higher for African Americans in 1995. (The rate was 40% lower for Asian Americans: stroke is the only leading cause of death for which mortality is higher for Asian-American males than for white males.)

Infant mortality is another important measure of a nation's health and a worldwide indicator of health status. Although infant mortality in the United States has declined steadily over the past several decades and was at a record low of 7.2 per 1,000 live births in 1996, the United States still ranks 24th in infant mortality compared with other industrialized nations because infant mortality rates (IMRs) vary substantially among and within racial and ethnic groups.

Infant death rates among African Americans, Native Americans, Alaska Natives, and Hispanics in 1995 or 1996 were all above the national average of 7.2 deaths per 1,000 live births. IMRs are 2.5 times higher for African Americans and 1.5 times higher for Native Americans. The overall Native American rate (9.0 per 1,000 live births in 1995) does not reflect the diversity among Native American communities, some of which have infant mortality rates approaching twice the national rate. Similarly, the overall Hispanic rate (7.6 per 1,000 live births in 1995) does not reflect the diversity among this group, which had a rate of 8.9 per 1,000 live births among Puerto Ricans in 1995.

Childhood immunizations are at a record high for the nation as a whole, with the most critical vaccine doses reflecting coverage rates of more than 90%. The 1996 immunization coverage targets for all five vaccines (measles, mumps, and rubella; polio; diphtheria, tetanus, and pertussis; *Haemophilus influenza* type B; and hepatitis b) were exceeded. However, immunization rates have been lower in minority populations compared with the white population. Although minority rates have begun increasing more rapidly, the gap has only narrowed, not closed.

There are approximately 604,200 adults and adolescents reported with acquired immunodeficiency syndrome (AIDS) in the United States, and roughly 62% (375,000) of them have died of the disease. For the first time since the epidemic began, human immunodeficiency virus (HIV) and AIDS rates are falling. Although the epidemic is decreasing in some populations, the *number* of new AIDS cases among African Americans is now greater than the number of new cases among whites. Racial and ethnic minorities constitute approximately 25% of the total U.S. population, yet they account for nearly 54% of all AIDS cases. Although the number of AIDS diagnoses among gay and bisexual men has decreased dramatically among white men since 1989, the numbers of diagnoses among gay and bisexual African American men have increased. In addition, AIDS cases and new infections related to injecting drug use appear to be increasingly concentrated in minorities; of these cases, almost 75% were among minority populations (56% African American and 20% Hispanic). Of cases reported among women and children, more than 75% are among racial and ethnic minorities.

Cancers also affect minority groups disproportionately. For example, African American men under 65 suffer from prostate cancer nearly at twice the rate of white men in the same age bracket. Vietnamese women suffer from cervical cancer at nearly five times the rate of white women. Latinos have two to three times the rate of stomach cancer as do whites.

Table 21.1 summarizes statistical evidence for health disparities among U.S. minorities, measured by six health status indicators. These disparities are alarming, and they demand dramatic action. In this era of unprecedented technological advancement, how can we use the new tools at our disposal to purge the American population of its health disparities?

Information Technology Solutions: An Overview

Technology is increasingly relevant in both health care and in everyday life. In the management of chronic disease, information technology has begun playing a vital role in a variety of intervention and prevention programs, and it has vast potential for application in the area of racial/ethnic health disparity. Databases, algorithms, decision support, expert systems, and clinician/consumer education are a few possible technology applications, although the inherent complexity of the issues related to racial and ethnic health disparities clearly requires an integrated system. Information harvested from such a system should, at minimal cost, furnish the needs of communication, audit, research, and management. This result will facilitate remarkably flexible evidence-based medicine.

Enabling education is a particularly valuable capability of technology applications. Technology can promote more comprehensive clinical education, both in terms of scientific and technical knowledge and of less quantifiable forms of knowledge like empathy and intuition, which are needed to develop sensitivity to the array of racial and ethnic issues in this country. E-health technologies can be used to provide educational information to patients and facilitate the storage and transmittal of clinical data between patients and clinicians.

Technology is an adjunct that will serve health care well if it is incorporated as a part of a multidimensional patient care environment. With the introduction of home-based technology, which provides an efficient way for doctors and patients to communicate, the question of the effectiveness of clinical decisions must be addressed. Lingering issues like these must be addressed through continuing research, development, and evaluation.

TABLE 21.1. Health Disparities among U.S. Minorities.

Health status indicator	Whites (non-Hispanics)	Blacks (non-Hispanics)	Hispanics	Native American/Alaska Native	Asian American/Pacific Islander
Infant mortality: 1996 infant mortality rates per 100,000	6.1	14.1	6.1	10.1	5.2
Breast cancer screening: 1994, women 50+ receiving clinical breast examinations and mammograms within the preceding 2 years, in percent	58	58	50	53	46
Cardiovascular disease: 1996 coronary heart disease deaths per 100,000	102.1	140.1	72.7	74.5	56.7
Diabetes: 1993–1996 diabetes-related end-stage renal disease per 1,000	2.8	5.5	Not available	5.4 (1992 data only)	Not available
HIV infection/AIDS: 1997 AIDS cases in persons 13 years of age or older per 100,000	12.4	107.2	50.6	13.6	5.6
Immunizations: 1996 immunization rates per 100,000	80	76	73	81	81

Sources: CDC/NCHS National Vital Statistics System, Linked Birth and Infant Death Data Set, Centers for Disease Control & Prevention, National Center for Health Statistics, National Health Interview Survey; Health Care Financing Administration, Program Statistics; Centers for Disease Control & Prevention, National center for HIV, STD, and TB Prevention; Adult/Adolescent AIDS Reporting System, Centers for Disease Control & Prevention, National Immunization Survey (1994–1996).

State Health Initiatives

Many advances in health have emerged from the use and implementation of technology solutions. The Health Delivery organizations and IDNs have implemented solutions that track the patient from infancy to death. These organizations typically are for-profit organizations or well-endowed academic medical institutions. State and community hospital organizations do not have the same level of funding, and they serve a population that frequently is uninsured or underinsured. As a result, they lack funds for investing in leading-edge technology or even staying current with applications that would improve access to care. To help some of these state healthcare providers, the Department of Health and Human Services has provided assistance through grants for breast cancer detection and screening, community-based outreach for training and technical assistance, nutritional studies, and immunization tracking.

Many states have taken advantage of these programs and are implementing strategies that will lead to a decrease in diseases that adversely affect multiple populations within the state. Texas, for example, is one of 20 states to receive a public health infrastructure grant to develop an integrated approach to capturing local health data and reporting this information to headquarters. Kansas has taken a grassroots approach through a privately funded public health collaboration to resolve data reporting and surveillance issues of local health providers. Florida, on the other hand, has developed a very robust WAN that connects 67 of its counties with high-speed data transfers. The Florida Department of Health has collected data in a standard format so that many of the diseases that plague minorities can be studied by age, morbidity and mortality rates, chronic diseases, immunizations, dental health, and communicable diseases. This form of data collection will allow Florida to develop programs that are focused on specific positive outcomes, thereby reducing the cost of health care and improving the health of all populations.

Montana has taken a different approach, one that involves a public/private partnership. This mode truly represents a "best in class" action, because it looks at the whole picture of health care in the state. The Montana Public Health task force tackled critical public health issues, eventually recognizing that the development of guidelines and policies required the involvement of all state/local/federal parties, and that the outlined responsibilities would need constant refinement based on actual outcomes. This recognition was a first for the state of Montana, and the task force is still actively engaged in improving infrastructure and processes such as the delivery and payment of healthcare services. The major goals for the public health improvement initiative are these:

- Increasing the Montana public health system's capacity
- Supporting public health collaboration

- Increasing accountability
- Building capacity at the community level

The level of data found in the Montana public health database allows for easy process improvements across all entities within the state, focused, and targeted programs. Studying the demographics and diseases by ethnicity will greatly improve their ability to improve health disparities for minorities.

The HHS Action Plan

In February 1998, President Clinton announced an initiative aimed at closing the racial and ethnic gaps in health status. The President's Initiative on Race asserts that the United States should fulfill its role as a leader in diversity by setting an example for other countries. This plan mobilizes the resources and expertise of the private sector, local communities, and each federal department to eliminate these disparities. President Clinton's approach, rooted in broad-based participation and multisector planning consistent with international models, recognized that health problems in underserved communities stem from poverty—not from the poor themselves.

To achieve the President's goals, the Department of Health and Human Services (HHS) would provide leadership by conducting research, expanding and improving programs to purchase or deliver quality health services, implementing programs to reduce poverty and provide children with safe and healthy environments, and expanding prevention efforts. As part of the plan, the HHS selected six areas of focus in which racial and ethnic minorities experience serious disparities in health access and outcomes:

- Cancer screening and management
- Cardiovascular disease
- Child and adult immunizations
- Diabetes
- HIV infection/AIDS
- Infant mortality

These six disparity areas must be addressed within a comprehensive framework that addresses broader issues. Any discussion of health disparities must include the larger issues of poverty, violence, substance abuse, mental health, discrimination, immigrant health, the breakdown of communal bonds, lack of education, increasing social fragmentation, and the inequity throughout the healthcare delivery system. Poverty is closely associated with poor health status among minorities; therefore, inequities in economic opportunity are an important consideration. Discrimination is another variable, with its own measurable impact on health status.

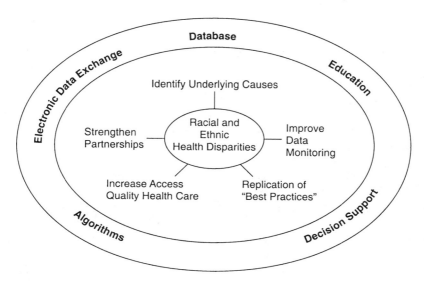

FIGURE 21.1. HHS IT Strategies.

An awareness of these larger issues is critical as we develop strategies to address minority health disparities. To move forward strategically, it is important to approach the problem in a comprehensive manner, understanding the necessity of vision. This need makes the challenge for the HHS even greater.

To begin to address these issues, the HHS has proposed several specific and strategic actions. These are shown in Figure 21.1 and summarized in the subsections that follow, along with some discussion on information technology approaches.

Identify Underlying Causes

The literature does not yet permit a clear understanding of underlying structures and processes that give rise to health disparities. Although it is fully recognized that poverty, lack of access to quality health services, environmental hazards, and less than effective prevention programs may play a role, additional research is needed to identify reasons for higher levels of disease and disability in racial and ethnic minority communities.

To achieve this goal, the HHS will direct attention to improvements in monitoring and developing the local and national data necessary for determining priorities and designing programs. Information technology can help key players electronically organize information for efficient retrieval. Improving and standardizing data collection will identify all high-risk populations and help assess the general health status of the targeted communities.

The HHS has begun examining current programs to see if they focus on opportunities to reduce health disparities and make full use of available knowledge on effective delivery of clinical and preventive services. Eventually, gaps in knowledge will be identified through the development of accurate baseline data, and research agendas will be developed to address those gaps. New programs or modifications to existing programs will be recommended.

Strengthen Partnerships

Next, the HHS will broaden and strengthen its partnerships with state and local governments, with national and regional minority health and other minority-focused organizations, and with minority community-based organizations—those which have the greatest access to and knowledge of the communities. The HHS vision will bring together foundations, corporations, government, universities, and other organizations that believe in the importance of this cause. Several of these organizations already have instituted innovative and productive programs to improve healthcare quality, delivery, and access in their communities and systems, sometimes in very difficult circumstances. Many of these organizations possess ample resources and are available to participate in this effort.

Clearly, it will be easier to access these resources if the organizations understand why eliminating disparity is important. These partnerships should be structured in a way that continually encourages partners to learn from one another. The goal is to provide a national framework for public and private sector collaboration to eliminate health disparities through Healthy People 2010, the nation's health action agenda for the twenty-first century. Improving the flow of information and communication is vital to the success of these partnerships. Community leaders and advocates must be helped to increase awareness and establish ongoing linkages with entities that will move the effort forward.

Optimal, cost-effective communication is a crucial aspect of strengthening partnerships for the HHS initiative. Information technology enablers include electronic data exchange, or the replacement of paper documents with standard electronic messages conveyed from one computer to another without manual intervention. Emerging technologies promise to improve communication between those segments of the public and private sectors that are being called to address health disparities.

Improve Data Monitoring

The HHS will improve monitoring and develop the local and national data necessary for determining priorities and designing programs. High-quality, thorough, and uniformly reported data on all racial and ethnic subgroups must accurately reflect the needs of the community. Definitions of each subgroup within racial/ethnic categories will enhance the quality of this data at the federal, state, and local levels.

Baseline measures must be clearly defined. Involving the community (particularly minorities) in this process will help ensure that the data are complete and accurate, as will training the individuals who gather and measure the data. Effective process and outcome measures must also be developed to monitor progress and to ensure accuracy. Although all these requirements can take time, the improved outcomes are invaluable. These data will be important in evaluating progress and allocating resources.

Increase Access to Health Care

To address the six disparities, all Americans must have access to the highest quality health care, either through universal coverage or another medium. To achieve this goal, policy makers, communities, healthcare providers, funders, and the media must recognize that this is an issue that affects all Americans, not only those who cannot afford health insurance.

Attracting more members of ethnic and racial groups to healthcare professions will help reduce disparities over the long term. Academic health centers must be part of the action, and universities, government agencies, and the private sector must all develop partnerships that will increase the numbers of minority healthcare professionals. Healthcare organizations also must make the best possible use of their available resources through clinical resource management, a four-stage process of identifying opportunities for improvement, developing an effective resource management team, implementing process improvement activities, and measuring the impact on care outcomes.

A wide range of information technology approaches will serve this strategic action.

- Computer-based clinical decision support tools, such as automated direct-from-patient information collection and disease-reporting/procedure-reporting programs, can improve physician performance in ambulatory care settings.
- ComputerLink, a specialized computer network, serves as a convenient, efficient, and enduring vehicle for delivering services to patients at home.
- Computer-based techniques for improving the day-to-day care of patients, such as computer-based interactive simulators and educational video games, may offer a means of training more healthcare professionals to deliver improved care.
- Internet applications can be used to locate information and identify and address barriers to care in a timely, convenient manner. A majority of

public health departments are technically capable of connecting to the Internet.

- Direct backups of medical activity can aid in epidemiological tasks and facilitate preventive follow-up with patients.

Replicate Best Practices

The communities must drive changes themselves. Education will play a major role in the elimination of health disparities with efforts targeted at the general public, public officials, community decision makers and leaders, and members of ethnic and minority groups themselves.

Information technology approaches include the following:

- Telephone-Linked Care (TLC), a telecommunications technology that enables computer-controlled telephone counseling with patients in their home, increases the medical care system's effectiveness in modifying behavior of individuals—ensuring patient compliance with medication regimens, healthy diets, regular physical activity, regular health screening, and the avoidance of substance abuse. It has been successfully applied to the task of improving a number of different health behaviors. Future uses involve applying the technology to other important health behaviors, targeting use of TLC to the most appropriate patient groups, incorporating new computer and telecommunications technology into the system, and interfacing TLC into the healthcare delivery system.
- Clinical databases that use all available information sources to analyze the outcomes of improvements in care quality create high potential for generalization and clinician participation.
- Internet applications as resources for healthcare information and new methods create partnerships between healthcare providers and patients.

Conclusion

Many people, processes, behaviors, and systems are required to improve access to care and reduce health disparities. Partnerships, community involvement, outreach, and strategic alliances will all play an important role in closing the gap. The federal sector programs have stimulated valuable thinking and are lending both financial and technical help. Many of the states that were briefly discussed in this chapter have taken serious and proactive steps to help care for their people.

Even with these advances duly noted, health care is only beginning to take advantage of the technologies available in this rapidly changing world. Because information must be delivered and received in a timely manner, the public health delivery and outreach organizations will have to embrace such technologies as e-health to improve access to health and promote wellness. This new way of conducting business enables stronger and more effective communication among patients, doctors, employers, payors, laboratories, pharmacies, hospitals, and suppliers. Employing this technology in the form of enterprise-wide solutions, data warehousing, and data mining can shorten the time needed to reduce disparities in health care for minorities. Properly aligned health initiatives embracing technologies will foster improved disease management and operational efficiency, lower transaction costs and increase capacity, and forge a stronger sense of connection among patients, physicians, and other caregivers.

Readings

Alexander, G.R., Kogan, M.D., Himes, J.H., Mor, J.M., Goldenberg, R. 1999. Racial Differences in Birthweight for Gestational Age and Infant Mortality in Extremely Low Risk US Populations. *Paediatr Perinat Epidemiol* 13(2):205–217.

Baehring, T.U., Schulze, H., Bornstein, S.R., Scherbaum, W.A. 1997. Using the World Wide Web—A New Approach to Risk Identification of Diabetes Mellitus. *Int J Med Inf* 46(1):31–39.

Black, S.A., Jakobi, P.L., Rush, R.D., DiNuzzo, A.R., Garcia, D. 1999. Ethnic Variation in the Health Burden of Self-Reported Diabetes in Adults Aged 75 and Older. *Ethn Dis* 9(1):22–32.

Bozzo, J., Carlson, B., Diers, D. 1998. Using Hospital Data Systems to Find Target Populations: New Tools for Clinical Nurse Specialists. *Clin Nurse Spec* 12(2):86–91.

Centers for Disease Control and Prevention. 1999. Decrease in Infant Mortality and Sudden Infant Death Syndrome Among Northwest American Indians and Alaskan Natives—Pacific Northwest, 1985–1999. *JAMA* 281(15):1369–1370.

Choi, K.H., Catania, J.A., Dolcini, M.M. 1994. Extramarital Sex and HIV Risk Behavior Among US Adults: Results from the National AIDS Behavioral Survey. *AM J Public Health* 84(12):2003–2007.

Corti, M.C., Guralnik, J.M., Ferrucci, L., Izmirlian, G., Leveille, S.G., Pahor, M., Cohen, H.J., Pieper, C., Havlik, R.J. 1999. Evidence for a Black-White Crossover in All-Cause and Coronary Heart Disease Mortality in an Older Population: The North Carolina EPESE." *Am J Public Health* 89(3):308–314.

Cytryn, K.N., Patel, V.L. 1998. Reasoning about Diabetes and Its Relationship to the Use of Telecommunication Technology by Patients and Physicians. *Int J Med Inf* 51(2–3):137–151.

Diaz, T., Chu, S.Y., Buehler, J.W., Boyd, D., Checko, P.J., Conti, L., Davidson, A.J., Hermann, P., Herr, M., Levy, A., et al. 1994. Socioeconomic Differences Among People with AIDS: Results from a Multistate Surveillance Project. *Am J Prev Med* 10(4):217–222.

Friedman, C. 1996. Progress Towards the Year 2000: Assessing the Health Status of Minorities in Texas. *Tex Med* 92(10):53–58.

Friedman, S.R., Young, P.A., Snyder, F.R., Shorty, V., Jones, A., Estrada, AL. 1993. Racial Differences in Sexual Behaviors Related to AIDS in a Nineteen-City Sample of Street-Recruited Drug Injectors. NADR Consortium. *AIDS Educ Prev* 5(3):196–211.

Fuller, J.H. 1998. Methods of Assessing the Quality of Diabetes Care. *Horm Res* 50(suppl. 1):64–67.

Goodwin, J.S., Black, S.A., Satish, S. 1999. Aging Versus Disease: The Opinion of Older Black, Hispanic, and Non-Hispanic White Americans about the Causes and Treatment of Common Medical Conditions. *J AM Geriatr Soc* 47(8):973–979.

Haverkos, H.W., Turner, J.F., Jr., Moolchan, E.T., Cadet, J.L. 1999. Relative Rates of AIDS Among Racial/Ethnic Groups by Exposure Categories. *J Natl Med Assoc* 91(1):17–24.

Lai, D., Tsai, S.P., Hardy, R.J. 1997. Impact of HIV/AIDS on Life Expectancy in the United States. *AIDS* 11(2):203–207.

Larson, E. 1997. Social and Economic Impact of Infectious Diseases—United States. *Clin Perform Qual Health Care* 5(1):31–37.

Lehmann, E.D. 1997. Interactive Educational Simulators in Diabetes Care. *Med Inform* (Lond) 22(1):47–76.

Liao, Y., McGee, D.L., Cooper, R.S. 1999. Prediction of Coronary Heart Disease Mortality in Blacks and Whites: Pooled Data from Two National Cohorts. *Am J Cardiol* 84(1):31–36.

Lillie-Blanton, M., Parsons, P.E., Gayle, H., Dievler, A. 1996. Racial Differences in Health: Not Just Black and White, But Shades of Gray. *Annu Rev Public Health* 17:411–448.

Louisiana State University Medical Center, New Orleans, USA. 1999. Cervical Cancer Screening Knowledge, Behaviors, and Beliefs of Vietnamese Women. *Oncol Nurs Forum* 26(5):879–887.

Mondragon, D. 1993. No More 'Let Them Eat Admonitions': the Clinton Administration's Emerging Approach to Minority Health [editorial]. *J Health Care Poor Underserved* 4(2):77–82.

Mueller, K.J., Ortega, S.T., Parker, K., Patil, K., Askenazai, A. 1999. Health Status and Access to Care Among Rural Minorities. *J Health Care Poor Underserved* 10(2):230–249.

Namboodiri, K.K., Fisher, J.B., Harris, R.E. 1993. The Ohio Cancer Information Service: Technology Transfer on Clinical Trials and Other Measures of Cancer Control. *J Cancer Educ* 8(3):227–237.

Parker, S., Tomaselli, M.B. 1996. Streamlining Breast Disease Management. *J Health Resour Manage* 14(7):23–26.

Piette, J.D., Mah, C.A. 1997. The Feasibility of Automated Voice Messaging as an Adjunct to Diabetes Outpatient Care. *Diabetes Care* 20(1):15–21.

Potter, S.J., Mauldin, P.D., Hill, H.A. 1996. Access to and Participation in Breast Cancer Screening: A Review of Recent Literature. *Clin Perform Qual Health Care* 4(2):74–85.

Saha, S. 1999. Patient-Physician Racial Concordance and the Perceived Quality and Use of Health Care. *Arch Intern Med* 159(9):997–1004.

Sanders-Phillips, K., Davis, S. 1998. Improving Prenatal Care Services for Low-Income African American Women and Infants [editorial]. *J Health Care Poor Underserved* 9(1):14–29.

Sayegh, A.J., Swor, R., Chu, K.H., Jackson, R., Gitlin, J., Domeier, R.M., Basse, E., Smith, D., Fales, W. 1999. Does Race or Socioeconomic Status Predict Adverse Outcome After Out of Hospital Cardiac Arrest: A Multi-Center Study. *Resuscitation* 40(3):141–146.

Seipel, M.M. 1998. Health for All: Is There Health Parity Between Blacks and Whites? *J Health Social Policy* 10(3):53–69.

Sexton, K., Gong, H. Jr., Bailar, J.C., Ford, J.G., Gold, D.R., Lambert, W.E., Utell, M.J. 1993. Air Pollution Health Risks: Do Class and Race Matter? *Toxicol Ind Health* 9(5):843–878.

Snowden, L. 1997. An Investigation into Whether Nursing Students Alter Their Attitude and Knowledge Levels Regarding HIV Infection and AIDS Following a 3-Year Programme Leading to Registration as a Qualified Nurse. *J Adv Nurse* 25(6):1167–1174.

Topping, S., Hartwig, L.C. 1997. Delivering Care to Rural HIV/AIDS Patients. *J Rural Health* 13(3):226–236.

Van der Veen, W.J. 1998. Comment on 'Compromised Birth Outcomes and Infant Mortality Among Racial and Ethnic Groups' [comment]. *Demography* 35(4):509–517.

Yi, J.K. 1998. Acculturation and Pap Smear Screening Practices Among College-Aged Vietnamese Women in the United States. *Cancer Nurs* 21(5):335–341.

State Information

Montana
Public Health Improvement, Montana Turning Point Imitative
Montana County Health Profiles
Strategic Plan for Public Health Systems Improvement in Montana (Draft)
Summary of the 1997 Public Health Improvement Plan

Texas
Population Data, Texas State Data Center, Texas Population Estimates and Projections Programs, Texas A & M University, 1998
Facts About the Bureau of State Health Data & Policy Analysis

Kansas
Kansas Health Data Resources
Health Care Governing Board
Policy Analysis
Evaluation & Monitoring
Data Development and Analysis Communication

Missouri
Missouri Department of Health Integrated Strategic Plan 2000–2005
Missouri Department of Health Missouri Information for Community Assessments

22
Telehealth

CAPT C. Forrest Faison III, Jay Sanders, James Smith,
and David Dimond

The federal sector has been advancing telehealth initiatives for many years, and with great success. The process of integrating telehealth, however, has not been easy or smooth. Issues related to planning, funding, and staffing these projects have introduced challenges and obstacles, and in our efforts to surmount these, we have collected a catalog of valuable lessons. In this chapter, we share some of those lessons and experiences for the benefit of other organizations interested in using telehealth to improve business and clinical processes.

History of Telehealth and the Federal Government

Telehealth, as defined by the federal government, is the use of computers and communications technology to deliver health care independent of time and distance. As such, the government has been conducting telehealth for the past 20 years. For the purposes of this chapter, we primarily discuss telehealth that improves access to care in remote places where, and in cases in which, care would not otherwise be available. We briefly discuss distance learning and other initiatives, but the primary focus is on access to care. Likewise, although they are worthy of enthusiastic study, state initiatives like telehealth provided to prison populations are not addressed here.

Some of the government's earliest telehealth initiatives began in the early 1990s and were conducted by the Department of Defense (DoD), the Department of Commerce, and the Department of Health and Human Services (HHS). Initially, the DoD's initiatives focused on providing medical support to operationally deployed units in remote areas around the world. Initiatives in the Commerce Department and the HHS focused on providing specialized medical services to remote, underserved populations within the continental United States. These initiatives had different funding sources: those for the DoD were primarily derived from research and development funds, whereas those for the Department of Commerce and the HHS were funded through grants.

Most early telehealth prototypes used synchronous, interactive communications for medical consultations and were essentially technological automations of the existing doctor–patient interaction. Because there was little if any reengineering associated with these early initiatives, they were expensive and difficult to sustain over the long term. Furthermore, utilization rates for most of these early prototypes were low, because most prototypes did not include training for physicians or other healthcare providers. These low utilization rates, combined with the high costs of communications, made it difficult (if not impossible) to achieve a positive return on investment (ROI) or realize tangible, quantifiable benefits.

In the mid-1990s, store-and-forward communications were used to control costs and ensure the long-term viability of telehealth projects. However, few of these early initiatives had any comprehensive programs to collect data and demonstrate a positive ROI. This lack became a significant hurdle in the mid-1990s, when federal funding decreased. Because no ROI data were available, it was difficult for these projects to compete for scarce dollars in an increasingly competitive healthcare market.

At the time, the government had few tools to measure return on investment, and it did not have a standardized, comprehensive methodology for needs assessment, metrics planning, equipment standardization, networks planning, or implementation. This limitation mirrored what most civilian programs with similar interests experienced, and it precluded long-term planning or support for these early telemedicine prototypes. For the most part, early government efforts were technology centered and focused on "proving" the concept with little regard for business case analysis or planning, both of which would help ensure the long-term viability of these telemedicine efforts.

Until 1996, collaboration within the federal government on telehealth initiatives was limited. Within the DoD, telehealth was managed by the individual services: Army, Navy, and Air Force. Separate funding lines and organizational structures made collaboration between the services difficult. Collaboration between constituencies within the Commerce Department and HHS was limited, as most telemedicine prototypes were created by means of grants given to academic centers. Budgetary and staffing constraints within these departments also deflected resources that could have offered levels of project oversight and management, which would have helped avoid duplicate efforts and disseminate lessons learned throughout the organization.

In summary, early efforts within the federal government focused on "proof-of-concept": an attempt to confirm that medical care could be effectively distributed to remote, underserved populations by means of information technology. Sporadic funding, disorganization, insufficient collaboration between the organizations involved, and the lack of a standardized business planning methodology severely diminished the chances of success for most of these prototype telehealth projects.

Collaborative Efforts: The Vice-President's Joint Working Group on Telehealth

As part of the Clinton Administration's commitment to build a national "information superhighway," Vice President Al Gore convened a working group in 1995 composed of key leaders from each federal organization involved in telehealth. The purpose of the workgroup was to promote the sharing of resources, greater collaboration between federal agencies, and the use of the evolving information superhighway as a means of providing better access and delivery of health care to the diverse communities of the United States. The participants selected the Department of Health and Human Services to serve as the first organizational "chair" of the workgroup.

The workgroup now meets on a biweekly basis to discuss current or planned telehealth initiatives within the government sector. It maintains, in collaboration with the U.S. Army Medical Materiel and Research Command at Fort Detrick, Maryland, a comprehensive website of all federal telehealth projects and research initiatives. The workgroup also publishes an annual compendium of all known federal and state telehealth projects. In the most recent compendium (1998), 43 states and the District of Columbia were noted to have one or more active, funded telehealth programs.

Role of the General Accounting Office

As watchdog for the U.S. Congress, the General Accounting Office (GAO) is responsible for monitoring most federal expenditures. The GAO ensures that telehealth expenditures meet congressional guidelines and are properly managed within the mandates of both statutory and regulatory guidance. To date, there have been three GAO audits of federal departments regarding telehealth initiatives. In general, the findings offered in these audits confirm previous experiences within the government and mirror findings typical of the civilian sector, including these points:

- Lack of coordination within and between federal departments
- Significant variety in funding sources and practices
- Lack of a uniform methodology for needs assessment, program planning, metrics, or business case analysis
- Significant duplication of efforts
- Difficulty in aligning current projects with department missions, goals, or objectives

These and other findings demonstrated the need to bring the rigor of business case analysis to all federal telehealth initiatives. Nearly all GAO reports recommend that the coordination for the telehealth initiatives of each federal department be centralized and that coordination between the federal departments be improved and enhanced. Follow-up reports to Congress have shown varying degrees of success in achieving these mandates.

The execution of the centralized coordination mandate has been left to the discretion of the individual federal departments, so long as it conforms to the centralized coordination plan. Properly administered, this brand of decentralized coordination should allow federal departments to leverage a rapidly evolving commercial market. The departments will also be able to preserve field autonomy in designing and implementing custom-tailored telehealth solutions for local constituencies, all without undue administrative delay or burden. The advantages and disadvantages of these efforts, which are numerous, are discussed in a subsequent section.

Funding Federal Telehealth Projects

With the exception of the Department of Defense, most telehealth projects within the federal government have been (and continue to be) funded by means of federal grants. Most often awarded as a result of some form of competitive assessment, they usually support proof-of-concept demonstrations. In general, they are awarded to private or academic institutions. Within the DoD, 80% to 90% of past and current telehealth projects are or have been funded from "Program Eight" budgets, the military name for general healthcare operating budgets. Approximately 15% are funded with research and development dollars ("Program Six"), while the remaining 5% are funded with military operational support dollars ("Program Two").

One survey revealed that by the late 1990s, the total cumulative federal investment in telehealth was approximately $600 to $700 million (GAO 1997). Approximately 60% of that amount has been expended by the DoD in support of global military operations. Of the remainder, approximately 30% are grants to academic institutions, and the remaining 10% has gone toward grants to private foundations, corporations, or other entities.

Funding patterns within the DoD significantly differ from those of other federal agencies and of corporate entities. The DoD has funded the majority of its telemedicine investments from daily operating funds, vice grants, or research funds, mainly because local commanders have been granted rather generous thresholds for procurement. In general, and with few exceptions, local commanders may purchase any medical equipment they wish so long as the price is less than $100,000. As the price of most telemedicine packages falls well below this threshold, local commanders have used excess operating funds to purchase telemedicine equipment.

Virtually all these investments have been initiated without complete business case analyses. With the best of intentions, these local commanders have simply attempted to increase the level of care available to their remote beneficiaries. A critical examination of such spending patterns reveals a strong correlation between the brand of equipment purchased by the local commander and the manufacturers that have been most visible in the locality. Local personnel have become enamored with technologies with little consideration of the business planning aspects that should accompany any capital investment. The result has been a DoD telemedicine investment portfolio largely determined by vendor marketing skills and travel.

Telehealth and the Department of Defense

The DoD's earliest telehealth initiatives began in 1994 in the research and development community. The United States Army Medical Research and Materiel Command, under Brigadier General Russ Zajtchuk, established an office specifically dedicated to telemedicine research and utilization. The Medical and Advanced Technology Management Office (MATMO), established at Fort Detrick, Maryland, comprised officers and researchers from all services and from prominent academic institutions in the Washington, D.C., metropolitan area. With the aid of cooperative agreements with Georgetown University and others, MATMO became the DoD's first telehealth testbed.

The first operational deployment of telehealth was performed by MATMO in support of operational ground forces in Bosnia and Macedonia in 1996 (Operation Joint Endeavor and Operation Joint Guard). The hypothesis was that telehealth technologies could be used to deliver quality health care—otherwise unavailable—to remote areas in support of Operations Other Than War (OOTW). The deployment, code named Operation Primetime, consisted of three discrete phases, shown in Table 22.1 with the activities and technologies associated with each phase.

An independent evaluation was done by the Army Medical Department Center and Schools, and by Northrup Grummann. The cognizant surgeon for the European Commander-in-Chief (EUCOM) established several objectives:

- To maintain seamless patient accountability
- To provide rapid, definitive response to trauma
- To deliver highest quality care to soldiers, leveraging remote specialty medical support
- To provide medical leadership with overall theater command and control view of assets

In general, the patient population consisted of young and healthy active duty personnel; all deployed personnel were screened for significant medical conditions and were disqualified if their medical requirements exceeded in-theater capabilities. A smaller population of older DoD contractors was not screened before entering the theater (to avoid potential

TABLE 22.1. Three phases of Operation Primetime.

Phase	Dates	Activity	Technology/capability

1	Jan 96–
	Apr 96
		Connect CONUS
		with Landstuhl AMC,
		67th CSH, 212th
		MASH
			• High-resolution remote video
			  communications equipment
			• Digital examination scopes
			• Diagnostic digital scanners for radiographs
			• Medical information systems:
			• Composite Healthcare System (CHCS)
			• Theater Army Medical Management
			  and Information System (TAMMIS)
			• Patient Accounting and Reporting
			  Realtime Tracking System (PARRTS)

2	Apr 96–
	Nov 96
		Connect FOBs,
		BOBs with CSH,
		MASH
			• High-resolution remote video
			  communications equipment (did not
			  include standardized software packages)
			• Digital examination scopes

3	Nov 96– Jan 98	Finish connectivity with FOBs, BOBs	• Store and Forward computer equipment • Digital examination scopes

AMC, Army Medical Center; CONUS, continental United States (Walter Reed AMC, Washington, D.C.); CSH, Combat Support Hospital; MASH, Mobile Army Surgical Hospital; FOB, Forward Operating Base; BOB, Brigade Operating Base.

violations of the Americans with Disabilities Act); it is possible that some of these individuals could have been chronically ill.

During the deployment, the conditions most often treated by medical personnel were orthopedic, sports-related injuries, and food poisoning, for which intestinal disorders (diarrhea) was the most common complaint. Trauma was relatively rare, as were other traditional nonbattle illnesses (infectious diseases, veneral diseases, etc.). The total number of medical encounters between April 1 and October 12 of 1996 was 7,046; approximately 90% of these encounters were conducted in an outpatient setting, and less than 1% resulted in a telemedicine consultation. The total number of telemedicine consultations during the deployment was more than 50,000.

An evaluation was conducted by the EUCOM surgeon, who checked findings against the project objectives. Outcomes are described in the subsections that follow.

Maintain Seamless Patient Accountability

Overall, telemedicine allowed for 85% patient accountability during the deployment, a substantial improvement over previous paper tracking methods. Frequent unit movements and other factors make tracking a patient particularly difficult in an evolving operational scenario, especially because medical units generally do not maintain their own communications bandwidth and must rely on operational bandwidth being available between uses. Previous deployments in Operation Desert Storm and elsewhere had yielded a patient accountability between 50% and 70%.

Although the 85% figure was a dramatic improvement, it fell far short of the 100% goal desired by the EUCOM surgeon. For inpatients, there was a 16% discrepancy between verified paper records and what was available in medical databases in theater. For outpatient encounters, there was an 85% to 90% concurrence between databases. The largest source of error was that of human, manual error, mainly caused by a lack of training, multiple concurrent taskings for data operators, and infrequent data verification. Compounding this problem was the lack of a Master Patient Index (MPI), the absolute criticality of which was reinforced by this project's results.

Provide Rapid, Definitive Response to Trauma

Because trauma was infrequent, few data were available to validate telemedicine's impact on this goal. However, two factors would have clearly impeded its efficacy:

- Dependence on a keyboard and terminal: Trauma providers are far too busy stabilizing the patient to pay sufficient attention to the computer designed to guide patient care.
- Discrepancy between on-site telemedicine capabilities and on-site staffing and supplies: Even if telemedicine could be used for trauma care, most forward facilities did not have appropriate staffing mixes or sufficient supplies to provide definitive care. The typical patient would have been evacuated after being stabilized, diminishing the potential role of telemedicine in such a setting.

When trauma did occur, telemedicine was not used in the "golden hour," as most providers were more concerned with patient stabilization and unable to leave the bedside to initiate a teleconsultation. Of the 200 documented trauma cases, none had an associated teleconsultation within the first hour of treatment.

Deliver Highest Quality Care with Specialized Remote Support

There was some evidence that telemedicine helped professionals avoid having to order medical evacuations. In total, there were more than 80 clinical videoteleconferences, 650 teleradiology consultations, and 40,000 clinical e-mails. Exactly how many medical evacuations were averted is unclear, because the in-theater bed policy (the maximum number of days a patient could convalesce before a return to full duty) was 5 days at the mobile Army surgical hospital (MASH), and 7 days at the Combat Support Hospital (CSH). Longer theater-based bed policies could have resulted in fewer medical evacuations but would have also meant a larger medical logistics footprint for both the MASH and CSH.

Another fact regarding medical evacuations was that no process reengineering occurred while telemedicine was instituted. There was no incentive for the local provider to retain on-site patients and avoid evacuation. In fact, there were numerous incentives available for the professional to facilitate an evacuation rather than use telemedicine; these included increased local workload, inherent peer review, risk management policies that held providers accountable for patient outcomes, and other factors. Furthermore, there was no command policy to enforce the use of telemedicine before medical evacuation.

Because these incentives encouraged providers to evacuate patients who otherwise could have been treated locally, a number of inappropriate medical evacuations occurred. Many patients were evacuated to Germany, only to be returned to full duty almost immediately after arrival. Of those patients evacuated to Landstuhl, 52% were returned to full duty in less than 1 day, 87% within 5 days, and 97% within 13 days.

On the positive side, telemedicine did facilitate peer review and specialty consultation. In general, on-site providers were junior officers, most having completed an internship but not residency. They were augmented by corpsmen, who received the equivalent of Emergency Medical Technician training, and by junior nurses. Having a telemedicine system allowed on-site providers to interact with seasoned colleagues in the rear echelons regarding second opinions and medical education. In fact, according to a National Guard (NG) report on consult breakdown, a large percentage of telemedicine consultations were for such second opinions. When medical evacuations did occur, the majority of patients were referred to inpatient Internal Medicine, Family Practice, or General Surgery wards.

Telehealth Oversight: Lessons Learned

Oversight of telehealth projects within the federal government varies widely among departments. Those that operate primarily by funding civilian projects may employ periodic in-process reviews, whereas others may employ more rigid, formal oversight. Most lessons learned by the DoD in this area come by virtue of its extensive experience.

Within the DoD, three groups are primarily responsible for oversight: the research and development community, centralized control by the Assistant Secretary of Defense (Health Affairs), and the individual services. Of these three, the research and development community had oversight of approximately 15% of the projects, while the services had oversight of the remainder. Health Affairs exerted little direct oversight in this arena because the large majority of projects (98%) were funded by the services. As in most instances, the source and level of oversight reflected the amount and source of funding. Coordination and resource sharing were extremely limited. There were distinct advantages and disadvantages to this arrangement.

Telehealth is an electronic solution to shortfalls in staffing and unbalanced medical skill sets. In the DoD, such staffing patterns are extremely fluid and change quickly. In one area, shortages and staffing inadequacies may not persist, depending on retention, recruitment, and other factors. Therefore, telehealth planning and deployment must be equally fluid and adaptable. Control by the services allows for greater flexibility and control over rapidly changing staffing patterns, which the services also control. Contrast this with Health Affairs, which uses government acquisition procedures that tend to unfold over several years and are not flexible enough to fit rapidly changing needs.

Mutiple layers of review and funding challenges also pose risks to timely and complete telehealth deployments for the benefit of the field. For instance, there is usually a multimillion dollar shortfall in funding each fiscal year in information management and technology, the acquisition programs of which are then delayed. In this arena, and without approved requirements, telehealth could not effectively compete for funding or support, especially without defined mission requirements approved by higher leadership. Service-based funding and oversight lead to a complete avoidance of this issue.

There are several disadvantages to service control, the most prominent being the historical tendency of the services to not fully utilize collaborative or cooperative opportunities. The result typically involves the wide-scale deployment of multiple duplicative projects with little overall coordination. Service-based funding, along with limited coordination, often has prevented leaders from adequately addressing the coordination of infrastructure planning, such as uniform process and policy revision to ensure equity in healthcare benefits.

As of 1998, there were more than 100 separate telehealth projects in the DoD, 10% to 20% of which were duplicative and uncoordinated. None of the leaders involved in them had done an adequate assessment of infrastructure requirements or capacity planning from the start. None had adequately coordinated the change of clinical and other processes, resulting in a distinct inequity in the quality of health care offered in different regions. Because incentives were lacking to compel the necessary coordination, efforts to create, sustain, and fully utilize a control-coordinating office had limited success.

Despite this, based on the findings of the GAO report of 1997, the DoD created a Telemedicine Program Office to oversee all telehealth investments. This office was not adequately funded or staffed, and the services had no incentive to use this office or comply with its recommendations because the office did not control funding or have any enforceable oversight mandate. After 1 year in existence, the office had influenced less than 1% of the telemedicine investment, and there is no evidence that the levels of coordination or resource sharing among the services were altered in any way.

The goals of this oversight regime were to preserve enough flexibility to meet quickly evolving needs while establishing a clear oversight structure to compel greater coordination among the service organizations and to monitor compliance. These were admirable objectives that still needed to be addressed. For this reason, the Surgeons General formed the Technology Integration Board of Directors (TIBOD), discussed in detail in Chapter 6.

Operational Telehealth

Beyond the experience in Bosnia, the DoD has engaged in numerous telehealth initiatives, which range from proof-of-concept demonstrations in operational exercises to full-scale deployments on board U.S. aircraft carriers. The largest of these is the Multimedia Intregrated Digital Network (MIDN) project, a multiyear effort to install telehealth capabilities aboard all aircraft carriers of the Atlantic Fleet.

In the 4-year existence of the MIDN project, officers successfully deployed telemedicine and teleradiology capabilities to more than four carrier battle groups. A study by the Center for Naval Analysis showed that despite anecdotal data, potential return on investment for the deployment was significant. Standardized metrics plans are being developed to better document this assertion. Numerous prototype demonstrations throughout the fleet have demonstrated telemedicine's utility for supporting the operational forces while helping to minimize the medical footprint (amount of medical resources taken with the operational forces).

Another potential success story for Navy telemedicine has been its use in proof-of-concept demonstrations aboard submarines. Medical support on submarines is extremely limited and consists of an independent duty corpsman (the military equivalent of a highly trained Emergency Medical Technician) with limited diagnostic and therapeutic capability. Medical spaces in submarines are roughly the size of a small bathroom. In these austere environments, telemedicine was used as an alternative to expanding medical skills and services. Using store-and-forward concepts and burst transmission, telemedicine significantly expanded medical capabilities.

Within the United States Air Force, telemedicine has been used to support flight nurses on aeromedical evacuation routes. The average aeromedical evacuation takes about 6 hours. Medical support aboard planes consists of a nurse with some corpsman support; usually no physician support or supervision is provided because of staffing constraints. Historically, if a patient's condition worsened in flight, the only alternatives were to try to communicate with a physician on ground through the pilot or to perform an emergency landing at a location where medical treatment was available. Both options suboptimized support for the patient. However, through a program called "Care in the Air," the Air Force Medical Service developed an intrinsic store and forward telemedicine capability. This solution allowed flight nurses to communicate with ground physicians and in-flight patients to have their vital signs transmitted electronically to physicians for interpretation and therapeutic intervention.

A constant theme throughout all operational uses of telemedicine has been a heavy reliance on proof-of-concept demonstrations without long-term or life cycle planning for either wide-scale deployment of successful prototypes or sustainment of current prototypes. Most projects have lacked a comprehensive metrics plan to demonstrate return on investment. These telemedicine projects mirror similar prototype efforts seen in the civilian sector and academia and underscore the need for comprehensive metrics planning and life cycle management planning at prototype inception.

Sustaining Base Telemedicine

The theme of absent metrics planning or life cycle management was also consistently found in the sustaining base (brick and mortar medical facilities). There was much interest in telemedicine as a potential alternative to increasing patient access and care, but few prototypes had the requisite metrics, life cycle management, or business case analysis to support long-term sustainment. The Surgeons General, acting through the Technology Integration Board of Directors (TIBOD), discovered this when they reviewed the status of DoD telemedicine projects in spring of 1999. Of the more than 100 known active telemedicine projects throughout the world, none were found to have all the elements of a valid business case. Three showed promise, but they needed more than anecdotal data collection to demonstrate a return on investment.

The DoD initially lacked a way to coordinate actions between prototype efforts, yielding much duplication of effort. (A primary goal of the TIBOD was to eliminate duplication and optimize collaboration among disparate efforts.) Also, as was consistently found in civilian and academic settings, the DoD lacked a smooth, well-defined methodology to transition products from a research/development focus to clinical focus for wide-scale deployment. As a result, several promising telemedicine prototypes never made it to wide-scale deployment. This situation was worsened by DoD funding guidelines, the long Program Objective Memorandum process, which precluded quick funding and deployment of promising telemedicine technologies.

Congressionally Directed Telemedicine

Congress has been involved in funding specific telemedicine projects since at least 1992. The best known of these efforts is the Akamai Project. Located at Tripler Army Medical Center in Honolulu, the project's goal is to use telemedicine to extend medical care and specialty availability throughout the Pacific Rim. The project, sponsored by Senator Daniel Inouye of Hawaii, receives annual funding in excess of $20 million and typically sponsors numerous individual efforts each year. Success stories have included establishment of a telemedicine-supported remote tumor board with oncology patients in Micronesia and development of clinical protocols to support general telemedicine use throughout the Pacific.

A separate project, funded by the Assistant Secretary of Defense for Health Affairs, was to establish telemedicine capabilities at the clinics in Diego Garcia and in mainland Japan, connecting them with the Naval Hospital in Yokosuka, Japan. This development allowed cessation of medical evacuations from these remote locations to Yokosuka at considerable cost savings to local commands. While Akamai was permitted to initially install this equipment, long-term sustainment was given to the services because Akamai's charter precludes long-term sustainment or life cycle management of projects they develop and deploy. Within the constraints of the current program objective memorandum (POM) process, this results in potential financial difficulties and risk for early project termination, as Akamai is unable to support projects until they can be funded through the normal POM process. In this case, however, the services reaped the immense return on investment by sustaining this individual project after Akamai support ceased.

The issue of long-term sustainment pervades many congressionally directed telemedicine projects, as it does with any special interest project. Funding is sustained so long as the individual congressman remains interested and committed to the project. However, in budget discussions and elections, such projects are at risk unless the services are able to arrange long-term support through the POM process. Lack of comprehensive metrics for most of these projects has precluded this from happening. In response to this, the DoD developed, through the TIBOD, a uniform telemedicine project planning methodology that was adopted by all services to ensure comprehensive planning for all future projects. Nonetheless, compliance with this methodology remains sporadic in Akamai and other congressionally directed projects. Working with the project officers will help reverse this trend.

Civilian Collaborations

The DoD has a long history of civilian collaborations in the field of telemedicine, dating back to at least 1994. Most prominent among these is a cooperative resource sharing agreement between the United States Army Medical Research and Materiel Command and Georgetown University for telemedicine research at Fort Detrick. This cooperative agreement was directly responsible for the Army's ability to deploy telemedicine in support of operational forces in Bosnia. Technical consultation/support and clinical guidance from Georgetown enabled this project to occur on schedule.

Another cooperative agreement is currently being developed between the United States Navy and NCHICA in North Carolina to develop a telemedicine network for DoD facilities in North and South Carolina. The goal of this effort is to batch telemedicine consults at one medical center, allowing that medical center to charge a per-patient consultation fee less than the TRICARE maximum allowable charge, a cost savings for the government. At the same time, patients can be treated on site, without travel. Initial planned projects include telemedicine to support dermatology, infertility, and otolaryngology evaluations.

The DoD also has a long-standing relationship with the American Telemedicine Association (ATA), jointly cosponsoring the ATA Annual Conference. This collaboration initially started as a DoD Conference (Global Telemedicine Forum) but was merged with the ATA Annual Conference in 1998. These conferences enable cooperative information sharing and project planning in an effort to increase collaboratives as a cost-saving measure for the DoD. This relationship with the ATA has received high-level support, with annual attendance by the service Surgeons General and the Assistant Secretary of Defense for Health Affairs.

With the rapid expansion of civilian telemedicine and accumulation of telemedicine experience in the civilian sector, there will likely be a significant increase in collaborative efforts between DoD and civilian healthcare partners.

Conclusion

The history of telemedicine experience in the DoD is long and varied. Significant progress and success stories have demonstrated telemedicine's vast potential for helping accomplish the DoD's mission. Whether this can be done in a cost-effective, resource-efficient manner remains a critical question. The answer will be determined as uniform, comprehensive metrics plans are implemented and data are accumulated to show telemedicine's long-term potential for supporting and sustaining DoD health care as its mission evolves.

Reference

GAO (General Accounting Office). 1997. "Telemedicine: Federal Strategy is Needed to Guide Investments." Report to Congress. www.gao.gov.

23
E-Health: Future Implications

Lt. Col. (Ret.) Fred Peters, Lt. Col. Michael Perry, Stephen O'Dell, and David Pedersen

Beginning in 1969 with the introduction of ARPANET, parent to the Internet, the federal government and its agencies have pioneered the use of electronic interconnectivity to share information in more timely and efficient ways. Today, with society embracing e-commerce, Internet technologies have increasing potential to affect nearly every area of both public and private sector health care—an exciting and challenging prospect. Moving information and knowledge directly between caregiver and patient, between insured member and payor, and between regulatory agency and reporting organization poses remarkable possibilities for improved timeliness, accuracy, value, and effectiveness of information. This is the simple essence of e-health: it enables people to have greater participation in, knowledge about, and influence on their health, and it improves interactions with their health and wellness service providers.

The Dawning of E-Health: Definitions and Impacts

"Virtually everything in business today is an undifferentiated commodity except how a company manages information. How you manage information determines whether you win or lose."
— Bill Gates, 1998, regarding the digital nervous system (DNS)

In a world captivated by the potential of electronic commerce (e-commerce), the world of e-health is sometimes mistaken for or misdirected into the services and capabilities in the e-business arena. While there are similarities and even overlaps depending on definitions and an organization's directions, distinctions must be made.

E-Health Framework and Definitions

Adding "e" or "I" to the beginning of a word is the latest fad in industry jargon to make current processes seem new or exciting. To have meaning

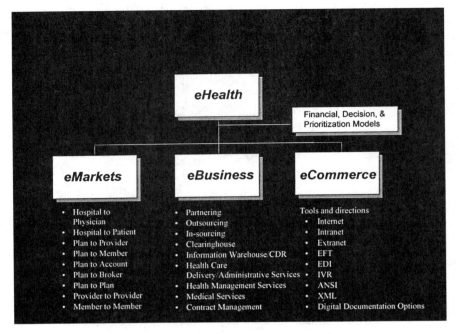

FIGURE 23.1. E-health framework.

and lasting impact, however, the jargon must be accompanied by real change on the part of people, processes, and technology. The first step in this process is defining and understanding the new terminology.

To help clarify how the definitions relate to each other, Figure 23.1 presents an e-health framework that identifies the relationships between the terms and each area's primary focus. Working definitions of each term follow.

- **Electronic Health (e-health or e-healthcare)**: any electronic exchange of data between individuals and healthcare providers or organizations across standard formats (EDI, Internet, e-mail, fax) for purposes of exchanging healthcare information through a network using technologies and tools, in either standard or nonstandard definitions related to the care, status, or results that affect a person's health. E-health is more service focused than typical e-commerce transactions, and it may not involve the exchange of dollars, only vital healthcare-related information. As the overall business or industry focus of the enterprise or unit within a government program, e-health requires new decision making, prioritization, metrics, and budgetary models. It should support senior-level executive and management leaders in making appropriate choices and in setting overall direction for programs in the rapidly evolving and radically changing federal "e-world."

- **Electronic Markets (e-markets)**: the set of connections/interactions available across stakeholders and the role an organization will perform for them. Because the federal sector serves as employer, provider, payor, and regulator, setting and managing stakeholder interactions in e-health is a critical success factor.
- **Electronic Business (e-business)**: any electronic exchange of data within or across enterprises, across a network through the use of technologies and tools, for purposes of conducting information exchange activities. E-business, the detailed examination of all business processes/services, is the directed effort to leverage the Internet and related digital technologies to radically streamline the organization's common tasks and core processes through the most direct and effective means. Government leadership in Internet and web-based services is being modeled by private business; that leadership in the effective use of technologies must accelerate in e-health areas as well.
- **Electronic Commerce (EC or e-commerce)**: any electronic exchange of data between individuals and enterprises, across a network through the use of technologies and tools, for purposes of conducting daily business activities. E-commerce is the enabling set of technologies, services, mandates, and standards that allows the organization to perform e-business functions with the e-market focus within the e-health vision. The government sector has aggressively piloted e-commerce tools with areas of success and showcase results. These now must gain attention, momentum, and wider implementation to achieve the value they can potentially contribute to healthcare services within the federal/military health programs.

Related terms of interest include the following:

- **Electronic Data Interchange (EDI)**: the application-to-application exchange of business information in a standard format. EDI typically requires translation software at both the sending and receiving locations for business-to-business transactions.
- **Electronic Connectivity**: the physical network and enabling technology that provides the infrastructure that allows electronic commerce to occur.
- **Business to Business (B2B)**: any electronic exchange of data between business organizations that streamlines the operations and business processes of either organization using direct electronic means and available tools, networks, standards, and processes.
- **Business to Consumer (B2C)**: any direct electronic exchange of data between business organizations and consumers that streamlines business processes and operations by providing access to new or changing information using direct electronic means and available web-based tools, networks, standards, and processes.

TABLE 23.1. Projected technological progress, 1999–2002.

Technology/environment	1999	2000	2001	2002
PC "standard configuration"/ cost	450 mhz 32 bit <$2,000	600 mhz 32 bit <$2,000	800 mhz 64 bit <$2,000	1 ghz 64 bit $2,000+/−
Network bandwidth/cost per user	100 mbps <$50/month	500 mbps <$50/month	800 mbps <$50/month	1 gbps <$80/month
Database capacity/cost	100 gbytes @ $50/gb	500 gbytes @ $40/gb	1 Tbyte @ $20/gb	5 Tbytes @ $10/gb
Internet personal users/% of U.S.	50 m/20%	70 m/25%	90 m/33%	120+ m/45%
Internet businesses as users/% of U.S.	3 m/30%	4 m/40%	5 m/50%	7 m/70%
Level of e-commerce standardization	<10%	20%	40%	60%

Numbers represent end-of-year projections based on expected "averages" for those technologies within that timeframe. Estimates are drawn from a variety of vendors and sources and are intended to show the dramatic increases that are projected in technology improvements during the next 3–4 years. Estimates have been developed for planning purposes only.

Technology Environment to Support E-Health

The pace of technological change in health care has never been greater. New technologies and their impact on our daily lives evolve faster with each generation of new products and tools. In times of rapid and even radical change, it is often difficult to plan because it is hard to predict what the world will look like when the developments, process changes, or system implementations are completed. As a result, it is important to look forward and project the technological platforms, performance capabilities, and cost/availability of devices and services in the future. Based on those predictions, we can consider new models of development, deployment, and services that leverage the new world and the enabling technologies we expect to be available.

Table 23.1 offers a glimpse of how technology may progress in the early years of the twenty-first century. Organizations should consider what they would do differently in the future if these environmental changes were in place.

E-Health in the Twenty-First Century

The technological shift that occurred during the final years of the 1990s has set the stage for even greater impact on the workforce and the workflows of most businesses. People now buy such items as groceries, cars, medicines, books, music, products, insurance, and mortgages over the Internet. Distance learning, online universities, and remote job sharing are now a reality and are gaining in popularity. As new models for delivering information are developed and promoted, new processes and services will evolve and expand. Clearly, the Internet may be the same "revolutionary" communications tool that the printing press was 500 years ago and that the telephone, radio, and television have become during this past century. It is truly bringing the world closer together and is accelerating the way we share information. Table 23.2 encapsulates some of the more significant trends associated with Internet technologies and their impacts on the way we share information.

The government sector knows the population it must serve and the healthcare needs it must meet. It can use rapidly evolving e-health services to address that population and their healthcare needs in new ways through more efficient and effective technologies. Although the Digital Revolution is just beginning, technology is becoming better, faster, and cheaper. Many of the obstacles that prevented the full realization of the potential of e-health within government healthcare are either disappearing or reducing in size and strength. E-health's evolutionary process will continue at a revolutionary pace, resulting in the improvements described in Table 23.3.

Progressing toward an e-health model, one that represents a convergence of communications, information, and technology, is both logical and practical. In today's healthcare world, an examination of communications among organizations and units within organizations highlights the major interactions required to complete a single healthcare event or visit. Ideally, each communication could have one or more e-health capabilities to simplify and support it.

TABLE 23.2. E-trends and impacts.

Trend	Results of the evolution	Impact
Start of the web and movement toward knowledge management	Information is readily available; knowing where to get it and how to use it is the critical skill	Information and services come to the user, at home or wherever needed
Intelligent consumers	The "average" user has access to more information than did the worldwide experts of the the prior generation	Users "armed" with information will expect more from services organizations
Availability of information	"Online, real-time" information has become the norm; anything less is considered second rate	All organizations will move toward real-time databases and transaction processing systems
Telecommuting	People do not go to the job site to get information; information flows to people wherever they are	The "virtual office" is a daily reality for more people worldwide because of the Internet
Use of Internet	Any communications medium (high-resolution images, media, audio, video, etc.) can be delivered via the Internet	Most products and services will be delivered or impacted by this medium of exchange

TABLE 23.3. Potential results and impacts of e-health applications.

What work is offset by its future use?	Results	Impact
Patient scheduling	Patients can self-schedule with access to physician's/clinic's calendar	More dynamic and responsive scheduling for both physicians and patients
Medical history assessment	Patients can complete self-assessments before visits and can route copies to multiple physicians	No redundant forms to fill out; history can be updated rather than recreated each visit
Review of lab results	Physicians and patients can log into the same site and view the results (e.g., lab tests, radiology exams) and can communicate via e-mail the questions or interpretations	No lost labs, faxes, copies, or repeated procedures because the results could not be found; patients need not make a second trip just to get the results read and reported
Claims status checking	Patients can review services, costs, and the process and progress of filing or settling their financial responsibilities for any services not covered under the benefits plan	No customer service calls, wait time, callbacks, delays in receiving statements or letters requesting additional information; faster settlement, more timely review and updates by the patient/provider
Demographics updates online	Patient information will remain more accurate and up-to-date as changes take place	Reduced cost in filling out and entering forms information; reduced keying errors; increased speed in processing from electronic information

E-health will impact every area of healthcare development and delivery. Some have even called the computer the "microscope of the 21st century" due to its impacts on medicine. From gene mapping projects to improved computerized tomography scans (CT scans) to vast data calculations and tabulations from clinical data, the PC computers and networks will reshape health care in our lifetime.

Current Strategy: Getting By Versus Getting Ahead

Although the late 1990s have been characterized as the beginning of e-commerce, using EDI in business is not new. Electronic data interchange (EDI) has been used in various areas of manufacturing, transportation, banking, etc. for the past 20 years. It progressed within the limitations of the existing technology and has been built on the tools and techniques from the past 30 years of computing. The Internet both accelerates and changes the cyber landscape by providing flexible, graphic-intensive, easy-to-use applications that anyone, anywhere can access and use.

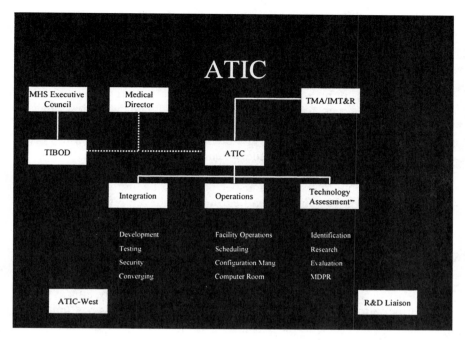

FIGURE 23.2. ATIC process of evaluation.

Healthcare programs within the government sector have effected various levels of incremental development in the areas of EDI and the Internet. These developments have demonstrated both progress and direction, but they must accelerate if they are to match the levels of growth and leadership that will be needed and expected as Internet usage expands. Figure 23.2 reflects the expected number of U.S. Internet users during the next several years. This growth curve may be steeper in some market segments, including the government sector, as individuals may have greater access to the Internet or have needs for wider distribution of information based on the wide geographic coverage for military and government personnel. Therefore, it is both appropriate and necessary that the e-health programs within the government progress at an advanced pace.

Driving Forces

The move toward e-health is based on a number of driving forces. Individually and collectively, these forces are changing people's perspectives and expectations about using technology to support and enable more effective care delivery, communications, information, and results. Examples of these driving forces include the following:

- More care is being delivered on an outpatient, home, or remote (telemedicine) basis
- Consumerism of health care and direct-to-consumer advertising are increasing
- Health delivery organizations are seeking economies of scale in operations and marketing, improved workflow, and effective processes
- Patients want access to medical information and medical professionals as well as more control in booking their own appointments
- Alliances and consolidations are creating a need for disparate, often remote, systems to work together to share information
- The Internet is evolving to define and serve virtual communities related by a common interest, such as a specific medical condition
- The Internet is becoming a battleground for developing and retaining physician allegiances. The emphasis is on persuading the physician to use the desktop as the preferred source for healthcare information
- Capitation reimbursement models are proactively driving toward community health and wellness, focusing on increased education, prevention, early treatment, and chronic disease management
- Internet-accessible medical information is creating a more educated and informed group of patients, which means that the providers, administrators, and regulators need to be better equipped with information to meet new patient expectations

Developing Internet Strategies

A number of themes and strategies are being embraced for their potential and benefits within an Internet or e-health set of strategies:

- A focus on excellence in an area of service
- World-class content/services delivered to a global community
- Specialty care services delivered where and when required
- A focus on building customer/patient relationships within the local community of medical providers
- Healthcare content and services tailored to the needs of the local community
- Primary care services easily identified and delivered in a cost-effective manner
- A focus on operational efficiency and effectiveness—value-based service delivery
- Quality care delivered at a "best" price to a regional community

These strategies are already part of the vision and direction within the Military Health System and other federal healthcare programs. Directives taken from internal policy letters indicate strong directional commitment toward operating in an e-commerce/e-business environment. A policy letter dated March 11, 1999, states that ". . . it is the policy of the DoD to achieve efficiency and economy wherever possible through the widespread application of EB/EC [e-business and e-commerce]." The letter includes such directives as the following:

- Employ EB/EC concepts and technologies in the conduct of all business process improvements and reengineering efforts.
- Plan, develop, and implement EB/EC from a DoD-wide perspective.
- Apply EB/EC processes to interoperate with the DoD's trading partners.
- Ensure that all EB/EC operations employ continuous process improvement.
- Cooperate with other Federal Government departments and agencies to develop and implement an EB/EC operational architecture.
- Utilize end-to-end standards-based solutions for EB/EC security.
- Describe and adhere to an EB/EC architecture.
- Comply with the standard DoD acquisition policies.

With these directives, all areas of military and federal programs are aggressively and progressively moving into a framework and architecture that will embrace more e-commerce and e-business tools and techniques.

E-Health in Action

Government healthcare programs have a number of current e-health initiatives and infrastructure projects that are positioning for future e-health initiatives. Although it is not practical to showcase or even mention all the work that is being done now, it is important to demonstrate a variety of important and exemplary projects to reinforce the trend, direction, and future of e-health in the governmental healthcare sector. This section discusses recent efforts in these programs:

- Defense Medical Logistics Support System (DMLSS)
- DoD's Commercial Off the Shelf (COTS) Pharmacy Application of e-health
- Enterprise-wide Immunization Tracking System (ITS)
- The Command Core System
- Collaborative Healthcare Environment (CHE)
- Military Healthcare System (MHS) Web Strategy
- The Advanced Technology Integration Center (ATIC)

Although these cases are only briefly discussed, many have websites containing more lessons that can be applied to other projects and programs within the federal healthcare sector.

Defense Medical Logistics Support System (DMLSS)

DMLSS is the Department of Defense's (DoD) worldwide medical logistics system, designed to support all three branches of the military services' medical logistics needs. Its progressive approach includes building on existing tools and technologies and aggressively replacing or extending capabilities with Internet and web-based tools. These strategies are designed to streamline processes and improve accuracy/timeliness of information.

The DMLSS project was awarded the DoD's first Electronic Commerce Pioneer Award in recognition of its effective use of technologies to enable and bridge the gaps in supply services. Its current focus is on three major areas:

- Electronic Catalog: ordering supplies from civilian vendors
- EC/EDI Processes: processing pharmacy supplies through Med/Surg Prime Vendors
- Electronic Bill: payment procedures for ordering supplies

DoD's Pharmacy Application of E-Health

This project is the direct application of the DoD's worldwide pharmacy systems, designed to partner with civilian pharmacies and drug manufacturers/suppliers. With the rapid increase in use of medicines for treatment, maintenance, and prevention, pharmaceutical costs in health care are rising the fastest. Health care needs to become more efficient to lower these escalating costs. By taking both the tactical and practical view of immediate needs, this approach positions for greater use of e-health-related tools and technologies in the future. Its primary focus has been in the following areas:

- Drug utilization reviews: tracks patients' prescribed drug therapy across military and civilian pharmacies
- Drug inventory (EDI): allows maintenance of appropriate stock levels
- Patient eligibility checks: performed by electronic communication between the Medical Treatment Facility (MTF, military hospital or clinic) and the Defense Enrollment Eligibility Report System (DEERS)
- Alerts and patient tracking: notifications sent to healthcare providers by pharmacy or outside agencies concerning patients who are noncompliant with their prescribed drug therapy
- Order processing: allows the pharmacy system and other individuals or organizations to support orders and maintain patient records during and after treatment

Enterprise-Wide Immunization Tracking System (ITS)

The ITS tracks adult and childhood immunizations to support the military health services contingency and peacetime mission. This project provides a portable method to record vaccine delivery in remote and mass immunization scenarios. Its capabilities include these:

- Providing multiuser access/log-on from local or remote sites
- Populating immunization records in real-time mode but over long patient histories

- Supporting high volume for both active updates and long-term history, trending, and reporting

The Command Core System: Infrastructure Component to Support Future E-Health Needs

This system provides a relational database to enable central access to data associated with managing environmental and health-related information. This system is one of several database initiatives positioning current data into new structures, a process that will enable faster linkages and greater use of information within e-health. These projects are not often counted as "new"; rather, they are considered part of a new architecture and technical infrastructure designed to support a more flexible and functional approach toward information sharing across the federal and military health services programs.

Collaborative Healthcare Environment (CHE)

The CHE establishes a virtual medical environment that allows healthcare providers and other healthcare professionals to meet in a virtual (cyber) hospital and discuss such information as patient status and management information. This pilot operation allows medical professionals and information specialists to determine what is needed and what works best in a virtual healthcare information-sharing environment. Lessons learned and new ways of working are the product and by-product of these early projects. Initial emphasis was placed on the following primary services:

- Reviewing patient's charts located at any CHE portal
- Consulting with medical specialists throughout the world
- Moving medical information to other participants throughout the world
- Actually viewing the telemetry of patients through the Internet

The Military Health System (MHS) sets up a strategic vision of how websites will be used and how they will incorporate many medical applications, such as making clinical appointments over the Internet and filling out forms. These early projects in CHE are establishing direction for future projects and are pushing the boundaries of how far technology can go to enable services and information exchange in health care. These strategic projects within MHS will become the blueprint for the next generation of systems, tools, standards, and processes that will be required to fully implement e-health.

The Advanced Technology Integration Center (ATIC)

The ATIC is using the Internet to work with industry, national laboratories, and other technology agencies to share the government's technology results. This cooperative effort begins to define the new synergies and areas for cross-functional service line developments. As the ATIC explores and introduces new technologies, the results of their assessments are published on the military healthcare system's website.

This process takes into consideration the technology needs of the government healthcare system and tries to align the strategic direction of government health care, current gaps in healthcare delivery, and compliance and constraint issues associated with the use of technology and the practice of medicine. The enabling technologies defined by the ATIC support the goals of MHS while ensuring that patient information can be accessed by military hospitals quickly and easily. The ultimate goal is better patient information at the site of service.

The ATIC has two forms of information published on their website. The first is geared toward how well a new technology performs, as stated by its marketers. In this case, just the facts are presented in the form of a "white paper," and the government takes no position; rather, the white paper speaks for itself. This general assessment adheres to standard testing protocols. In this effort, the ATIC has requested that it be considered the military's certification agency for the National Voluntary Laboratory Accreditation Program.

The second type of information published on the Web states the government's position on a type of technology being used by one of its medical agencies. The ATIC scrutinizes technology, focusing on matching capabilities to its strategic needs, improving its processes, and adhering to associated compliance and constraints. In this case, the information is intended for use by any government medical agencies that may be in the process of pursuing some initiative and require a better understanding of how their initiative fits into the enterprise's future plans. Developments created through this project include the Technology Assessment Model, which is tied to the Internet to allow all outside agencies and MTFs to search for and review the results of the assessment. Such information sharing can be extended to other types of data and services.

The ATIC process of evaluation is depicted in Figure 23.2.

Long-Term Strategy: Bridging Health Care into a Better World

The potential for e-health development is in its infancy. As e-health grows, develops, and matures, new opportunities will surface and new challenges will be discovered and conquered. At this point of great discovery, it is safe to proceed in new directions, knowing that each venture can open up creative and exciting possibilities. Every interaction today can be considered for change, and every change allows for improved interaction and dramatically greater levels of information and knowledge exchange.

Table 23.4 highlights a few of the areas that will be explored in future generation(s) of e-health developments. Some will be dropped because they no longer apply. New ones will be added as ideas create new models of service and support. It is a time of great development and great demand from skilled and committed staff. It is the right time to make a difference in the world of health care.

The future growth and development of e-health within the federal healthcare sector will depend on how individual programs, departments, or segments of health care view their roles and responsibilities. It is common that organizations choose one of three main strategies (listed at the end of this paragraph) and then build the content and infrastructure to support that strategy. Each has a progressively larger cost and requires more time and skill to develop. It is at these levels that government programs and projects have the opportunity and obligation to take a leadership role in e-health. This leadership would not operate only in favor of the government sector, but would also benefit the industry at large. Excellence in both content and in structure and format should be the hallmark of future projects and developments in the e-health area of governmental developments.

- Center of Excellence Presence (highest order value): information flow is bidirectional; user profiles are actively collected and "mined" to better provide information, products, and services
- Information Resource Presence (primary services/value): information is centered on the needs of a defined audience; it is easy to find, access, and use content; e-mail feedback mechanisms are actively monitored; some discussion groups exist
- Basic Presence (basic services/value): information is centered around sponsoring organization; few or no feedback mechanisms exist

Goals for Healthcare Organizations Using the Internet

Just as the Internet is opening new opportunities for processing healthcare information in streamlined ways, organizations are setting goals that will leverage this potential for their future. It is a new world, and higher goals will be required to take advantage of the next several years of pioneering health care on the Internet. Some of the new goals that will emerge are the following:

- **Market presence.** Tri-Care is taking an aggressive approach to marketing its existence and capability. In addition to mass mail-outs, the use of its website has made its presence known and its programs understandable. Anyone with access to the Web can see what programs are offered by the government and how they can participate.
- **International exposure.** Through one MHS website, we serve beneficiaries worldwide. Changes in information, policy, and guidance can be

TABLE 23.4. Current and future areas of focus for e-health.

Area of focus	Current actions/future actions	C/F
Patient support	Websites may be developed to allow patients to book their own appointments and fill out their own medical history before the appointment. It is not uncommon for patients to spend 30 minutes or more filling out paperwork, during which they are usually taking limited parking space. This is a chronic issue in the military; on many occasions, patients have missed appointments or arrived late because they could not park. Also, while patients fill out paperwork, they often do not have all the information they would have at home or the office. Through the use of web technology, we could populate demographic information from several sources, resulting in less paperwork.	F
Guided health risk appraisal process	Current extended health risk appraisal computer application may be updated to leverage Internet capabilities to extend the direct input and shared output to other programs in the future.	F
Telehealth/ telecare	The Army is the lead agency on telehealth. They have an extensive program that covers many aspects of telehealth, from plain televideo conferencing to telesurgery, whereby a surgeon can perform surgery remotely.	C
Clinician decision support	True clinical decision support is difficult to accomplish. We are providing reference material, online interaction checking for orders, the ability to put in decision support information in line with documentation templates, and the ability to use PKC, problem knowledge couplers. Tools and technologies will continue to expand in the future.	C
Clinical pathways support	Clinical pathways actually are met similarly via the above capabilities in clinical decision support and via order sets that match, etc.	F
Health plan outcomes information dissemination	DoD Health Affairs uses its website to disseminate its information; this includes policy, operational procedures, and timely news releases.	C
Clinical–patient communications	Currently, the healthcare provider decides whether he wants to communicate with patients through this method. There is no formal mandate in place to do this. In the future, this will be an option based on patient needs and preferences.	F
Interactive scheduling	An initiative is under way. The process is scheduled to work in the following manner. Provider gives patient a website URL and an appointment code. The patient accesses the website and searches for an appointment based on the availability of both the provider and the patient. Once a selection is made, the patient enters the appointment code and arrives at the scheduled time using the code as identification.	F
Patient–support group communications	Some mental health organizations have started this. Support groups provide patients with other sources of reliable information, counseling, and assistance beyond the direct medical professional community. This will be a valuable part of the rehabilitation and maintenance approach in the future.	F

TABLE 23.4. *Continued*

Area of focus	Current actions/future actions	C/F
Prescription refills	The DoD has implemented two major programs over the Internet. One uses the Internet to order refills, the other uses it to check for drug interactions and patient profiles. Each time a patient goes to a military pharmacy, the pharmacy system goes through the Internet to a clearinghouse and checks against other pharmacies in the area.	C
Online collaboration	The Military Health Service is pushing hard to develop a system called CHE (Collaborative Healthcare Environment). CHE will allow a medical provider to meet with consultants in a virtual hospital to discuss patients. In this environment, the physicians can share X-rays, lab results, and other information.	C
Reference to online health administration resources	Generally, the government is cautious about pointing to any outside agency for fear that it will be construed as an endorsement. If we do point, we have to point to all similar agencies to ensure fairness among citizens. Drawing from shared sources will be easier and less costly in the e-health world.	F
Communication with other healthcare professionals	This is done routinely now, but more as a "grassroots" process than an edict. Quick e-mails, instant messages, general electronic bulletin board postings, etc. help establish linkages between people with similar needs for information.	C
Monitoring health policy and legislation	Gathering empirical and comparative statistics is routinely done over the Internet. Often, however, the statistics are suspect. Therefore, one would more likely see the government using information gathered by a third party such as Gartner Group.	C
Access to patient records	Although we do not yet have a "true" computer-based patient record, much of our clinical information is stored on our Composite Health Care System (CHCS). A patient can arrive at a clinic 100 miles away and much of his clinical information will be available. Still, this is not a universal capability; the clinics that share information with other clinics must be within the same area, and there are limitations based on data elements differing among military treatment facilities. This issue continues to be addressed with some success, and military treatment facilities within certain areas can now share more of their information. There remain limitations, however, as one crosses regions.	C
Purchasing goods and services	The military has for many years used "just in time" purchasing of goods. This ability has been extended to both the Internet and intranets. Reorder has been taken down to the point of use. Through this method, the supply "pipe" has been reduced to basically 1 day. Savings in time, cost, and paperwork are paying off in various areas of the military and other federal programs.	C

C, current; F, future. "Future" means potentials for development, not yet committed.

rapidly shared and expanded upon to provide patients with information at any point of care anywhere in the world.

- **Education.** The military healthcare system is incorporating several e-health techniques. It started with kiosks and has moved to the Internet. Each branch of the service develops medical education programs that can be sent either through TV or over the Internet. These programs are aimed both at medical staff for continuing medical education and at the patient population so they can educate themselves about a variety of health issues.
- **Information and knowledge.** The military medical establishment understands the importance of having valid information for all its agencies and employees. Therefore, it has developed a system called Corporate Executive Information System (CEIS), which uses the Internet to gather logistics, human resources, and financial information from its enterprise. Once the information is consolidated, any level of management can access it over the Internet and use it to better manage operations.

Obstacles to E-Health

The healthcare industry has made significant progress toward Internet access, web-enabled applications, and connectivity and support in an "anytime, anywhere, anyone" model. However, a smooth transition to e-health is not going to happen quickly or easily. There are barriers to any form of change, and e-health is a set of ongoing changes. Table 23.5 covers some of the categories of obstacles and the solutions that both the government and private sector can use to overcome them.

Other Future Impacts to E-Health

The road to e-health is not yet a superhighway running at top speed. Because it is still under construction, we can expect some obstacles and rough spots ahead. Several pressing issues will impact the pace and speed with which e-health becomes the mainstream choice of users.

- **Immature technology.** With the rapid rate of new technology introductions and the significant increases in capacity and capabilities, there is a limited amount of good, comparative data. Benchmarks are just starting to emerge, and the comparative frame of reference will be essential for most departments that wish to embrace the new capabilities as total replacements for the tried-and-true platforms of the past 20 years.
- **Lack of experience.** With the ever-increasing rate of change in technology, there is a corresponding lack of experience with the new tools. Stovepiped, stand-alone applications are yielding to more enterprise and component models. As such, there are limited numbers of staff who have direct, relevant experiences from which to build the next generation of applications and enterprise-wide solutions.

- **Educating end users.** With the pace of technology and healthcare change increasing, the need to provide available, easy to use, and relevant end user education becomes a critical success factor. If users do not understand the tool or the purpose and impact of the new technology, they will not use it or will use it poorly, undercutting potential savings or indirectly subverting the intended changes. In the Information Age, where knowledge is the currency of commerce, education is the foundation for all e-health participants.
- **Security.** With the rapid migration toward e-commerce and EDI, security in all forms becomes the pivotal point of concern for expanding the use of e-health into all potential service areas. Because of the critical nature of security for healthcare information dissemination and sharing, its focus is expanded in the next section.
- **Fear of use.** Along with any change comes the fear of what it can do and how it will alter the way we work, communicate, interact, and contribute value through our services or products. There is no question that e-health can transform major areas of healthcare service delivery, financing, processing, and reporting. Instead of fearing it, it is important to understand it, harness its potential, and put it to work to improve what we do and how we do it. It has been said, "no one can predict the future," and that is especially true with the power and pervasiveness of the Internet, but we can help direct and shape it through our choices and priorities.

Security: A Special Concern

The fact that the Internet/World Wide Web (WWW) connects networks, universities, businesses, and governments poses a significant number of new and challenging security concerns. The use of firewalls, Virtual Private Networks, and encryption all begin to address the issues, but within health care, the nature of the personal data and its potential uses and abuses bring all aspects of security under the microscope of public scrutiny. Until there are stronger standards and assurances of consistency across all participants and trading partners, there will be limitations on what is transmitted. Security is being addressed in other industries beyond health care, so there are many options that could be adopted by or altered for the healthcare field. This conern is the largest obstacle currently impacting the speed of adoption and acceptance of EDI and e-commerce initiatives.

Health Insurance Portability and Accountability Act of 1996 (HIPAA)

Security has a prominent role within the HIPAA mandates, guidelines intended to address all stakeholders and establish a "security mindset" as it relates to the electronic exchange of medical or healthcare-related information. It covers physical security, user level security, confidentiality/privacy

TABLE 23.5. E-health obstacles and solutions.

Obstacle	Solutions
Physical: Many physicians/clinicians do not have easily accessible computers from which to send EDI transactions or participate in EC opportunities.	• Provide low cost/no cost options with software, connectivity, etc. • Leverage other initiatives (HIPAA, BBA, etc.) to provide multiple reasons with a single solution to make the move now. • Partner with others to set the minimum desktop standard. • Centralize to fewer capture points, if possible.
Connectivity: A large percent of those providers with computers do not have reliable connections to clearinghouses or gateways to get electronic transactions to their destination organizations in a timely or cost-effective manner.	• Establish relationships with multiple clearinghouses, routers, etc. (Use the "postal service model": users can drop the data in any "box" and it will be picked up and delivered.) • Establish metrics, audits, and controls to assure that all transactions are getting the priority and that the throughput options exist. • Start the flow as input but look for opportunities to send back. • Overreport to alleviate the doubts and concerns about EC
Software: Of the organizations with connections, most do not have current versions of software or formats that make the transmission useful or effective.	• Provide low cost/no cost options with software that is compliant with program needs and industry standards. • Package software for easy access and installation. • Partner with others to set the minimum desktop software versions as the standard. • Centralize distribution to fewer points of contract, if possible. • Aggressively promote it and follow through.
Training: Of the organizations submitting claims or information updates, the office staff generally does not have the training or skills to perform these tasks in the most effective or efficient manner.	• Establish relationships with local firms, drug companies, or others who have access to and contact with physician offices. • Establish supporting tools, helps, online training, etc. • Offer refreshers frequently; reduce staff turnover and keep all staff moving toward EC. • Overemphasize the value of training and the rewards—personally, professionally, and for the industry. Make it special to be part of it.

TABLE 23.5. *Continued*

Obstacle	Solutions
Incentives: In most organizations, there are generally not sufficient financial incentives or specific directives to invest in reaching EDI/ EC connectivity under current terms. In fact, at times physicians are *dis-incented* to use EDI due to rejections, poorly designed error handling processes, and delays.	• Provide low cost/no cost pricing for sending in current EDI transactions. • Pay for transition to new EDI transactions or formats for a 12-month time period. • Offer extra services, free or low cost, if they achieve or maintain an increasing level of EDI submissions. • Make the payments noticeable; not just back-end credits or discounts. • Aggressively promote it and follow through with every media contact and communication.
Feedback: In most organizations, there is not the level of communications, feedback, and mutual benefit that would draw physicians to EDI/EC on a purely voluntary basis.	• Offer new services frequently; make them practical and appealing to physicians and office staff (preauthorizations, electronic rosters, etc.) • Overemphasize the value of EDI and EC to every part of the healthcare industry. Emphasize HIPAA compliance rules. Share information and ideas to assist them. • Survey and drill down from the metrics to the weak areas; fill the gaps.

and the use of data, and even the use of encryption or digital certificates and electronic signatures. For the wide variety of potential users/viewers of healthcare information to perform their functions within the guidelines without risking unauthorized dissemination of information, all these levels of security are necessary. In many ways, e-health will become much more secure than current paper charts, claims, and encounters routed through the mail, fax, or other manual processes.

As HIPAA becomes the new "standard for health care" in early 2002 and beyond, the common use and exchange of electronic information will become as prevalent as the use of credit card information is in the banking industry. Although the safeguards and protections must be built, monitored, and enforced, there eventually will be no turning back to the problems of paper-based processes in the federal and military health sectors of the twentieth century.

Future Benefits and Value

It is impossible to fully outline or predict all the benefits e-health will create in the future. Examples of projects and early successes in deploying the Internet and intranets offer just a glimpse of the possibilities. As technologies continue to improve, costs will continue to drop, access will become easier, availability will become universal, and potential uses will explode into all areas of daily life. Health care needs to take a leadership position to ensure both productive and constructive use of e-commerce and e-health in promoting wellness and early intervention for disease management.

Other issues to be considered include the following concerns:

- **ROI.** The initial investment in the Internet Architecture and Infrastructure does not show positive return on investment in either the private/commercial sector or the federal sector. Without it, however, organizations cannot achieve the desired results in e-business or e-health. The challenge is to look beyond the initial ROI and to focus on the new foundation of services and information made possible within the e-health architecture.
- **Costs.** "Better, Faster, and Cheaper" is the by-line of e-commerce in the beginning of the twenty-first century. It is important to make steady or increasing investments in the tools and services of e-health. They may be cheaper in the future, but organizations must learn as they go. Selective purchasing of proven tools and technical capabilities is cost-effective today and provides the foundation for future growth and expansion.
- **Benefits.** The benefits of e-health are difficult to fully qualify at this point because it is still new and largely untested in large-scale use. The potential for immediate access to vital, relevant information about patients when making medical and clinical decisions will dramatically improve outcomes and will lower the overall costs of care within the system; this applies to military programs and to the other federal healthcare programs as well. Using enabling tools and technologies to improve quality of care and services to patients will be the ultimate benefits.
- **Investment.** Although the movement into the world of e-health will require some level of investment, it is an investment in a future of enabling technologies, processes, and solutions that will have dramatic impacts on health care at military facilities around the world. Investing in a well-trained, healthy military population and their dependents will be vital to preserving a strong and ready force.

Time will tell about the duration and long-term impacts of the change e-health will bring. For now, it is enough to know that e-health is not a fad. It will change our future, and we in health care will have the opportunity to be a significant part of that change. We cannot predict the future, but we can help create it through the choices we make and the support we offer through our prioritizations and efforts. For instance, the government and private industry are supporting new and expanded options in the Internet 2 that will create virtually unlimited bandwidth, faster speeds, improved reliability, and new security options. It will be the backbone of the next levels of communications, telecomputing, and medical information interactive exchange.

Although e-health will eventually touch every area of healthcare delivery, medical management and reporting, quality of care, and patient access and satisfaction, it is important to remember that not every pilot project will yield instant success. New technologies will require changes in policy, changes in process, and, most importantly, changes in behavior. Some will come easily, but most will take time to adapt, shape, evolve, and adopt before they achieve their full and desired impact.

Conclusion

The emphasis on e-health in this chapter has placed special focus on the Military Health System and its related processes. This approach in no way minimizes the major advances or accomplishments that are in process or are planned in other federal healthcare programs like Medicare, Medicaid, or the Federal Employees Program (FEP). Many of these are highlighted in case studies or examples throughout this volume. Their emphasis and direction toward e-health may be developing at slightly different paces, but all are focused on the value and benefits e-health can provide to their constituents.

A simple but insightful saying summarizes our duties in the twenty-first century: "You have to use the tools to use the tools." Health care must pledge active commitment to the e-health world, using its tools and technologies to improve processes and deliver better information and services. This is a challenge we must take seriously and aggressively pursue to ensure excellence in our healthcare services to all military personnel and their dependents. If we maintain a tight focus on this goal, the journey into the e-world of the twenty-first century will be exciting, challenging, and rewarding.

Readings

DoD Electronic Business/Electronic Commerce Strategic Plan. 1999. Policy letter signed by the Office of the Assistant Secretary of Defense, DoD Senior Civilian Official Arthur L. Money, May 15.

DoD CIO Guidance and Policy Memorandum No. 2-8190–031199, Defense wide: Electronic Business / Electronic Commerce. 1999. Policy letter signed by Office of the Assistant Secretary of Defense, DoD Senior Civilian Official Arthur L. Money, March 11.

Index

Contributors

RADM(s) Donald C. Arthur
U.S. Navy, Chief, Bureau of Medicine and Surgery (BUMED),
Washington, DC, USA

Marion J. Ball, EdD
Adjunct Professor, Johns Hopkins University School of Nursing,
Baltimore, MD, USA; formerly Vice President, First Consulting Group,
Baltimore, MD, USA

Gina Barhoumy, RN, MS
Senior Manager, First Consulting Group, Beltsville, MD, USA

David Beaulieu, BA
Vice President, Managing Director, First Consulting Group, Avon, CT, USA

Martin Belscher, EdD
Vice President, First Consulting Group, Lexington, MA, USA

COL Frank Berlingis
U.S. Army, Chief, Surgeon General's Initiatives Group, Office of the
Surgeon General, Falls Church, VA, USA

Lori B. Blades, AS
Director, First Consulting Group, Lexington, MA, USA

COL Daniel Blum
U.S. Army, Health Affairs, Falls Church, VA, USA

COL Thomas Broyles
U.S. Army, Washington, DC, USA

COL Raymond Burden
U.S. Army, Director, Managed Care/TRICARE Division, Office of the
Surgeon General, Falls Church, VA, USA

Kathryn A. Burke, BS
Reengineering Coordination Team/Program Coordinator, Axiom
Resource Management, Falls Church, VA, USA

Wendy Carter, MLS
Co-Director, Health Information Resources Service, Veterans Health
Administration, Kensington, MD, USA

Col. Sue Chiang
Director, Information Management, TRICARE Management Activity,
Health Affairs, Office of Assistant Secretary of Defense, Department of
Defense, Falls Church, VA, USA

Morris F. Collen, MD
Director Emeritus of Research, Kaiser Permanente, Oakland, CA, USA

Col. Leo Cousineau
Col. Director, Health Informatics and Technology Insertion, Air Force
Medical Operations Agency, Bolling Air Force Base, Washington, DC, USA

CAPT Charles Davis
U.S. Navy, Director, Clinical Operations Division, Bureau of Medicine
and Surgery (BUMED), Washington, DC, USA

Jim Demetriades, MS, PE
Albany Chief Information Officer Field Office, Department of Veterans
Affairs Veterans Health Administration, Albany, NY, USA

David Dimond, MS
Vice President, First Consulting Group, Lexington, MA, USA

CAPT C. Forrest Faison III, MD
Director, TIBOD Support Office, Director, Department of Defense
Telemedicine, Bethesda, MD, USA

Cynthia Fodor, MPH
Manager, First Consulting Group, Lexington, MA, USA

COL James D. Fraser
U.S. Air Force, Washington DC, USA

CAPT James Garvie
Acting Associate Director, Office of Information Resource Management,
Indian Health Service, Division of Information Resources, Rockville, MD,
USA

W. Todd Grams, BA
Deputy Chief Financial Officer, Department of Veterans Affairs,
Washington, DC, USA

Peter Groen, MPA
Deputy Associate Chief Information Officer, Business Enterprise
Solutions and Technologies (BEST), Department of Veterans Affairs,
Veterans Health Administration, CIO Field Office, Martinsburg, West
Virginia, USA

Maj. Julie Hall
Deputy Director, Financial Development, Office of the Assistant
Secretary of Defense for Health Affairs, TRICARE Management
Activity, Resource Management Directorate Office of Financial Analysis
and Integration, Department of Defense, Falls Church, VA, USA

Capt. Robert Hardie
Executive Officer, Headquarters Air Combat Command, Office of the
Command Surgeon, Langley Air Force Base, Hampton, VA, USA

CAPT William M. Heroman
Chief of Staff, TRICARE Management Activity, Washington, DC, USA

Barbara Hoehn, MBA
Vice President, First Consulting Group, New York, NY, USA

Ginny Houghton, BSc
Director, First Consulting Group, Beltsville, MD, USA

Beth Ireton, MS
Director, First Consulting Group, Lexington, MA, USA

W. Paul Kearns III, FACHE, FHFMA, MBA, CPA
Deputy Director of Resource Management, TRICARE Management
Activity, Department of Defense, Falls Church, VA, USA

Cyndi Kindred
Chief Information Officer, VA Central Plains Health Network, Lincoln,
NE, USA

Kenneth W. Kizer, MD
President and Chief Executive Officer, The National Quality Forum,
Washington, DC, USA

Lt. Col. Edward Kline
Chief, TRICARE Management Activity ATIC Field Operations, Langley
Air Force Base, VA, USA

Robert Kolodner, MD
Associate Chief Information Officer, Veterans Health Administration, Department of Veterans Affairs Washington, DC, USA; University of Maryland School of Medicine, Baltimore, MD, USA

Col. (Ret.) Robert A. Leitch, MBE, RGN
Senior Research Associate, Uniformed Services University of the Health Sciences, Casualty Care Research Center, Bethesda, MD, USA

Col. Patricia Lewis
Hospital Administrator/Support Squadron Commander, Langley Air Force Base, VA, USA

John Manson, MBA
Director, FCG Doghouse, Denver, CO, USA, and Associate Professor, Uniformed Services University of the Health Sciences, USA

Lt. Col. Janet Martino, MD
IT Architecture & Standards Implementation Manager, Military Health System, Falls Church, VA, USA

CAPT James McCain, RPh
Medical Informatics Consultant, Indian Health Service, Tucson, AZ, USA

MSgt. James Mendes
U.S. Air Force, Functional Design, Composite Health Care System (CHCS) II, Medical Defense Partnership for Reinvention, Chantilly, VA, USA

Kimberly Miller, BA
Senior Consultant, First Consulting Group, Alpharetta, GA, USA

Alex Mustafaraj, RN
Director, First Consulting Group, Tampa, FL, USA

Stephen O'Dell, MS
Vice President, FCG Doghouse, Denver, CO, USA

Col. Bruce Oksol, MD
Commander, 1st Medical Group, Langley Air Force Base, VA, USA

Maj. David Parker
U.S. Air Force, Functional Design Lead, Composite Health Care System (CHCS) II, Medical Partnership for Reinvention, Chantilly, VA, USA

Col. Michael D. Parkinson
U.S. Air Force, Associate Director, Medical Programs & Resources, Office of the Surgeon General, Washington, DC, USA

David Pedersen, MA
Vice President, First Consulting Group, Chicago, IL, USA

Lt. Col. Michael Perry
Chief, Advanced Technology Integration Center, Office of the Assistant Secretary of Defense for Health Affairs, U.S. Air Force, Medical Service Corps, Falls Church, VA, USA

Lt. Col. (Ret.) Fred Peters
Director, Operations/Advanced Technology Integration Center, Office of the Assistant Secretary of Defense OASD (Tricare Management Activity), U.S. Air Force, Medical Service Corps, Falls Church, VA, USA

Steven J. Phillips, MD
Assistant Director for Research and Education, Office of the Director, National Library of Medicine, Bethesda, MD, USA

Don Pratt, MBA
Staff Director in the VHA Revenue Office, Department of Veteran Affairs, Alexandria, VA, USA

Maj. Roger Price
Chief Information Officer, Keesler Medical Center, Keesler Air Force Base, MS, USA

Peter Ramsaroop, MBA
Chairman and Founder, HealthCPR.Com, Inc., Alexandria, VA, USA

Todd A. Ritter, MS
Director, Business Development and Product Deployment, Idaho Technology Inc., Salt Lake City, UT, USA

Lt. Gen. (Ret.) Charles H. Roadman II
President and Chief Executive Officer, American Health Care Association, Washington, DC, USA

LT Edwin Rosas
TRICARE Management Activity, Falls Church, VA, USA

Jay Sanders
President and Chief Executive Officer, The Global Telemedicine Group, McLean, VA, USA

Brig. Gen. Klaus Schafer
Assistant Surgeon General—Science, Readiness and Technology, U.S. Air Force Surgeon General Office, Bolling Air Force Base, Washington, DC, USA

William L. Sheats, MHA
Vice President, First Consulting Group, Lexington, MA, USA

Col. John S. Silva, MD
Program Manager, Defense Advanced Research Projects Agency (DARPA), and Communications Expert, National Cancer Institute, Eldersburg, MD, USA

Maj. Detlev Smaltz
Chief Information Officer, TRICARE GulfSouth, Keesler Air Force Base, MS, USA

James Smith
Senior Consultant, First Consulting Group, Long Beach, CA, USA

Selina Smith, PhD
Director, Research & Collaborative Studies, Minority Health Professions Foundation, Atlanta, GA, USA

CDR Wyatt Smith
TRICARE Management Activity, Falls Church, VA, USA

Mary Walker, BS
Director, First Consulting Group, Alpharetta, GA, USA

COL Sandra Wilcox
U.S. Air Force, Washington, DC, USA

Col. Robert L. Williams
Member and Senior Consultant, Practical Data Solutions, Humphreys, MO, USA

Lt. Col. James Williamson
TRICARE Management Activity (Clinical Operations), Department of Defense, Falls Church, VA, USA

Col. Paul Williamson
Executive Director, Department of Defense Health Services Region IV, Information Management Chair, Keesler Air Force Base, MS, USA

Lt. Col. (Ret.) Harry Young, RN, MSN
Senior Clinical Consultant/Project Manager, Navy Medicine Technology
Integration Support, Naval Medical Information Management Center
(NMIMC), New Market, MD, USA

Maj. J. Zarate
Information Management, Flight Commander, 1MDG, Langley Air Force
Base, VA, USA

Vice Adm. (Ret.) James A. Zimble, MD
President, Uniformed Services University of the Health Sciences,
Bethesda, MD, USA

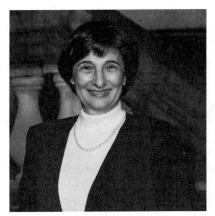

Marion J. Ball

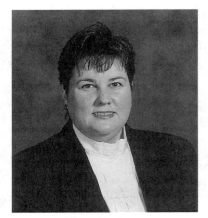

Gina Barhoumy

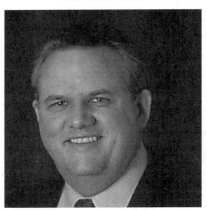

David Beaulieu

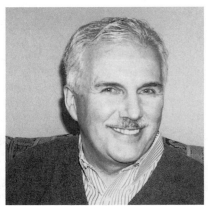

Martin Belscher

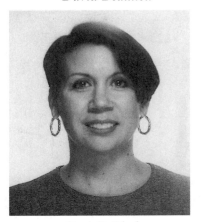

Lori B. Blades

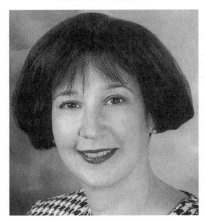

Wendy Carter

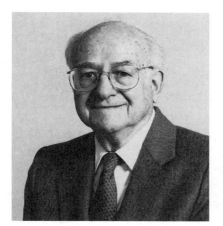

Morris F. Collen

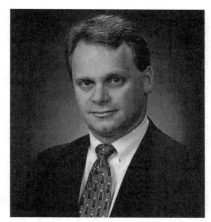

David Dimond

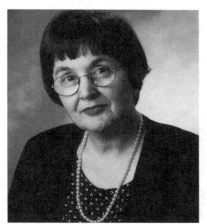

Judith V. Douglas

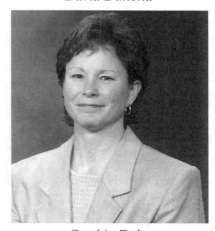

Cynthia Fodor

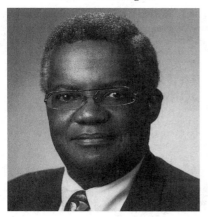

Henry W. Foster, Jr.

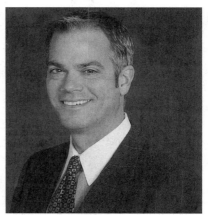

W. Todd Grams

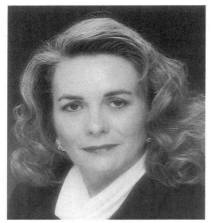

Barbara Hoehn

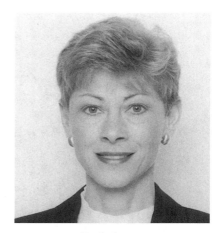

Beth Ireton

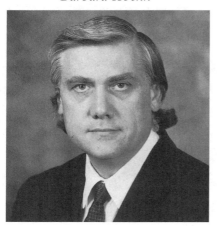

Kenneth W. Kizer

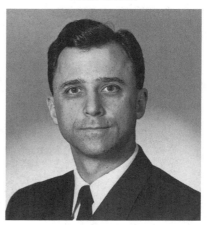

Edward Kline

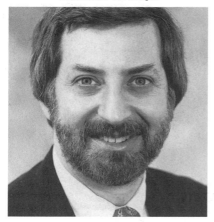

Robert Kolodner

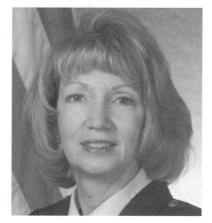

Patricia Lewis

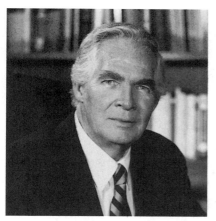

Donald A.B. Lindberg

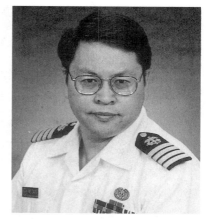

James McCain

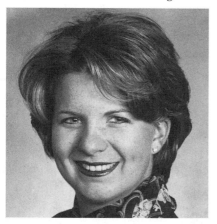

Kimberly Miller

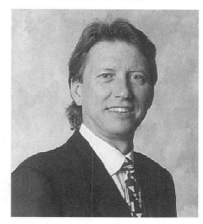

Stephen O'Dell

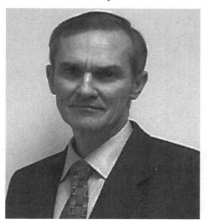

Fred Peters

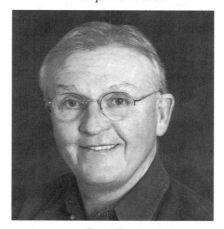

Don Pratt

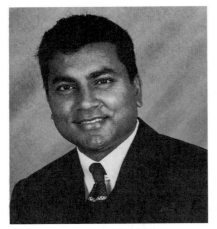

Peter Ramsaroop

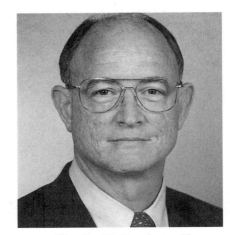

Charles H. Roadman II

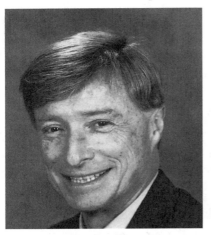

Jay Sanders

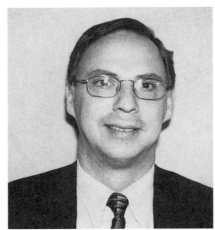

William L. Sheats

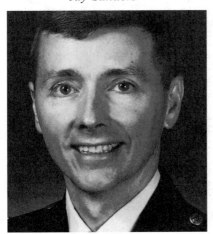

James Williamson

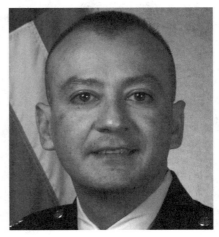

J. Zarate

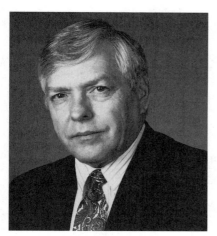

James A. Zimble

Health Informatics Series
(formerly Computers in Health Care)